D1029004

WILLIAM F. MAAG LIBRARY
YOUNGSTOWN STATE UNIVERSITY

Abnormalities of Respiration During Sleep

Abnormalities of Respiration During Sleep

Diagnosis, Pathophysiology, and Treatment

WITHDRAWN

Edited by

Eugene C. Fletcher, M.D.
Assistant Professor of Medicine
Baylor College of Medicine
Houston, Texas

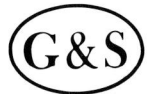

Grune & Stratton, Inc.
Harcourt Brace Jovanovich, Publishers
Orlando   New York   San Diego   Boston   London
San Francisco   Tokyo   Sydney   Toronto

Copyright © 1986 by Grune & Stratton, Inc.

All rights reserved. No part of this publication
may be reproduced or transmitted in any form or
by any means, electronic or mechanical, including
photocopy, recording, or any information storage
and retrieval system, without permission in
writing from the publisher.

Grune & Stratton, Inc.
Orlando, Florida 32887

Distributed in the United Kingdom by
Grune & Stratton, Ltd.
24/28 Oval Road, London NW 1

Library of Congress Catalog Number 86-81333
International Standard Book Number 0-8089-1812-5
Printed in the United States of America
86 87 88 89   10 9 8 7 6 5 4 3 2 1

RC
737.6
.A26
1986

Dedication

To my wife Joyce and son Patrick.
In memory of my father, Eugene C. Fletcher.

WILLIAM F. MAAG LIBRARY
YOUNGSTOWN STATE UNIVERSITY

Contents

10 Breathing Disorders During Sleep in Other Medical
Diseases   **203**
Eugene C. Fletcher and J. Warren Schaaf

11 Sudden Infant Death Syndrome: Respiratory
Mechanisms   **229**
Mary Anne McCaffree

Index   241

Foreword

Only 15 years ago, the thought of publishing an entire book about breathing during sleep would have seemed ludicrous. So little was known about the subject that physicians had no reason to be interested in such a topic. Nevertheless, we do spend a third of our lives sleeping. Evidence accumulated during the past 15 years has conclusively shown that breathing is not even and regular during certain sleep states. In the late 1960s gross abnormalities in the regularity of breathing during sleep were labeled as "the sleep apnea syndrome." Since then, the literature on this subject has been voluminous and its very volume has determined the need for a book entitled *Abnormalities of Respiration During Sleep.*

Not only has the volume of literature related to sleep and breathing increased, but the numbers of patients and the numbers of diseases in which irregularity of breathing occurs have also increased. How one breathes during sleep and the consequent effects on tissue oxygenation are important in the understanding of numerous neurologic, cardiac, pulmonary, and psychiatric illnesses. Even in the general population, some variations of "normal" intelligence, weight, sleepiness, and personality may be related to breathing during sleep.

This book is timely, relevant, and comprehensive. It covers an extremely important area and is written by young investigators with active research interests in the area. I predict that it will not be the last book written on this subject because we are just beginning to understand respiration during sleep. The youth of the authors is thus heartening, and future editions of the text will be awaited with great anticipation.

A. Jay Block, M.D.
Professor of Medicine and
    Anesthesiology
Chief, Pulmonary Division
University of Florida
College of Medicine
Gainesville

Preface

Compared to the many specialty fields of medicine, the diagnosis and treatment of sleep related respiratory disorders is in its infancy. It was only 16 years ago that Kuhlo described the first successful treatment of obstructive sleep apnea. Many important advances have been made in the short time since. Sleep laboratories have become nearly as commonplace in the hospital setting as cardiac catheterization or pulmonary function laboratories. A plethora of therapies has been proposed to cure or ameliorate such breathing disturbances. It has been recognized that abnormalities of breathing during sleep are probably very common in the general population. With these important gains have come more questions than answers.

The movement away from invasive techniques, the development of simple, accurate, noncumbersome methods of monitoring breathing and sleep, and a widespread interest in sleep related breathing disorders both among professionals and the lay public have promoted the growth of sleep disorders clinics and laboratories. As with many advances in medicine, this proliferation of sophisticated techniques has come with a high price tag, and we are now faced with the dilemma of whom to study, how often, and what is "enough" information upon which to make diagnostic and therapeutic decisions. Many short cuts to the more traditional (if that word can be applied to this infant specialty) clinical methods are being sought to solve this problem. Some of these include home monitoring devices, abbreviated nap studies, computer scoring of studies, etc. One purpose of this volume is to inform the clinician of basic techniques available for diagnosing patients with such disorders and to provide useful information to aid in making therapeutic decisions.

It can often be said of medicine that the more therapeutic options open to the clinician, the less we know about the disease and the less successful are the therapies. The past 10 years have seen the application of a range of therapies from simple prosthetic devices such as tongue retainers and nasal pharyngeal airways, to an alphabet soup of nonsurgical treatments including CPAP, EPAP, and CNA, and finally, a host of tongue twisting surgical procedures such as uvulopalatopharyngoplasty and midline sagital mandibular osteotomy among others. It is not enough to know that these treatments are available. The clinician must know what is tried and tested fact, what is research, and what is theory, another goal of this volume.

Sleep researchers have determined sleep-breathing disorders to be related to age, gender, weight, and many major categories of illness. Having realized that there are so many people with abnormalities of breathing during sleep, investigators are now attempting to define what is normal and what is pathologic. Hopefully, new ambulatory and home monitoring devices will allow accurate epidemiologic studies to identify populations with disordered breathing, to relate symptoms to polysomnographic findings, and to follow the natural history of some of these disorders, determining if they indeed, do need treatment. Along with this we must take a closer look at the more feared consequences of these sleep-breathing disorders: hemodynamic sequellae and sudden death. Again, this volume will give the reader insight into these controversies.

I wish to clarify two points about the title of this book. First, in deference to those with formal training in polysomnography, I wish to make the distinction between "sleep disorders" and "breathing abnormalities during sleep." Whereas the former term denotes the entire field of behavior during and resulting from normal and abnormal sleep, the latter applies directly to abnormalities of breathing during sleep. This volume is a compilation of fact, theories, and, in some cases, opinions about the diagnosis and treatment of sleep related breathing disorders. It does not deal with sleep disorders in the broader sense and for that, the reader is referred to one of the general texts on sleep disorders. Second, according to Webster, "respiration" refers to the act of inhaling and exhaling air and the "processes by which a living organism or cell takes in oxygen from the air, distributes and utilizes it in oxidation, and gives off products of oxidation." I chose to use the term "respiration" in the title rather than "breathing" because I would like the reader to think of respiratory disturbances in the broader sense. Current research is beginning to show that abnormal respiration during sleep results not only in problems of oxygen uptake and carbon dioxide elimination, but disturbance of delivery and perhaps even oxygen utilization.

The goal of this book is to provide the practitioner of medicine with a comprehensive guide to sleep related breathing disorders. The authors have tried to provide sufficient detail so that the physician can approach the more practical aspects of recognition of clinical sleep-breathing disorders along with basic physiology and pathophysiology of the upper airway during sleep. A great deal of attention is devoted to cardiac and pulmonary hemodynamic consequences of apnea as well as nonapneic sleep desaturation because as clinicians, decisions concerning aggressiveness of treatment should be influenced by subjective clinical symptoms as well as objective signs of cardiovascular dysfunction. Three chapters have been devoted to the treatment of sleep apnea because of the numerous alternatives (often with little objective data backing efficacy) now available to clinicians. Several chapters have been devoted to the interaction of sleep and lung disease, a topic which will, in my opinion, assume increasing importance in the field of pulmonary medicine. Finally, attention is given to an extremely timely topic, that of respiratory death in infants.

I wish to thank Christina Hartse, Ph.D., Clifford Zwillich, M.D., and A. Jay Block, M.D. for their contributions in reviewing sections of the text.

Contributors

Martin A. Cohn, M.D.
Assistant Professor of Medicine, University of Miami, and Chief, Sleep Disorders Center, Mount Sinai Medical Center, Miami Beach, Florida.

Eugene C. Fletcher, M.D.
Assistant Professor of Medicine, Baylor College of Medicine, Houston, Texas.

David W. Hudgel, M.D.
Associate Professor of Medicine, Case Western Reserve University, Cleveland, Ohio.

Samuel T. Kuna, M.D.
Assistant Professor of Medicine, The University of Texas Medical Branch, Galveston, Texas.

Richard J. Martin, M.D.
Associate Professor of Medicine, University of Colorado Health Science Center, Denver, Colorado.

Mary Anne McCaffree, M.D.
Associate Professor of Pediatrics, University of Oklahoma Health Sciences Center, Oklahoma City, Oklahoma.

John E. Remmers, M.D.
Professor and Director, Respiratory Research Group, University of Calgary, Calgary, Alberta, Canada.

J. Warren Schaaf, PA-C
Baylor College of Medicine, Houston, Texas.

John W. Shepard, Jr., M.D.
Associate Professor of Medicine, St. Louis University School of Medicine, St. Louis, Missouri, and Director, Sleep Evaluation Laboratory, Veterans Administration Medical Center, St. Louis, Missouri.

Abnormalities of Respiration During Sleep

Eugene C. Fletcher

1

History, Techniques, and Definitions in Sleep Related Respiratory Disorders

HISTORY OF SLEEP RELATED RESPIRATORY DISORDERS

While our knowledge about the role of sleep in health and disease has blossomed in the past two decades, even ancient men were aware of an association between sleep, somnolence, and disease. Some early reports about sleep and respiration have appeared throughout history in memorable characters. Many of these are quite accurate descriptions. Others, although not so accurate, provide colorful names such as "Ondine's Curse" and "Pickwickian Syndrome," giving the modern student of sleep related respiratory abnormalities insight into earlier clinicians' understanding of such disorders. These accounts are part of a fascinating history that is still evolving in sleep clinics and laboratories throughout the world.

The earliest cited description of a man who may have had sleep apnea is that of Dionysius of Heracleia, from the 4th century B.C. His dyspnea was described by Aelianus: "I am informed that Dionysius . . . through daily gluttony and intemperance, increased to an extraordinary degree of corpulency and fatness, by reason whereof he had much adoe to take breath."[1,2] Even early therapy is described in this account. "Because of his obesity, he was afflicted with shortness of breath and fits of choking. So the physicians prescribed that he should get some fine needles, exceedingly long, which they thrust through his ribs and belly whenever he happened to fall into a very deep sleep."[2,3] Athenaeus also describes Magas, King of Cyrene, who suffered a fate similar to that of Dionysius, in 258 B.C.[4]

A school of medicine known as iatrophysics expressed new interest in sleep around 1685. "The iatrophysicists . . . in evaluating therapy or arriving at a prognosis paid considerable attention to disturbances in the sleep rhythm. Sleep was regarded as the reparative time of the body, and, in nervous affectations, the indications were for regeneration of "nerve-fluid."[5]

In 1822, William Wadd[3] published several elegant descriptions of sleep apnea. His publication bore the lengthy title *Cursory Remarks on Corpulence: or Obesity*

ABNORMALITIES OF RESPIRATION DURING SLEEP
ISBN 0-8089-1812-5

Copyright © 1986 by Grune & Stratton, Inc.
All rights of reproduction in any form reserved.

Considered as a Disease: With a Critical Examination of Ancient and Modern Opinions Relative to its Causes and Cure. It contained a variety of anecdotes from colleagues and from his own medical practice. In some detail he discussed obesity, somnolence, and an example of improvement with weight loss. Apnea during sleep was not mentioned and apparently never suspected as being a cause of the problem.

Although probably not recognized at the time, a reasonably accurate clinical description of sleep apnea was published in 1877 by W.H. Broadbent.[6] This account alluded to the pathophysiology as well.

> When a person, especially advanced in years, is lying on his back in heavy sleep and snoring loudly, it very commonly happens that every now and then the inspiration fails to overcome the resistance in the pharynx, of which stertor or snoring is the audible sign, and there will be perfect silence through two, three, or four respiratory periods, in which there are ineffectual chest movements; finally, air enters with a loud snort, after which there are several compensatory deep inspirations. . . ."[6]

One of the earlier, but unrecognized descriptions of obesity-hypersomnolence syndrome appeared in a mid 19th century novel by Charles Dickens, *The Posthumous Papers of the Pickwick Club.*[7] In that book, Dickens described a famous character by the name of Joe the fat boy. His obesity, plethora, snoring, psychological changes, and nickname, "young dropsy," elegantly describe advanced right ventricular failure resulting from obesity-hypoventilation and most likely, associated obstructive sleep apnea. Burwell published a now famous account of obesity, hypersomnolence, and cor pulmonale in which he uses the term "Pickwickian syndrome"[8] but the connection between the patient's symptoms and respiratory pathology during sleep was not made. Breathing abnormalities during sleep were noted by Spitz in 1937 in connection with some features of the syndrome, including improvement with weight loss.[9] However, no connection with Pickwickian syndrome was made. Indeed, credit for the association of this syndrome with disordered breathing during sleep goes to Gastaut et al[10] and Jung[11] publishing independently in 1965.

Scientific research into sleep in the late 1800s revolved around measurement of physiologic functions during behavioral ("observed") sleep since no objective method of assessing the sleep state was in general use. Early studies involved measuring the threshold to arousal[12,13] and the response of blood pressure, respiratory rate, and heart rate to sleep.[14] Even though the first electroencephalographic (EEG) recordings of brain activity were made in animals as early as 1875, the first EEG data identifying a recognizable electrical pattern in humans was not published until 1929.[15,16] The study of sleep physiology gained momentum with the description of distinct EEG stages in 1935[17] and the description of rapid-eye-movement (REM) sleep in the mid 1950s.[18,19] These articles related REM sleep to dreaming and changes in autonomic functions such as respiration.

It was not until the 1960s that clinical reports concerning respiration and sleep appeared. In 1963, Bulow published a classic article dealing with respiration during sleep in normal individuals.[20] Although this group was asymptomatic, he found irregular breathing patterns to be present, particularly at sleep onset and during REM sleep. His attempts to describe normal and disturbed sleep respiration as well as the mechanisms underlying respiratory control provoked a new interest in studying respiration during sleep. However, the current high level of interest in the cardiovascular sequelae of respiratory disorders during sleep began with the first reported successful treatment of sleep apnea by tracheostomy in 1969.[21] Since then, the growth of clinical sleep centers and centers for research into sleep disorders has mushroomed such that knowledge of the existence of sleep pathology is now widespread among medical as well as lay persons. Explanation of the pathophysiology and mechanics of obstructive apnea have been described[22] and with this knowledge, new treatments based upon scientific theory are now being tested.[23]

MONITORING TECHNIQUE

Monitoring respiratory abnormalities during sleep is now common practice in many hospitals and teaching institutions throughout the world. Indeed, some unique methods of adapting commonly used intensive care monitoring devices to the measurement of sleep respiration have also been described but leave much to be desired in comparison to formal sleep studies.[24] Outpatient home monitoring systems for apnea screens are now in use and may have a place in screening large populations for epidemiologic data.[25] This chapter is not intended to be a comprehensive manual on how to perform sleep studies, and for that, the reader is referred to additional sources for excellent descriptions of sleep monitoring techniques.[26]

Basic to all formal sleep studies are the recording of the electroencephalogram (EEG), the electro-oculogram (EOG), and the electromyogram (EMG) to aid in the identification and staging of sleep. Recording of these electrophysiological variables is necessary to assure that the patient indeed slept, to assess the quality of sleep, and to observe the effect of the breathing disturbances on the normal distribution of sleep stages (sleep architecture). Many laboratories routinely include a recording of the anterior tibialis EMG to detect nocturnal myoclonus and other leg movements that produce arousals and sleep fragmentation. Current standards recommend the placement of at least two EEG electrodes (one on each side of the midline) in the central vertex area, most commonly C_4 or C_3 (Fig. 1-1). Occipital electrodes may be applied to aid in the visualization of alpha activity. The EEG electrodes are referenced to neutral sites (A_1, A_2) on the earlobes or over the mastoid bones. These EEG placements allow detection and recording of alpha activity, sleep spindles, K complexes, and vertex sharp waves, all used to classify sleep stages. Two electro-oculogram leads, one at the outer canthus of each eye, record the slow, rolling eye movements of Stage 1 sleep and the phasic bursts of rapid-eye-movement characteristic of REM sleep. Two electromyographic leads are placed over the chin and referenced to each other. The EMG signal is essential to identify the chin muscle atonia of REM sleep (see illustrations). Chart recorder paper speed is usually set by convention at 10 to 15 mm/s and pen deflection is set at 7.5 to 10.0 mm per 50 microvolts.

The electrocardiogram from a single chest lead should accompany all studies to detect arrhythmias and to observe cyclic changes in heart rate. One author has proposed that apnea can be strongly suspected just from cyclic bradycardia-tachycardia on a Holter monitor report.[27] Multiple leads may be needed to distinguish arrhythmias resulting from disturbed breathing during sleep. Rate and rhythm must always be reported since arrhythmias during apneic periods may have a significant impact upon prognosis and recommended therapy.

To detect apneas, it is essential to monitor expiratory airflow at the mouth and

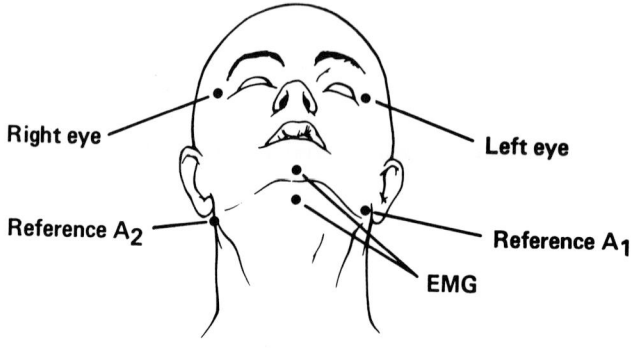

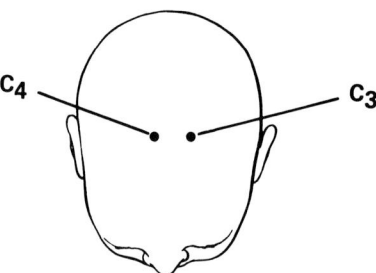

Fig. 1-1. Drawing of typical lead placement used for nocturnal polysomnography. Two leads are placed along the vertex to monitor EEG activity (C_3,C_4); two over the chin to monitor genioglossus EMG, one over the outer canthis of each eye to monitor EOG; and two reference placements on the earlobes or over the mastoid bones (A_1,A_2).

nose. The two commonly used devices are heat sensitive thermistors and the rapid response CO_2 analyzer (capnograph). The thermistor, which detects changes in temperature between room air (cooler) and expired air (warmer), is the most commonly used flow detector. The capnograph continuously removes small samples of air from a face mask or nose piece and measures expired carbon dioxide tension. Inspiration causes a fall in CO_2 to zero while expiration causes a marked upward deflection (Fig. 1-2). If properly calibrated, some estimate of the effect of apnea on end tidal CO_2 can be measured by this technique.

In order to differentiate between the types of apnea, respiratory effort must be monitored. There are many methods available for doing this. The most accurate technique is to measure negative deflections in esophageal pressure by a balloon-tipped catheter swallowed prior to sleep.[28] This is a highly sensitive method since esophageal balloons detect virtually any respiratory effort, no matter how small, in any patient, no matter how obese (see Fig. 3-5). The disadvantage of this technique is that it is relatively uncomfortable for the patient and requires some technical skill to calibrate and place. Other, less invasive measures that are more comfortable for the patient have been adapted to the clinical sleep laboratory. The simplest, but perhaps the least accurate, is to measure diaphragmatic and intercostal muscle EMG in a

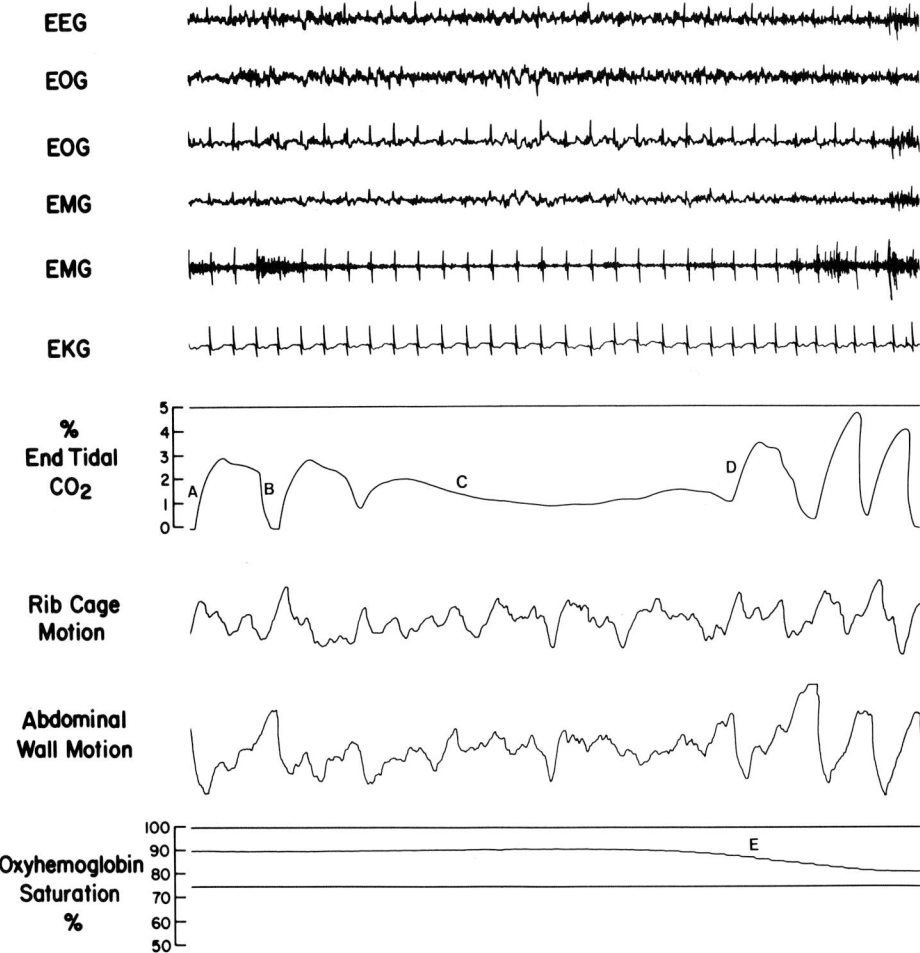

Fig. 1-2. Example of a tracing using the capnograph to display expiratory airflow. Two normal expiratory-inspiratory cycles [upward deflection is expiration (A) and downward is inspiration (B)] followed by an obstructive apnea (C). During the apnea, the sharp inspiratory descent is absent and end tidal CO_2 slowly drifts downward as expired air dissipates from the face mask. At the termination of the apnea, the inspiration of fresh air is not obvious but expired air from the next normal breath is now seen (D). Note the delay in fall of oxyhemoglobin saturation due to the circulation time between the lung and earlobe and intrinsic delays in the computer (E). EKG artifact is seen in all leads.

manner similar to that described above for chin EMG recording. Respiratory effort reflected by electrical activity in these muscles during ineffective breathing (apnea) signifies an obstructive event and lack of electrical activity signifies a central event. There is, however, some question as to whether apnea types are accurately differentiated by this method.[29] Mercury strain gauges, pneumatic devices, and magnetometers[30] positioned around or on the chest and abdominal wall may be used to detect motion. Stretching or separation of the devices (mercury strain gauge, magnetometers) causes a change in electrical resistance or magnetic field, which is detected and amplified. Although these measures are not quantitative, they are usually adequate for the differentiation of obstructive versus central apneas. It is important that both the abdomen and chest wall are monitored so that motion in either area will be detected.

In recent years, a more quantitative method of measuring respiratory effort has been adapted to the study of respiration during sleep. Two inductance vests (Respitrace, Ardsley, NY) encircle the rib cage and abdomen. Using a spirometer and various respiratory maneuvers, measurements of rib cage and abdominal motion are quantitated and the amplifier calibrated so that changes in thoracic and abdominal circumference are translated to volume. In order to achieve truly accurate calibration in all positions, computer calibration is available and almost necessary.[31,32]

In addition to devices for the detection of apnea, some measure of oxygenation is essential to nocturnal respiratory monitoring. Ear oximetry is now widely used to measure oxyhemoglobin saturation during sleep. Some early oximeters such as the Hewlett-Packard 47201A ear oximeter (no longer manufactured) were extremely accurate[33] and easy to calibrate but were uncomfortable because of the large size of the ear piece and the necessity to heat the ear to improve capillary circulation (Fig. 1-3A). Patients often became uncomfortable wearing the ear piece overnight. The newer models do not require heating, are less affected by skin pigmentation, and are, in general, more comfortable because of their smaller size and ease of application.[34] A small clip containing a light sensor is placed on the ear lobe (Fig. 1-3B). Changes in the transmission of two wavelengths of light through the vascular bed of the earlobe allow rapid detection of the severity of the desaturation following apnea. There is always some delay between the apneic event and the resulting desaturation because of the circulation time required to carry poorly oxygenated blood from the lung to the ear lobe plus small delays within the oximeter itself.

Prior to the use of oximetry, indwelling radial and brachial arterial lines were used to monitor blood gas changes induced by apnea. This method involves intermittent sampling of gas tensions rather than continuous recording of changes in saturation, and therefore may not be as useful because trends are less obvious and profound changes in oxygenation may be missed. There are, however, advantages in that the equipment needed is much less expensive than that of ear oximetry, and changes in $PaCO_2$ and acidosis may be recorded by this method. Surprisingly, these invasive lines, if correctly and painlessly placed prior to sleep, bother the patient very little and usually do not prevent sleep. Personal experience has shown that patients can sleep with radial artery as well as flow-directed pulmonary artery catheters in place with minimal discomfort.[35]

The laboratory time and expense involved in performing polysomnography has prompted investigators to search for less demanding methods of detecting apnea that will allow screening of large populations for epidemiologic data. Several machines designed for home monitoring are now in use. One of these (Vitalog Inc., Redwood City, CA) has been used for collecting such data.[36,37] This device employs chest wall and abdominal wall inductive coils to measure breathing excursions which are summed to approximate tidal volume (Fig. 1-4). Central and obstructive apneas are then separated by the absence (central) or presence (obstructive) of paradoxical wall movement. Used with an ear oximeter, the device can incorporate oxyhemoglobin saturation into the final data printout as well as fluctuations in heart rate accompanying the apneas. A mercury switch attached to the patient's wrist detects body motion. The usefulness of this device for clinical purposes (primary diagnosis and treatment of sleep apnea) remains to be determined. However, its obvious application now is for the determination of apnea frequency among various

ISI Citation Databases

Patrons of OhioLINK institutions now have World Wide Web access to citations from more than 8,000 science, social science, and arts and humanities journals. Known for their ability to allow for **cited reference searching** (using a known paper to find other, more recent papers that cite it), these are the most comprehensive, multidisciplinary databases covering scholarly literature available:

SciSearch - over 5,300 of the leading science and technical publications from all over the world

Social SciSearch - 1,700 of the world's leading social sciences journals in a broad range of disciplines

Arts & Humanities Search - over 1,100 of the world's leading arts and humanities journals

Access these databases from your library's home page or connect directly to OhioLINK from your home, office or dormitory at:
http://www.ohiolink.edu

Bringing a world of information to your fingertips... **OhioLINK**

OhioLINK Announces....

Biological Abstracts

Biological Abstracts provides worldwide coverage to citations from more than 6,000 journals, representing nearly every life science discipline, including:

agriculture	microbiology
biochemistry	molecular biology
biotechnology	neurology
botany	pharmacology
ecology	public health
environment	zoology
genetics	

Other OhioLINK research databases that may be of interest: *Applied Science & Technology*, *BioethicsLine*, *Biological & Agricultural Index* and *History of Science & Technology*.

Access these databases from your library's home page or connect directly to OhioLINK from your home, office or dormitory at:
http://www.ohiolink.edu

Bringing a world of information to your fingertips... **OhioLINK**

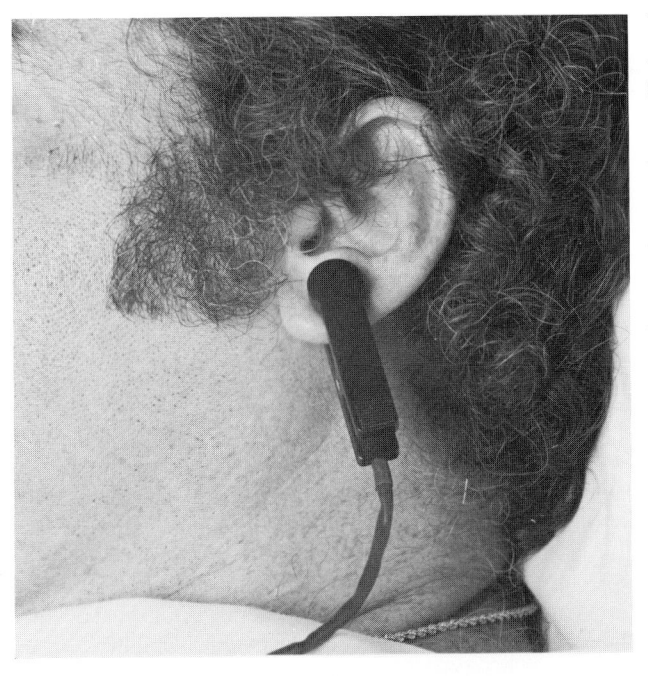

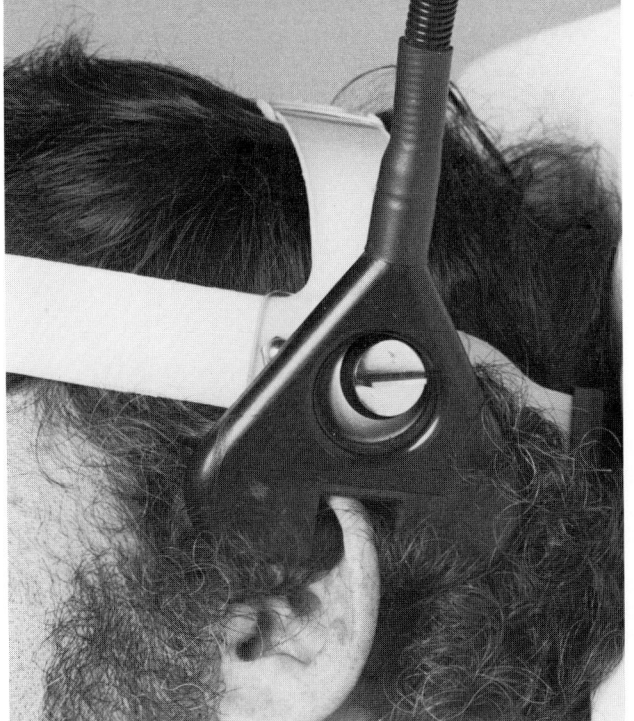

Fig. 1-3. Ear pieces used in monitoring oxyhemoglobin saturation. Left: Hewlitt-Packard 47201A heated, fiber-optic ear piece with head harness. Right: Biox IIA ear piece.

WILLIAM F. MAAG LIBRARY
YOUNGSTOWN STATE UNIVERSITY

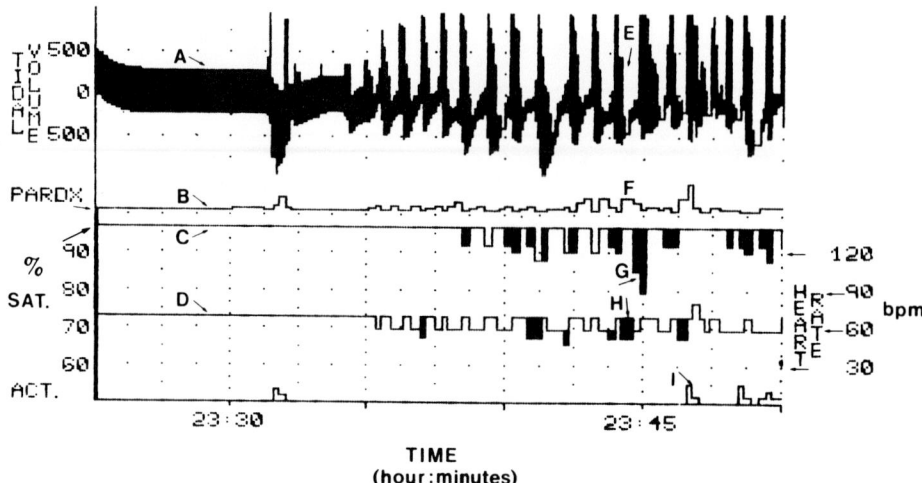

Fig. 1-4. Example of a home monitoring device tracing in a patient with severe obstructive sleep apnea (Vitalog Inc., Redwood City, CA). The tracing shows transition from normal unobstructed breathing (A–D) to obstructive apneas (E–H). The top channel is the sum of two inductance vests (chest and abdomen) and if properly calibrated, approximates tidal volume (no measure of airflow is used). Quiet, regular, tidal breathing is reflected by the smooth tidal volume signal (A). Apnea is reflected by alternating hyperpneas followed by segments with little or no tidal volume signal (E). Obstructive apnea is separated from central apnea by the presence of chest/abdominal wall paradox (B = no paradox, F = paradox). No variation in oxygen saturation (C) by ear oximeter or heart rate (D) is seen during quiet, unobstructed breathing. During obstructed breathing, the high to low saturation is recorded every 10 seconds (G). In example apnea at G, the patient desaturates from 96 percent to 80 percent. Motion is detected by mercury switches attached to the wrist (I). Abbreviations: Paradx = paradoxical rib cage/abdominal wall motion; Sat = O_2 saturation; bpm = heart rate in beats per minute; act = body activity (measured by wrist motion).

populations and subgroups (the aged, sleeping pill users, etc.) as well as long term followup of these populations.

SLEEP ARCHITECTURE

Sleep architecture refers to the pattern and distribution of sleep stages as judged by standard sleep stage scoring.[38] Sleep is divided into nonrapid-eye-movement (NREM) and rapid-eye-movement or "dreaming" sleep. NREM sleep contains four stages. Stage 1 or light sleep is usually the first sleep stage experienced at sleep onset, and is often seen during transitions between wakefulness, NREM, and REM sleep. The EEG is characterized by a mixed voltage, low amplitude tracing with slow rolling eye movements in the EOG (Fig. 1-5). The respiratory pattern during stage 1 sleep is often irregular with cyclic waxing and waning of ventilation. This may be related to oscillation between awake and asleep breathing control mechanisms including variations in the CO_2 set point, which may change with levels of arousal.[39] Apneas are frequently seen at sleep onset and are not necessarily considered pathologic. Stage 2 is usually the most abundant stage (Table 1-1) and is defined by the presence of short bursts of 12–14 cycles per second activity (sleep spindles) and/or

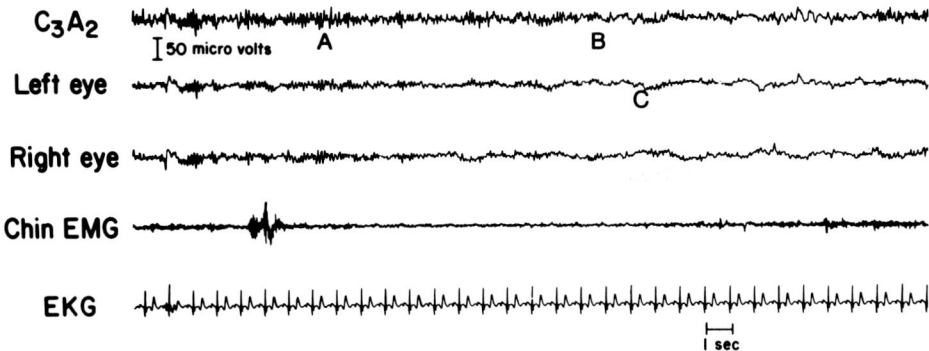

Fig. 1-5. Typical example of the transition between wake and Stage 1 sleep. Alpha waves (A) and low-voltage, mixed-frequency activity characterize the waking EEG. Loss of alpha activity with a mixed-frequency, low-amplitude EEG (B) accompanied by slow rolling eye movements (C) characterize Stage 1 sleep.

Table 1-1
Average Values for Men of Different Ages

Report indices	20–29 years old		30–39 years old		40–49 years old		50–59 years old	
* Time in bed (minutes)	442	(12.2)	435	(20.5)	429	(39.2)	423	(44.9)
† Sleep period time (minutes)	425	(14.4)	428	(23.2)	414	(36.9)	407	(45.9)
‡ Total sleep time (minutes)	419	(14.5)	421	(21.9)	389	(46.5)	390	(49.5)
§ Sleep efficiency index	95%	(0.04)	97%	(0.02)	91%	(0.06)	92%	(0.04)
Stage 0 (percent of SPT)	1.3	(1.1)	1.5	(1.9)	6.2	(5.6)	4.3	(2.3)
Stage 1 (percent of SPT)	4.4	(1.6)	5.7	(3.4)	7.5	(3.0)	7.5	(3.9)
Stage 2 (percent of SPT)	45.5	(5.2)	56.9	(7.4)	54.7	(11.1)	61.7	(10.3)
Stage 3 (percent of SPT)	6.2	(1.4)	5.7	(1.46)	5.4	(3.3)	3.2	(4.8)
Stage 4 (percent of SPT)	14.5	(4.4)	6.8	(5.2)	3.2	(6.3)	1.6	(3.2)
Stage REM (percent of SPT)	28.0	(5.7)	23.5	(3.9)	22.8	(4.0)	21.4	(4.0)
‖ Sleep latency onset	14.5	(4.4)	5.8	(3.9)	10.0	(7.9)	11.9	(10.5)

NOTE: Numbers in parenthesis are ±1 standard deviation.
* Time in bed (TIB): The time from lights out at night until the subject gets out of bed in the morning.
† Sleep period time (SPT): The time from first sleep at bedtime until final awakening in the morning.
‡ Total sleep time (TST): SPT less any time that the subject spent awake during the night after falling asleep.
§ Sleep efficiency index: The TST divided by the TIB.
‖ Sleep onset latency: The time from lights out until the appearance of the first sleep stage, either Stage 1 or Stage 2.
Adapted from: William RL, Karacan I, Hursch CJ: Electroencephalography of Human Sleep: Clinical Applications. New York, John Wiley and Sons, 1974.

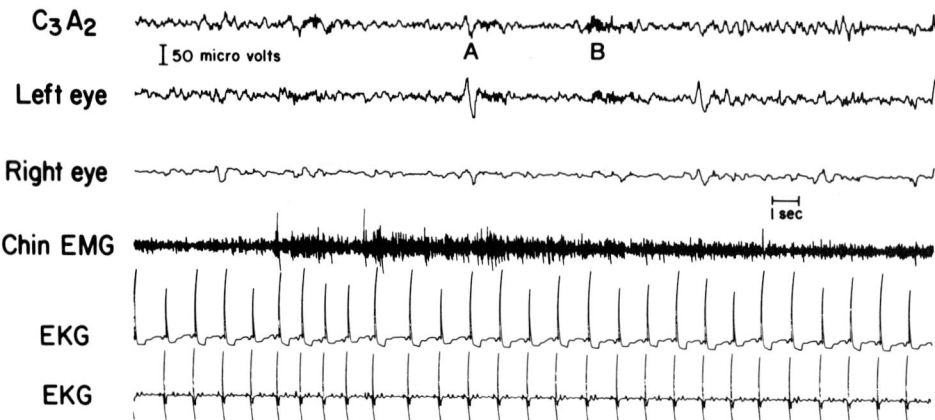

Fig. 1-6. Typical example of Stage 2 sleep characterized by high voltage, low amplitude EEG pattern with K complexes (A) and sleep spindles (B) superimposed on the underlying EEG rhythm.

K complexes (positive-negative waves) superimposed on the underlying EEG (Fig. 1-6). The respiratory pattern of stage 2 is usually regular but may show some of the same cyclic changes seen in stage 1 sleep. Stages 3 and 4 of NREM sleep are often called deep or slow wave sleep and are characterized by high amplitude, slow wave activity. The difference between stage 3 and 4 sleep is in the frequency of slow waves (delta waves). Stage 3 is composed of 20–50 percent slow wave activity and stage 4 shows greater than 50 percent slow waves. Respiration during Stage 3–4 sleep is more regular, and apneas are usually not present (Fig. 1-7).

The REM EEG looks much like that of Stage 1 but there are other important physiological characteristics of this stage (Fig. 1-8). The chin EMG is at the lowest level of the night reflecting a general loss of skeletal muscle tone. Phasic bursts of eye movement are present, and autonomic activity is altered with changes in heart rate, respiration, and blood pressure. Respiration during REM sleep shows increased frequency and decreased tidal volume and may be quite irregular. There may be short apneas during the bursts of rapid-eye-movement. The dramatic decreases in

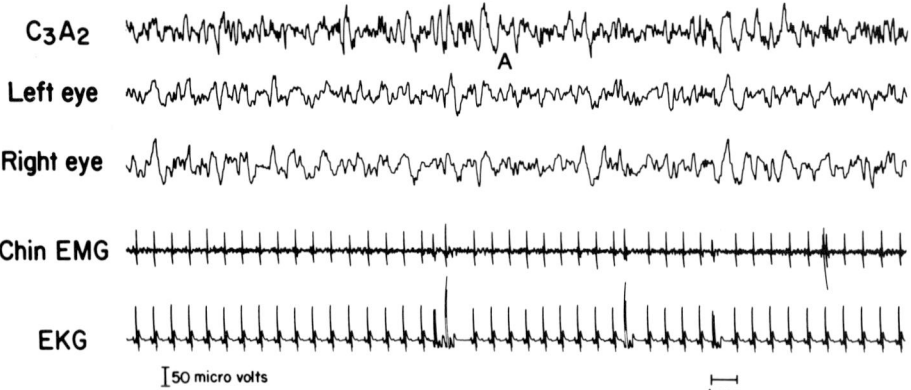

Fig. 1-7. Stage 3/4 sleep characterized by high amplitude slow waves (A). Stage 3 is composed of 20 to 50% slow waves and stage 4 greater than 50 percent.

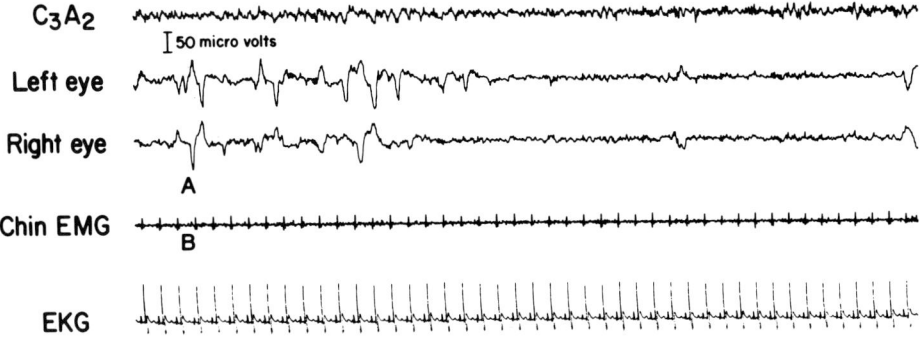

Fig. 1-8. Stage REM sleep is characterized by a low voltage, mixed-frequency EEG, bursts of phasic rapid-eye-movement (A), and loss of EMG activity (B).

muscle tone along with unstable respiratory and autonomic control make REM sleep periods more vulnerable to breathing problems such as apnea, hypopnea, and oxyhemoglobin desaturation. REM sleep appears periodically throughout the night, usually starting approximately 90 minutes after sleep onset and recurs at 90 minute intervals.

The sleep record should be scored for the percentage of time spent in each sleep stage. Sleep stage architecture changes with age and sex (Table 1-1) and is frequently abnormal because of various disease states that interfere with normal stage distribution such as sleep apnea syndrome, nocturnal myoclonus, and chronic obstructive lung disease. For example, patients with obstructive sleep apnea will have a marked increase in the number of arousals leading to sleep fragmentation and frequent stage shifts. They experience a shift toward more stage 1 and 2 sleep with less REM and almost no stage 3/4 sleep. They may have a short sleep onset latency (time from lights out to the first scorable sleep epoch) reflecting their usual state of hypersomnolence.

Polysomnographic reports include information on sleep onset latency, the percentage of total time spent in sleep, distribution of sleep stages (Table 1-1, Fig. 1-9) number, type, and duration of the apneas, and the presence of any myoclonus or arrhythmias (Fig. 1-10). Some measure of oxyhemoglobin desaturation associated with respiratory events should be included. Saturation is frequently expressed in the form of mean or lowest saturation reached during apneas or hypopnea. Newer methods of computer scoring of saturation during the entire night will aid in determining the beneficial effect of various treatment modalities available to clinicians.[40] All of the above information should be evaluated in light of the clinical symptoms, medical history, and physical condition of the patient in order to arrive at appropriate therapeutic decisions.

DEFINITIONS

As in any newly developed specialty field of science or medicine, confusion may exist about nomenclature and definitions. The field of sleep-related respiratory disturbances is no exception. Although most of the following definitions offer no problem to the clinician or researcher involved in the study of sleep, they are frequently

SLEEP SUMMARY SHEET

SUBJECT: PAUL BUFFALO   CHANNEL   3
STUDY : QUALITY   START TIME 10:27
NIGHT : 1   END TIME   6:40
DATE : 8-23-80   SCORED BY : CB

TOTAL RECORD TIME 1430\ 1430.0min.
TOTAL SLEEP TIME   1276\ 1276.0min.

WAKE DURING SLEEP   345\ 345.0min.
# of EPOCHS of SLEEP 931
SLEEP EFFICIENCY   65%
NUMBER of AWAKENINGS 28
DURATION of AWAKENINGS
(Epochs)
1= 34   2= 4   3= 22   4= 2
5= 13   6= 2   7=   2   8= 4
9=   7 10= 8 11=   3 12= 5
13= 1 14= 1 15= 48 16= 51
17= 2 18= 28 19= 2 20= 18
21= 2 22= 11 23= 7 24= 27
25= 26 26= 26 27= 6 28= 2

MEAN DURATION of AWAKENINGS 12.32min.   5.27= 6 28= 2
SD - DURATION   14.17min.   6 28= 2

SLEEP ONSET LATENCY 155.0min. from Beginning of RECORD
LATENCY TO STAGE 2= 2.0   3= -1.0   4= -1.0   REM= 374.0 min.
NUMBER of REM > 2eeochs   3   0 Epochs
DURATION of REM 5= 75   6= 89   7= 95   4= 0   8= 0   0 Epochs

MEAN DURATION of REM   86.33min.
SD - DURATION   10.263min.
REM PERIODICITY 1= 459.0   2= 326.0   3= .0   4= .0 min.
                 5=   6=   7=   8=

MEAN PERIOD.   392.50min.
SD - PERIOD.   94.045min.
INTER-REM INTERVAL 1= 384.0   2= 237.0   3=   4=   min.
NUMBER of STAGE SHIFTS   86
NUMBER of STAGE CHANGES   51
NUMBER of STAGE CHANGES   51
NUMBER of STAGE CHANGES   51

HISTOGRAM

SLEEP SUMMARY

	1st QTR		2nd QTR		3rd QTR		4th QTR		TOTAL	
STAGE WAKE	90	28%	119	37%	64	20%	72	22%	4098	321.2%
STAGE 1	21	6%	13	4%	9	2%	13	4%	2927	229.4%
STAGE 2	208	65%	111	34%	157	49%	139	43%	3628	284.3%
STAGE 3	0	0%	0	0%	0	0%	0	0%	3501	274.4%
STAGE 4	0	0%	0	0%	0	0%	0	0%	#####	#####
STAGE REM	0	0%	75	23%	89	27%	95	29%	#####	#####
STAGE MOVEMENT TIME	0	0%	1	0%	0	0%	0	0%	2	.2%
STAGE T1	0	0%	0	0%	0	0%	0	0%	2906	227.7%
STAGE T2	0	0%	0	0%	0	0%	0	0%	#####	#####
TOTALS	319		319		319		319		14885	1276

Fig. 1-9. Example of an extensive report of sleep architecture in a subject with severe, hypoxic COPD. This patient exhibited disturbed sleep architecture with poor quality sleep evidenced by the long sleep onset latency and a large portion of the night spent awake, frequent awakenings after sleep onset, frequent stage changes, and only a small amount of REM sleep.

12

Summary Sleep Report on John Doe

Name: John Doe
Age: 65
Date of Sleep Study: 6/15/85

TST: 300 minutes
Sleep efficiency index: 75%
Sleep onset latency: 3 minutes
# of awakenings: 33
Percent of SPT
    Stage 0: 20%
    Stage 1: 13%
    Stage 2: 57%
    Stage 3/4: 0%
    Stage REM: 10%

Summary: The patient had 150 obstructive apneas with an apnea index of 30 per hour. The average duration of apnea was 35 seconds with the longest duration being 55 seconds. The average sleeping baseline saturation was 94% with lowest apneic oxygen saturation of 84%. Occasional PVC's and a mild bradycardia/tachycardia were documented. There were 10 episodes of myoclonus causing 7 arousals. Frequent hypopneas were present with mild desaturation.

Fig. 1-10. Example of an apnea report in a patient with moderate apnea. The total number of apneas per night and apneas per hour (apnea index) of sleep give some indication of apnea frequency. An estimate of baseline saturation and average apnea desaturation along with average apnea duration gives in indication of the severity of the apnea. Finally, some indication of the cardiac rate and rhythm may be an important indicator of the tissue effect of hypoxia on the heart.

misused or misunderstood by some physicians. The reader should have a clear understanding of these terms in order to avoid confusion about their use in subsequent chapters.

Sleep Apnea is defined as a greater-than-ten second pause in respiration during sleep. This pause may take the form of obstructive apnea caused by closure of the pharyngeal airway during inspiration, central apnea caused by lack of central respiratory drive, or a combination of both (mixed apnea) with the central component preceding the obstructive component (see Chapter 3 for complete definition and examples). Apnea episodes that occur at sleep onset or during bursts of rapid eye movement in REM sleep should not be considered pathologic since they occur in normal populations.[39] These are of a short duration (10–20 seconds), central in origin, and usually not associated with EEG arousal.

Sleep Apnea Syndrome is defined as "a potentially lethal condition characterized by multiple obstructive or mixed apneas during sleep associated with repetitive episodes of inordinately loud snoring and excessive daytime sleepiness."[41] A frequently quoted publication defines sleep apnea syndrome as the presence of 30 or more episodes of apnea per 7 hour sleep period.[42] However, there is some evidence that this standard may be clinically inaccurate since there is a high false positive rate when applied to older populations (several studies have shown that disordered breathing during sleep is more common with increasing age in people who are otherwise asymptomatic[43]). For example, there are no prospective studies correlating severity of clinical symptoms or degree of hemodynamic dysfunction and apnea frequency. This dilemma is discussed in more detail below.

Excessive Daytime Somnolence (EDS) may be defined as the tendency to fall asleep during activities that would otherwise not be considered soporific and is a classic symptom of sleep apnea syndrome. This symptom in sleep apnea patients may result from sleep fragmentation, which occurs with the numerous arousals and awakenings associated with the termination of apnea episodes. Some authors, however, feel that hypersomnolence may be related to other factors such as the degree of hypoxemia created by the apneas.[44] Extreme examples of EDS include sometimes humorous reports of falling asleep during sexual intercourse, inability to watch television or read due to hypersomnolence, persistent drowsiness or falling asleep while driving, and falling asleep while talking to people. Indeed, the original patient Burwell uses in describing "Pickwickian Syndrome" finally sought medical advice following years of debilitating symptoms only after he fell asleep during a poker game in which he failed to bid his hand containing a "full house." It is important to remember that daytime somnolence may not always take the form of overt sleepiness. Brief instances of sleep waves interrupting the normal waking EEG (microsleeps) have been reported in patients with "automatic behavior" (performance of simple acts or thought processes for which the patient has no recollection.[45] Such cases have sometimes been misdiagnosed as temporal lobe epilepsy. There is wide variation in the degree of daytime sleepiness among apneic patients. It is not unusual to see patients with 200 or more apneas per night who steadfastly deny daytime hypersomnolence, either because they no longer recognize the limits of normal sleepiness or they actually are not hypersomnolent. The Multiple Sleep Latency Test (MSLT) was developed to overcome the subjective aspect of daytime hypersomnolence and quantitatively measure sleep onset latency. Using the EEG, EMG, and EOG techniques described above, the patient is given the opportunity to fall asleep during several daytime nap periods, limited to 20 minutes each.[46] Latency to sleep onset is defined as the first epoch of Stage 1 sleep or any single epoch of the other four stages. The presence of a rapid sleep onset is indicative of pathologic somnolence and may be used as an objective measure in comparing the patient to others as well as to himself after some treatment modality. In an interesting variation of this study, the patient is told to "stay awake" during the nap, presumably measuring the patients' ability to resist the hypersomnolent state.[47]

Narcolepsy is a distinct clinical syndrome consisting of irresistable daytime hypersomnolence associated with the several other symptoms. These include cataplexy (the sudden loss of skeletal muscle tone in response to strong emotions such as laughter, anger, or surprise), sleep paralysis (the inability to voluntarily move just as the patient is waking up or falling asleep), or hypnogogic hallucinations (vivid, life-like dreams at sleep onset).[48] Narcolepsy is diagnosed by the presence of at least two of four sleep onset REM periods (REM sleep occurring within 15 minutes of sleep onset) during the daytime MSLT. The definitive diagnosis of narcolepsy is important to the clinician interested in respiratory disorders during sleep since narcolepsy is in the differential diagnosis of disorders associated with daytime hypersomnolence. In patients diagnosed as narcoleptic, the incidence of overt sleep apnea is about 6 percent.[49,50]

Pickwickian Syndrome refers to the clinical syndrome discussed by Burwell in 1956.[8] As originally described, Pickwickian syndrome includes the clinical features of marked obesity, somnolence, twitching, cyanosis, periodic respiration, polycythemia, and right ventricular hypertrophy and failure (edema). Since no formal sleep studies were done at the time this syndrome was described, the etiology of the cor pulmonale remained obscure and was not related to sleep pathology by the authors. However, periodic respiration with alternating apnea and tachypnea was noted in Burwell's patient during short naps while undergoing physical examination. Several diverse mechanisms may cause a clinical picture similar to the Pickwickian Syndrome. These include obstructive apnea (frequently associated with obesity), idiopathic obesity-hypoventilation syndrome, and central apnea. Clinical use of the term "Pickwickian Syndrome" should probably be abandoned as it is frequently misapplied to describe sleep apnea syndrome in obese patients.

Ondine's Curse is an eponym used to describe alveolar hypoventilation due to apnea. In the French play[51] from which the syndrome takes its name, the hero spurns the love of a mermaid (Ondine) and finds that bodily functions are no longer automatic so that he must consciously effect such vital functions. Unfortunately, this interesting eponym has sometimes been misused as a term for obstructive apnea and equated with "forgetting to breathe." When awake, patients with Ondine's curse have normal blood gas tensions by voluntary effort and are rarely dyspneic. When asleep or sedated, they exhibit hypoventilation manifested by hypercarbia and hypoxemia. Daytime hypersomnolence may be a prominent part of this syndrome. The proper application of the term "Ondine's curse"[52] describes hypoventilation or apnea resulting from one of three mechanisms: (1) destruction of the central CO_2 receptors or interruption of their afferent pathways; (2) destruction of the medullary respiratory neurons; or (3) interruption of the descending respiratory motor axons in the spinal cord. These situations have been described in medullary compression due to tumors, bulbar poliomyelitis, and other neuropathies involving the phrenic nerves,[53] and after bilateral chordotomy.[54]

Alveolar hypoventilation is reduced alveolar ventilation due either to impairment of the respiratory apparatus or decreased central drive to breath. It is usually defined as a resting awake $PaCO_2$ above 44 torr along with arterial hypoxemia, usually below 70 torr. Alveolar hypoventilation is most commonly associated with chronic obstructive pulmonary disease, interstitial lung disease, and long standing, severe deformities of the chest wall such as kyphoscoliosis. It is frequently seen in obese patients with obstructive sleep apnea and sometimes in obese patients without apnea. When no obvious chest wall or parenchymal pathology is evident, the hypoventilation is termed *Primary* or *Idiopathic Alveolar Hypoventilation*.[53,56] When hypoventilation is present only during sleep and is traceable to one of the specific etiologies listed in the above paragraph, it could properly be called "Ondine's Curse." Dyspnea as a result of abnormal blood gases is *not* a feature of this syndrome and ventilatory challenges to hypercarbia are diminished or flat. Since primary alveolar hypoventilation is frequently accompanied by obesity, such patients are often labeled "Obesity-Hypoventilation Syndrome."[57] This syndrome is characterized by morbid obesity, hypercarbia ($PaCO_2 > 44$ torr), diminished CO_2 sensitivity, a propensity toward the male sex, lethargy, and hypersomnolence. Indeed, in the extreme form and accompanied by severe hypoxemia and signs of congestive heart failure, such a patient may be termed "Pickwickian." However, if the patient exhibits a large number of obstructive apneas during sleep, the term "obesity-hypoventilation syndrome with obstructive sleep apnea" is more accurate since it is unclear whether the etiology of the hypoventilation is obesity or recurrent nocturnal apneas. Treatment of primary alveolar hypoventilation is discussed in Chapter 6.

INCIDENCE AND PREVALENCE OF SLEEP APNEA

At the present time, it is not possible to state with any certainty the incidence and prevalence of sleep apnea in the general population. This is due in part to two problems. The first is the time and expense involved in surveying large populations of normals with formal polysomnography. The second is that a definition of apnea frequency based upon sound objective criteria correlated with clinical symptoms and other parameters of hemodynamic dysfunction is still forthcoming. Sleep apnea is any pause in breathing during sleep, lasting more than 10 seconds. Thus, anyone with a single apnea during the night may be defined as having "sleep apnea." A single apnea, however, does not imply the presence of hemodynamic sequalae nor sleep disturbances that may lead to typical apnea symptoms.

In an effort to quantify apnea, and in essence correlate the frequency of apnea with clinical symptomatology, Guilleminaul[42,58] studied two groups of asymptomatic men and women (age 18–28 and 40–60). None of these subjects exceeded 25 apneas per night whereas the lowest apnea frequency in a patient considered to have "sleep apnea" was 45. Thus, the definition of sleep apnea as five or less apneas per hour of sleep was derived. Berry[59] has recently challenged this assumption in light of the clinical definition of sleep apnea syndrome, that is, requiring the presence of clinical symptoms to make the diagnosis. He surveyed the literature to date (13 publications), which reported greater than five apneas per hour in otherwise normal (asymptomatic) individuals. Using the criterion of the presence of clinical symptomatology, he found that above the age of 60, an apnea index of 5 falsely diagnosed sleep apnea syndrome in the normal elderly population. Another author reported that in 20 elderly subjects observed for 3 years, an apnea index above 5 did not predict a higher than control risk of serious medical problems.[60] Similarly, in a study of 145 upper class, randomly chosen elderly subjects, 62 percent had an apnea index of 5 or more per hour but 80 percent of these reported satisfactory sleep. These authors state "our questionnaire results suggest that the criteria of five events per hour do not always indicate a syndrome of any clinical severity."[25]

Several generalizations can be made from the few studies that have thus far been done. First, the incidence of apnea increases with age and the definition of normal may have to be adjusted for age just as normal blood sugar is in diabetes mellitus and normal pressure is in systemic hypertension.[41,59] A longitudinal study by Bliwise[62] in 8 middle aged and 12 elderly patients showed a modest but definite increase in apnea index over an 8 year period. Because of this relation to aging, the impact on the current population will grow as the average age of the population rises. The danger of the growing use of hypnotics, particularly among these populations at risk, has been the source of some concern.[63,64] Second, apnea is strongly sex related and found predominately in males through middle age when menopause places women at a risk approximately equal to men.[39,64,65] Published studies show a male to female ratio from 6:1 to 10:1.[65] The correlation has been attributed to hormonal influences, particularly the role of progesterone as a respiratory stimulant. Most cases of sleep apnea in women occur among the post menopausal age group.[66]

Finally, the presence of sleep apnea is strongly related to obesity, although it must be emphasized that patients of normal or only slightly above ideal body weight may develop sleep apnea.[58]

We have only scratched the surface in our pursuit of knowledge about respiratory abnormalities during sleep. Now that the proper tools are available for diagnosing these disorders, some effort must be made to simplify methods and make such studies less expensive. Such methods must then be used to determine the importance of this disorder to the population in general. Furthermore, the proliferation of treatments (uvulopalatopharyngoplasty, tracheostomy, continuous positive airway pressure, etc.) that have developed in the past 15 years may be some indication that our effectiveness in treating this problem leaves something to be desired. Therefore, future efforts at research must be aimed at simple, effective, noninvasive treatment of apnea.

REFERENCES

1. Aelianus C: Various History: Book IX. London, Thomas Dung, 1666, Chap. 13, p 177
2. Kryger MH: Sleep apnea: From the needles of Dionysius to continuous positive airway pressure. Arch Intern Med 143:2301–2303, 1983
3. Wadd W: Cursory Remarks on Corpulence; or Obesity Considered as a Disease: With a Critical Examination of Ancient and Modern Opinions Relative to its Causes and Cure (ed 3). London, Gallow Medical Bookseller, 1822
4. Athenaeus: The Deipnosophists, Gulick CB (trans). Cambridge, Mass, Harvard University Press, 1933, vol 5, pp 491–497
5. Mettler CC: History of Medicine. Philadelphia, Blakiston Publishing Co., 1947, p 560
6. Broadbent WH: Cheyne-Stokes respiration in cerebral haemorrhage. Lancet 1:137–139, 1877
7. Dickens C: The Posthumous Papers of the Pickwick Club. London, Chapman and Hall, 1837
8. Burwell CS, Robin ED, Whaley RD, Bickelmann AG: Extreme obesity associated with alveolar hypoventilation—A Pickwickian syndrome. Am J Med 21:811–818, 1956
9. Spitz A: Das klinishe syndrom: Narkolepsie mit fettsucht und polyglobulie in seinen beziehungen zum morbus cushing. Dtsch Arch Klin Med 181:286–304, 1937
10. Gastaut H, Tassinari C, Duron B: Etude polygraphique des manifestations episodiques (hypniques et respiratoires) du syndrome de Pickwick. Rev Neurol 112:568–579, 1965
11. Jung R, Kuhlo W: Neurophysiological studies of abnormal night sleep and the Pickwickian syndrome. Prog Brain Res 18:140–159, 1965
12. Fechner G: Elemente der Psychophysik. Leipzig, Breitkopf & Hartel, 1860
13. Kohlschuter E: Z Ration Med 3 Reihe 17:209, 1863
14. Howell WH: A contribution to the physiology of sleep, based upon plethysmographic experiments. J Exp Med 2:313–345, 1897
15. Caton R: The electric currents of the brain. Br Med J 2:278, 1875
16. Berger H: Uber das elektroendephalogramm des menschen. Arch Psych Nervenkr 87:527–570, 1929
17. Loomis AL, Harvey EN, Hobart GA: Potential rhythms of the cerebral cortex during sleep. Science 81:597–598, 1935
18. Aserinsky E, Kleitman N: Regularly occurring periods of eye motility, and concomitant phenomena, during sleep. Science 118:273–274, 1953
19. Aserinsky E, Kleitman N: Two types of ocular motility occurring in sleep. J Appl Physiol 8:1–10, 1955
20. Bulow K: Respiration and wakefulness in man. Acta Physiol Scand 59:209, 1963
21. Kuhlo W, Doll E, Franc M: Exfolgreich behandlung eines Pickwick syndrome durch eine dauertracheal kanule. Dtsch Med Wochenschr 94:1286–1290, 1969
22. Remmers JE, deGroot WJ, Sauerland EK, Anch AM: Pathogenesis of upper airway occlusion during sleep. J Appl Physiol 44(6):931–938, 1978
23. Sullivan CE, Berthon-Jones M, Issa FG, Eves L: Reversal of obstructive sleep apnea by continuous positive airway pressure applied through the nares. Lancet 1:862–865, 1981

24. Riedy RM, Hulsey R, Bachus BF, et al: Sleep apnea syndrome: A practical diagnostic method. Chest 75(1):81–83, 1979

25. Ancoli-Israel S, Kripke DF, Mason W, Kaplan OJ: Sleep apnea and periodic movements in an aging sample. J of Gerontol 40(4):419–425, 1985

26. Carskadon MA: Basics for Polygraphic monitoring of sleep, in Guilleminault C (ed): Sleeping and Waking Disorders: Indications and Techniques. Menlo Park, CA, Addison-Wesley Publishing Co., 1982, pp 1–16

27. Tilkan AG, Motta J, Guilleminault C: Cardiac Arrhythmias in Sleep Apnea, in Guilleminault C, Dement W (eds): Sleep Apnea Syndromes. New York, Alan R Liss, 1978, 197–210

28. Lemen R, Benson M, Jones JG: Absolute pressure measurements with hand-dipped and manufactured esophageal balloons. J Appl Physiol 37(4):600–603, 1974

29. Sanders MH, Holzer BC, Reynolds CF: A tale of two polysomnographic techniques. Sleep Res 13:212, 1984

30. Sharp JT, Druz WS, Foster JR, et al: Use of the respiratory magnetometer in diagnosis and classification of sleep apnea. Chest 77(3):350–353, 1980

31. Chadha TS, Watson H, Birch S, et al: Validation of respiratory inductive plethysmography using different calibration procedures. Am Rev Respir Dis 125:644–649, 1982

32. Loveridge B, West P, Anthonisen NR, Kryger MH: Single-position calibration of the respiratory inductance plethysmograph. J Appl Physiol 55(3):1031–1034, 1983

33. Douglas NJ, Brash HM, Wraith PK, et al: Accuracy, sensitivity to carboxyhemoglobin, and speed of response of the Hewlett-Packard 47201A ear oximeter. Am Rev Respir Dis 119:311–313, 1979

34. Rebuck AS, Chapman KR, D'Urzo A: The Accuracy and Response Characteristics of a Simplified Ear Oximeter. Chest 83(6):860–864, 1983

35. Fletcher EC, Gray BA, Levin DC: Nonapneic mechanisms of arterial oxygen desaturation during rapid-eye-movement sleep. J Appl Physiol: Respirat Environ Exercise Physiol 54:632–639, 1983

36. Simmons FB, Guilleminault C, Miles LE: A surgical treatment for snoring and obstructive sleep apnea. West J Med 140:43–46, 1984

37. Nino-Murcia G, Bliwise D, Keenan S, et al: Respiration monitoring in sleep: Comparison of judgments based on conventional polysomnography and an ambulatory, microprocessor-derived recording. Sleep Res 14:274, 1985

38. Rechtschaffen A, Kales A (eds): A manual of standardized terminology, techniques and scoring system for sleep stages of human subjects. Washington D.C., NIH publication 204, 1968

39. Phillipson EA: State of the art: Control of breathing during sleep. Am Rev Resp Dis 118(5):909–939, 1978

40. Slutsky AS, Strohl KP: Quantification of oxygen saturation during episodic hypoxemia. Am Rev Respir Dis 121:893–895, 1980

41. Association of Sleep Disorder Centers. Diagnostic classification of sleep and arousal disorders (ed 1). Sleep 2:1–137, 1979

42. Guilleminault C, Dement WC: Sleep Apnea Syndromes and Related Sleep Disorders, in Williams RL, Karacan I (eds): Sleep disorders: Diagnosis and Treatment. 1978 p 11

43. Carskadon MA, Dement WC: Respiration during sleep in the aged human. J Gerontol 36:420–423, 1981

44. Orr WC, Martin RJ: Hypersomnolent and non-hypersomnolent patients with upper airway obstruction during sleep. Chest 75:418–422, 1979

45. Guilleminault C, Billiard M, Montplasir J, Dement WC: Altered states of consciousness in disorders of daytime sleepiness. J Neurol Sci 26:377–387, 1975

46. Mitler MM: The multiple sleep latency test as an evaluation for excessive somnolence, in Guilleminault C: Sleeping and Waking Disorders: Indications and Techniques 1982, p 145–155

47. Browman CP, Gujavarty KS, Sampson MG, Mitler MM: REM sleep episodes during the maintenance of wakefulness test in patients with sleep apnea syndrome and patients with narcolepsy. Sleep 6(1):23–28, 1983

48. Roth B: Narcolepsy and Hypersomnia, in Williams RL, Karacan I (eds): Sleep Disorders: Diagnosis and Treatment. New York, John Wiley and Sons, 1978, pp 29–59

49. Guilleminault C, Eldridge FL, Dement WC: Narcolepsy, insomnia and sleep apneas. Bull Physiopathol Respir 8:1127, 1972

50. Guilleminault C, Dement W: 235 cases of excessive daytime sleepiness: Diagnosis and tentative classification. J Neurol Sci 31:13, 1977

51. Girauddoux J: Ondine: A Romantic Fantasy in Three Acts. Valency M (trans). New York, Samuel Frach Inc., 1956

52. Severinghaus JW, Mitchell RA: Ondine's curse-failure of respiratory center automatically while awake. Clin Res 10:122, 1962

53. Goldstein RC, Hyde RW, Lapham LW, et al: Peripheral neuropathy presenting with respi-

ratory insufficiency as the primary complaint. Am J Med 56:443, 1974

54. Kreiger AJ, Rosomoff HL: Sleep-induced apnea: Part 1—a respiratory and autonomic dysfunction syndrome following bilateral percutaneous cervical cordotomy. J Neurosurg 39:168, 1974

55. Reichel J: Primary Alveolar Hypoventilation. Clinics in Chest Medicine 1(1):119–123, 1980

56. McNicholas WT, Carter JL, Rutherford R, et al: Beneficial effect of oxygen in primary alveolar hypoventilation with central sleep apnea. Am Rev Respir Dis 125:773–775, 1982

57. Rochester DF, Enson Y: Current concepts in the pathogenesis of the obesity-hypoventilation syndrome: Mechanical and circulatory factors. Am J Med 57:402–420, 1974

58. Guilleminault C, van den Hoed J, Mitler MM: Clinical overview of the sleep apnea syndromes, in Guilleminault C, Dement WC (eds): Sleep Apnea Syndromes. Alan R Liss Inc., New York, NY 1978, pp 1–12

59. Berry DTR, Webb WB, Block AJ: Sleep apnea syndrome—A critical review of the apnea index as a diagnostic criterion. Chest 86:529–531, 1984

60. Krieger J, Turlot JC, Mangin P, Kurtz D: Breathing during sleep in normal young and elderly subjects: Hypopneas, apneas, and correlated factors. Sleep 6(2):108–120, 1983

61. Webb P: Periodic breathing during sleep. J of Appl Psychol 37:899–903, 1974

62. Bliwise D, Carskadon M, Carey E, Dement W: Longitudinal development of sleep-related respiratory disturbance in adult humans. J Gerontol 39(3):290–293, 1984

63. Dolly FR, Block AJ: Effect of flurazepam on sleep–disordered breathing and nocturnal oxygen desaturation in asymptomatic subjects. Am J Med 73:239–243, 1982

64. Kreis P, Kripke DP, Ancoli-Israel S: Sleep apnea: A prospective study. West J Med 139:171–173, 1983

65. Block AJ, Boysen PG, Wynne JW, et al: Sleep apnea, hypopnea and oxygen desaturation in normal subjects—A strong male predominance. N Engl J Med 300:513–517, 1979

66. Block AJ, Wynne JW, Boysen PG: Sleep–disordered breathing and nocturnal oxygen desaturation in postmenopausal women. Am J Med 69:75–79, 1980

David W. Hudgel

2
Clinical Manifestations of the Sleep Apnea Syndrome

Our growing awareness of the major health consequences of respiratory and other physiologic disorders that occur principally during sleep has led to rapid development of sleep disorders centers specializing in the diagnosis and care of patients inflicted with these maladies. In spite of this concentrated effort, the true incidence of disorders such as sleep apnea syndrome is unknown. Although heavy snoring is estimated to occur in about 25 percent of the population[1,2] (higher in older individuals[3]), symptoms of sleep apnea were found in only 1–3 percent of an industrial working population.[4] Males have a higher incidence of sleep apnea than females,[5] but the incidence becomes more equal when examining older males and post-menopausal females.[6,7]

Although a significant incidence of sleep apnea syndrome likely exists in the middle-aged to older age groups, the disease has often gone unrecognized in the past primarily (1) due to the subtle and nonspecificity of symptoms and signs of sleep apnea and (2) the unavailability of the technology to readily make the diagnosis. Other disease entities are often thought to be present explaining the symptoms and signs that exist in a particular clinical situation. However, these symptoms and signs may really be indicative of sleep apnea. Although the diagnoses of these other disease entities may be correct; they, in fact, may be secondary to sleep apnea. For example, hypersomnolence and impotence may be thought to be secondary to mental depression in a given patient; but indeed the symptoms and the depression may be caused by sleep apnea. Another glaring realization has been that the most important symptom of sleep apnea, heavy snoring, cannot be ascertained in adequate detail, or sometimes even be recognized at all by the patient himself; this history *must* be obtained from the patient's bed partner or other family member. Without such history, the physician will be unable to relate such symptoms as hypersomnolence, impotence, and depression to the snoring and, thereby the potential diagnosis of sleep apnea may well be overlooked.

The purpose of this chapter is to review the clinical picture and laboratory findings of sleep apnea syndrome and to focus on associated illnesses.

ABNORMALITIES OF RESPIRATION DURING SLEEP
ISBN 0-8089-1812-5 Copyright © 1986 by Grune & Stratton, Inc.
All rights of reproduction in any form reserved.

MAJOR CLINICAL FINDINGS

The primary symptom of nearly all patients with sleep apnea is heavy snoring. Loud sonorous snoring that disturbs others occurs in obstructive apnea. Jokes are made about the snorer who "rattles the rafters" or keeps all his buddies awake while on the annual fishing expedition. However, it is not humorous when a patient's spouse files for divorce because of disruption of marital life due to the snoring. As mentioned above, an adequate snoring history needs to be obtained from family members; the patient is usually unaware of its severity or characteristics. Typically, the patient with obstructive apnea makes several, progressively more forceful inspiratory efforts against the obstructed airway. During this time he may be restless, but he will not be snoring since there is no air movement during apnea. When the apnea breaks, a loud snort occurs because of the high level of thoracic muscle and diaphragm inspiratory activity that has built up during the apnea. Snoring usually continues with each inspiration until obstruction occurs again. The cycle repeats itself hundreds of times throughout the night. Thus, bed partners of these patients are not only kept awake by the sonorous snoring but may be accidently injured by the restless, suffocating, apneic patient. Patients with partial obstructive sleep apnea and those with central apnea also may snore, but this snoring is not as loud as that produced by patients with complete obstructive apnea. The restlessness is also not present in these patients.

As indicated by the epidemiological studies mentioned above, patients with obstructive sleep apnea are usually, but not always, male and frequently obese. Obesity is surely an important component of the illness in many individuals, but the mechanism of the connection between obesity and apnea is presently unknown.

Another disabling symptom of sleep apnea is hypersomnolence. Obviously, some daytime sleepiness is normal. It is normal to feel somewhat sleepy in the early afternoon, but actual sleep is unusual, and if recurrent afternoon naps are a pattern, the individual should be considered hypersomnolent. Patients with sleep apnea have varying degrees of daytime hypersomnolence. Those individuals who fall asleep while talking with others (like their physician) or who lose their job or fail to receive a promotion because of their sleepiness, have disabling hypersomnolence requiring medical attention. Some patients can stay awake, albeit usually not fully alert, if they work on their feet. Sleep apnea patients should not hold a position where they are responsible for the safety of others. Of course, a very dangerous activity for these patients is driving a vehicle. Surely several traffic mortalities every year are the result of sleep apnea patients falling asleep at the wheel. In other situations such as meetings and social gatherings, sleep apnea patients often nod off to sleep while listening to a presentation or participating in small talk. Their snoring is disruptive and embarrassing to their spouse and friends. Other causes of hypersomnolence must be considered in the differential diagnosis (Table 2-1).

Sometimes, one must differentiate the hypersomnolence of narcolepsy from that of sleep apnea.[3,8] Narcoleptic patients can usually predict the times of their sleep attacks and sense their onset. They can resist the sleepiness by becoming physically active. However, patients with sleep apnea, who are severely hypersomnolent, usually cannot feel the episodes of sleep approaching; or they may be continuously sleepy. Of course, these generalizations do not apply to all patients. The presence of cataplexy in narcoleptic patients may be another differentiating factor. Cataplexic

Table 2-1
Differential Diagnosis of Daytime Hypersomnolence

1. Sleep apnea syndrome
2. Narcolepsy
3. Sleep pattern disturbances, insomnia
4. Hypometabolic states such as hypothermia, hypothyroidism
5. Uremia and other metabolic derangements
6. Cerebral vascular disease or other CNS degenerative diseases
7. Mental depression and other functional states
8. Sedatives or medications with sedating side-effects

patients know they have to sit down to avoid collapse before they laugh or become emotionally upset. The multiple sleep latency test may be used to differentiate patients with narcolepsy without cataplexy from patients with other causes of hypersomnolence.[8,9] Typically, narcoleptic patients will enter rapid-eye-movement (REM) sleep within 15 minutes of sleep onset. This is distinctly abnormal in that normally REM sleep does not occur until about 90 minutes of sleep has elapsed. Usually a good history and nocturnal polysomnography are enough to make the appropriate distinction between sleep apnea and narcolepsy.

Another complication of sleep apnea, primarily obstructive apnea, is hypoxemia. The degree of hypoxemia seen depends on the awake oxygenation and pulmonary function status, the length of the apneas, and the amount of "recovery time" between apneas and the sleep stage. Usually the most severe hypoxemia is seen during REM sleep. Hypoxemia may result in pulmonary and systemic hypertension.[10] Patients may be treated for essential hypertension for years as a primary diagnosis;[11,12] again, a history of snoring would lead one to suspect sleep apnea. Lugaresi et al found that more snorers had hypertension than an age, weight matched nonsnoring group.[2] When hypertensive patients are male, obese, and have other symptoms like snoring and/or hypersomnolence, sleep apnea must be considered as a diagnostic possibility.

Patients with isolated nocturnal hypoxemia may present with erythrocytosis and/or cor pulmonale. Sleep apnea patients may develop obvious right sided congestive heart failure; this is a sign of marked decompensation and indicates the need for immediate reversal of the situation, not only with treatment for erythrocytosis or heart failure, but primarily with institution of a program that will promptly reverse the sleep apnea. Occasionally, but not as often as might be anticipated with the extreme degree of hypoxemia observed, these patients experience significant cardiac rhythm disturbances.[13–15] Worrisome arrhythmias such as complete heart block, sinus arrest, or ventricular tachycardia may occasionally occur, even in patients with no arrhythmias during wakefulness. When these severe arrhythmias do occur, rapid treatment of the apnea and monitoring of cardiac rhythm in an environment where resuscitation equipment is available are paramount. Some patients will experience brady-tachycardia. In fact, this phenomenon was thought to be useful as a simple diagnostic screening tool. However, because this finding is not specific and because measurement of ventilation would be required in a patient with this finding to discern the type of apnea and its severity, the test is really not useful.

Other important complications of sleep apnea are likely secondary to sleep deprivation. Mental depression, mood swings, intellectual deterioration, and impotence occur in varying degrees in many sleep apneic patients. Occasionally psychoses can develop.[16] Sleep apnea and resultant hypoxemia or abnormal sleep stage distribution may cause pituitary hormone or CNS neurotransmitter secretory abnormalities, resulting in some of these secondary complications. Some patients may present nearly moribund. With successful treatment these abnormalities usually reverse rapidly. It also has been noted that sleep apnea present in adolescence may depress sexual maturation by preventing normal diurnal fluctuation of sex hormones responsible for puberty. In addition, these hypogonadal individuals are often obese, which surely amplifies the apnea.

Morning headaches may be secondary to hypoxemia or the hypercapnia that occurs as a result of the apnea. Enuresis can occur in some individuals. Because of the frequent awakenings and drowsiness of these patients, hypnagogic hallucinations can occur. Some patients cannot resume sleep after awakening and thus will actually present with insomnia. Therefore, sleep apnea must be included in the differential diagnosis of individuals presenting with disorders of maintaining sleep.

SLEEP APNEA SECONDARY TO OTHER DISEASE ENTITIES AND ANATOMIC VARIANTS

Sleep apnea, especially obstructive sleep apnea, is sometimes related to localized anatomical abnormalities of the upper airway or appears in conjunction with some systemic diseases (see Chapter 10). Resolution of the primary defect, be it a local anatomical problem or a systemic disease process, usually results in resolution of the apnea. A list of these entities known to date is given in Table 2-2. Any anatomical abnormality that leads to narrowing of the upper airway may contribute to obstructive sleep apnea. These examples point out that a compromised upper airway is potentially dangerous. For instance, an individual with heavy snoring without apnea may be converted to a person with severe obstructive sleep apnea by alcohol or sedative consumption.

PHYSIOLOGIC BASIS FOR SYMPTOMS OF SLEEP APNEA

Snoring

There are anatomical and physiologic components of snoring. During inspiration several muscles of the upper airway including alae nasi, genioglossus, positerior cricoaryteroid, cricothyroid, and geniohyoid are activated to maintain or increase airway cross-sectional area. This inspiratory activity stabilizes the airway against the collapsing effects of the negative intrapleural pressure produced during inspiration by diaphragm and chest wall muscle contractions. During sleep there is some loss of muscle tone and less inspiratory muscle activity of the upper airway muscles.[36] As a possible consequence of this relative inactivity, the upper airway resistance normally increases two to three times above that of wakefulness[37] (Fig. 2-1). Thus, the upper airway appears to be narrowed during normal sleep. With this amount of airway narrowing, any additional anatomical narrowing compromising the airway prior to sleep onset will have a greater impact. In addition to anatomical abnormalities, an abnormal physiologic state of suppressed inspiratory muscle activity may

Table 2-2
Abnormalities Complicated by Obstructive Sleep Apnea

Anatomical

 1. Adenoid and tonsillar hypertrophy in children and adults[17–19]
 2. Glottic web and vocal cord paralysis[18]
 3. Acromegaly[20,21]
 4. Lymphoma or Hodgkin's disease within pharyngeal lymphoid tissue[22]
 5. Microagnathia of various causes[17]
 6. Ectopic thyroid
 7. Upper airway radiation edema or fibrosis[23,24]
 8. Mandible retroagnathia (congenital or secondary to trauma), inadequate repair of fractures, or systemic diseases involving the mandible like rheumatoid arthritis[25]
 9. Correction of velopharyngeal incompetence in infants[17,26]
10. Severe kyphoscoliosis[27]
11. Cushing's disease or syndrome

Functional

 1. Poliomyelitis, muscular dystrophy, amyotrophic lateral sclerosis and other diseases with bulbar incoordination secondary to brain stem abnormalities[28]
 2. Acquired dysautonomia[29]
 3. Diaphragm pacing for primary alveolar hypoventilation[30]
 4. Hypothyroidism
 5. Flurazepam induced[31]
 6. Alcohol ingestion[32]
 7. Testosterone administration[33]
 8. Eplipesy[34]
 9. Encephalitis[35]

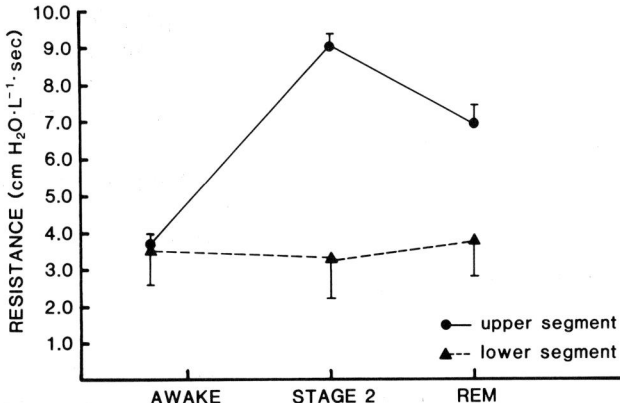

Fig. 2-1. Inspiratory airflow resistance in healthy adult male subjects during sleep. The resistance in the supralaryngeal airway (solid line) increases significantly while the resistance across the lungs and larynx (dotted line) remains unchanged. (From Hudgel DW, Martin RJ, Johnson B, Hill P: Mechanics of the respiratory system and breathing pattern during sleep in normal humans. J Appl Physiol 56:136, 1984. With permission.)

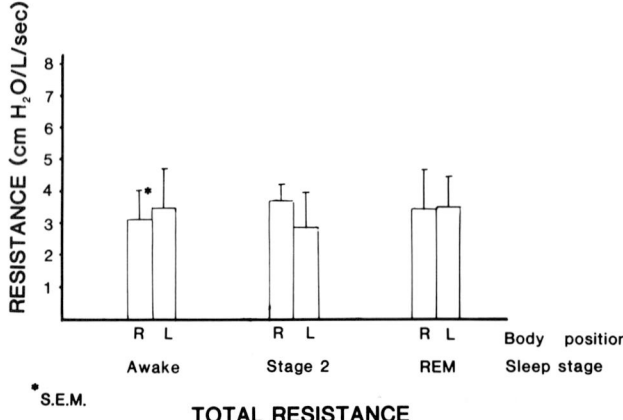

Fig. 2-2. Total nasal resistance in healthy adult male subjects during sleep. No significant changes in nasal resistance occur during sleep in either right (R) or left (L) lateral body position. (From Hudgel DW, Robertson DW: Nasal resistance during wakefulness and sleep in normal man. Acta Otolaryngol 98:134, 1984. With permission.)

exist and contribute to upper airway obstruction. Abnormal control of pharyngeal muscle activity may occur in hypothyroidism and in other states such as hyperoxia, where the control of inspiratory muscle activity is suppressed. It is possible that a combination of depressed central controls of ventilation and a narrow upper airway may be necessary for obstructive apnea to occur. At this time, uncertainty exists about the relative contributions of anatomic and physiologic abnormalities to obstructive apnea.

Airway narrowing occurs in the supralaryngeal region or at the level of the soft palate, or at both sites. Rubin reported soft palate and posterior faucial pillar vibrations appearing during snoring.[38] This has been observed cinegraphically also.[39] Most likely the primary site of narrowing is not located within the larynx or nose. However, increased total nasal resistance, which we have found does not normally occur during sleep[40] (Fig. 2-2) may occur in acute or chronic rhinitis. This would increase the negative inspiratory pressure within the pharynx, lower the pharyngeal inspiratory diameter, and possibly lead to inspiratory upper airway occlusion in some individuals. In fact, apneas and periodic breathing have been described in patients with chronic rhinitis.[41]

Hypersomnolence

The etiology of the hypersomnolence of patients with sleep apnea has been thought to be sleep disruption and the lack of deep stage 3 and 4 sleep. Usually, a short arousal occurs at the time of reversal of each apnea. These arousals, often several hundred per night, are thought to prevent the normal progression from stage 2 sleep into stage 3 and 4 sleep.[42] However, the data of Orr et al demonstrates that hypoxemia per se may contribute to the hypersomnolence of sleep apnea.[43] CNS neurotransmittor and mediator metabolism may be abnormal in sleep apnea. Lugaresi et al demonstrated increased levels of homovanillic acid (HVA) and 5-hydroxyindolacetic acid (5-HIAA) in the cerebral spinal fluid of two sleep apnea patients.[2] These elevations disappeared abruptly following tracheostomy. The authors concluded that both the serotoninergic and the dopaminergic systems may be altered by sleep apnea. Cramer et al[44] showed cyclic adenosine monophosphate (cAMP) elevation in CSF of apneic patients. This finding was not specific to sleep apnea since some patients with hypoxemia secondary to pulmonary disease also had elevated cAMP values. It is interesting that the pulmonary patients had daytime hypersomnolence, but they did not have sleep apnea. The immediate reversal of hypersomnolence after tracheostomy indicates the mechanism of hypersomnolence is short-acting and directly tied to the presence of apnea.

Pulmonary and Systemic Hypertension

Pulmonary hypertension is presumably due to the repetitive nocturnal hypoxemia these patients experience. Sleep hypoxemia has been demonstrated to result in an increase in pulmonary arterial pressure.[10] Improvement of the sleep apnea will reduce the extent of hypoxemia and pulmonary hypertension. The etiology of systemic hypertension is unclear, but again, this entity also improves or clears with successful therapy of the sleep apnea. (The hemodynamic consequences of sleep apnea are further discussed in Chapter 4.)

Depression, Memory Loss and Impotence

These important clinical manifestations of sleep apnea are considered to be secondary to sleep disruption and an abnormal sleep stage distribution. Hypoxemia per se is also a CNS suppressant. Secondary hypersomnolence itself could cause these complications. The impotence is usually physiologic and not anatomical since these patients can have erections during REM sleep. Recently, preliminary data were presented that showed serum testosterone levels were depressed because of hypothalamic-pituitary suppression in sleep apnea patients.[45] Impaired sexual maturation is also known to occur in adolescents with sleep apnea. This is thought to be due to lack of nocturnal elevation of luteinizing hormone (LH) and testosterone; the nocturnal elevations of these sex hormones are thought to be necessary for pubertal development.[46]

LABORATORY FINDINGS IN SLEEP APNEA

Are there any laboratory tests than can be performed during wakefulness that will be indicative of the presence of apnea during sleep? Disagreement exists about the value of such testing. However, there are no awake measurements that will *specifically* predict whether sleep apnea will be found in a given patient nor predict the severity of the apnea. If the pharynx is narrow in the sitting position, measurement of maximal expiratory and inspiratory flow rates may be decreased, and the flow-volume loop pattern will be consistent with extrathoracic airflow obstruction. In addition to flow limitation, "sawtoothing" may be seen on the forced expiratory and inspiratory flow-volume loop. This pattern has frequently been seen in groups of obstructive sleep apnea patients and is thought to be caused by vibration of redundant pharyngeal tissue.[47,48] This finding is by no means specific to these patients and may be seen in subjects without obstructive sleep apnea. This observation is also dependent on the mechanical properties of the spirometer and recorder used.

Table 2-3

Arterial Blood Gas Fluctuations During Sleep in
Obstructive Sleep Apnea

	Awake	Sleep Nonapneic	Apneic Period
pH	7.43	7.42	7.36
PCO$_2$ (mm Hg)	35	36	44
PO$_2$ (mm Hg)	56*	50	31
O$_2$ Saturation (percent)	92	89	67
CO$_2$ Content (mMol/L)	23	24	25

* Measurement made in asthmatic patient in Denver, Colorado—normal PO$_2$ = 69 ± 10 (2SD) mm Hg.

Erythrocytosis can be seen, and right ventricular hypertrophy or strain may be observed on the electrocardiogram of patients with sleep hypoxemia and pulmonary hypertension. Enlarged pulmonary artery trunks may be observed on the chest radiograph in such a setting. The absence of these findings does not exclude the possibility of significant sleep hypoxemia since there is individual variability in the severity and time course of the chronic cardiovascular response to hypoxemia.

Some patients with sleep apnea will experience alveolar hypoventilation during wakefulness. This hypoventilation may be due to (1) suppressed ventilatory drive

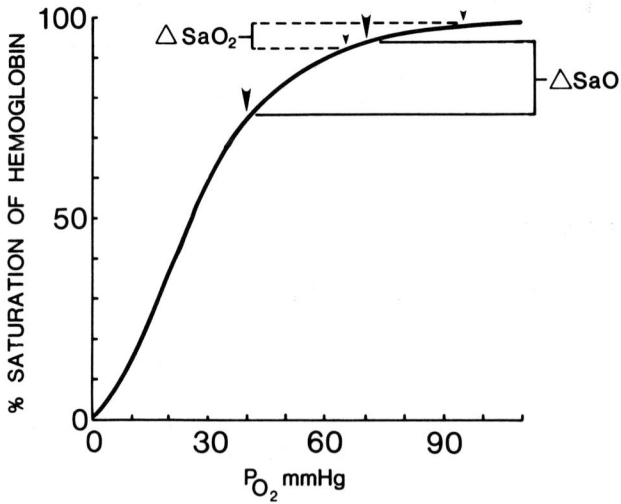

Fig. 2-3. Affect of initial PO$_2$ on amount of arterial oxygen desaturation seen. Because of the shape of the oxygen-hemoglobin dissociation curve, the amount of decrease in SaO$_2$ seen with equivalent decrease in PO$_2$ is different for different starting PO$_2$'s. When the starting PO$_2$ is near or below the "elbow" of the curve more desaturation is seen.

mechanisms, (2) increased mechanical load to breathing, such as occurs in obesity or severe upper airway narrowing, or (3) weak inspiratory muscles. Pure alveolar hypoventilation is manifested by hypercapnia and hypoxemia with a normal alveolar-arterial oxygen gradient. In addition to alveolar hypoventilation, patients may have a widened alveolar-arterial oxygen gradient because of maldistribution of inspired air into a small lung with airspace compression, usually due to obesity.

Arterial blood gas analysis in a sleep apnea patient is shown in Table 2-3. During wakefulness, a slightly increased alveolar-arterial oxygen gradient is present. During nonapneic sleep, the pCO_2 remains constant and the pO_2 decreases. This is possibly due to lung compression secondary to the chest wall muscle hypotonia of sleep. During the apnea, evidence of alveolar hypoventilation is present in that the pCO_2 increases and pO_2 decreases. Of course, an oximeter in place on the ear or finger will show a decrease in arterial oxyhemoglobin saturation (SaO_2), depending on the location of PaO_2 values on the hemoglobin-oxygen dissociation curve. If the initial PaO_2 is high, it can decrease considerably with only minimal changes in SaO_2. However, if the PaO_2 is approximately 65 mmHg or below, the SaO_2 drops almost linearly with a decrease in PaO_2 (Fig. 2-3).

POLYSOMNOGRAPHY

Once a practitioner suspects a patient of having a breathing problem during sleep, observation may often be adequate to make a tentative diagnosis. Obstructive apnea, central apnea, and hypopnea are sometimes distinguishable by educated observation. However, to watch a patient for several hours during sleep is quite impractical. Thus, with rather simple monitoring techniques not only can an accurate qualitative diagnosis be made, but a quantitative assessment of the severity of the problem can be accomplished. Rechtschaffen and Kales have developed the standards being currently followed for sleep staging.[49] Guidelines for the measurement of ventilation during sleep have recently been published.[50].

For sleep staging, one or two electroencephalographic patterns (vertex to opposite ear [C_3–A_2 or C_4–A_1]), one or two electrooculographic and one submental electromyogram recordings should be obtained. Paper speed should be at least 10 mm/second for adequate sleep stage scoring. Breathing pattern is monitored qualitatively with flow sensors, usually thermisters at the nose and mouth. It is important to monitor nasal and oral flow in case ventilation changes pathways during the study, as Figure 2-4 demonstrates. Of course, one thermister could be used inside a facemask, but most patients prefer the two thermisters instead of a mask. Snoring intensity can be measured with a microphone near the mouth or attached to the anterior chest. Flow detectors will assess the presence of apnea, defined as the cessation of airflow. An evaluation of ventilatory effort is needed to determine whether such apneas are due to complete or partial upper airway closure or secondary to a cessation of ventilatory activity. Ventilatory effort is best assessed with an esophageal balloon. In extremely obese patients the esophageal balloon is the only technique that will accurately assess ventilatory effort. In less obese individuals strain gauges around the thorax and abdomen or an inductance vest may be adequate. Inspiratory muscle activity can also be recorded from the chest wall with electrodes placed in the sixth and seventh intercostal spaces in the anterior axillary line. A precordial

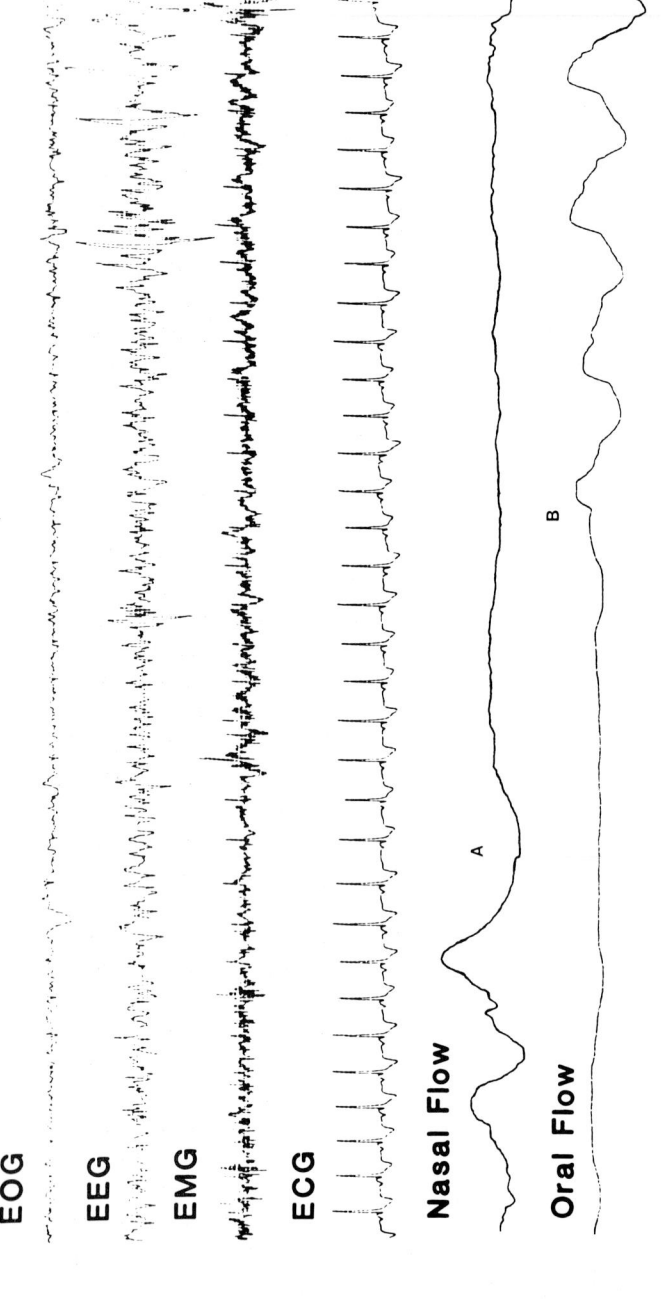

Fig. 2-4. Fluctuation between oral and nasal airflow during sleep. This fluctuation necessitates monitoring nasal and oral flow separately or simultaneously via a face mask (see Fig. 2-5). EOG, electrooculogram; EEG, electroencephalogram-C_4-A_1, or C_3-A_2; EMG, electromyogram of submental area; ECG, electrocardiogram precordial leads; SaO_2, oxygen saturation measured by a finger-pulse oximeter (same for all following figures). Nasal airflow ceases at point A but continues via the oral route at B. Nasal airflow monitored alone would have indicated the presence of complete apnea.

electrocardiogram is used to detect cardiac arrhythmias that might occur. Arterial oxygen saturation is monitored with an oximeter attached to the ear, a finger, or the bridge of the nose.

Care should be taken to calibrate the strip chart recorder with an electrical pulse for AC signals and with a mechanical signal for DC channels (oximeter or vest). The recorder should be calibrated for the range of saturation values predicted and linearity of the signal needs to be insured by having at least one calibration signal in between the maximum and minimum calibration level (only one oximeter available allows such calibration).

Patterns of polysomnographic findings. A typical obstructive apnea is shown in Figure 2-5. The thermistors show some minimal deflection related to expiratory flow often seen during an obstructive apnea. There is continued respiratory effort with increasing inspiratory pleural pressure swings during each successive obstructed breath. With breaking of the apnea, increased chin muscle activity, snoring, and resumption of airflow at the nose and/or mouth occurs. A severe degree of arterial oxygen desaturation is seen. Desaturation follows the apnea primarily because of

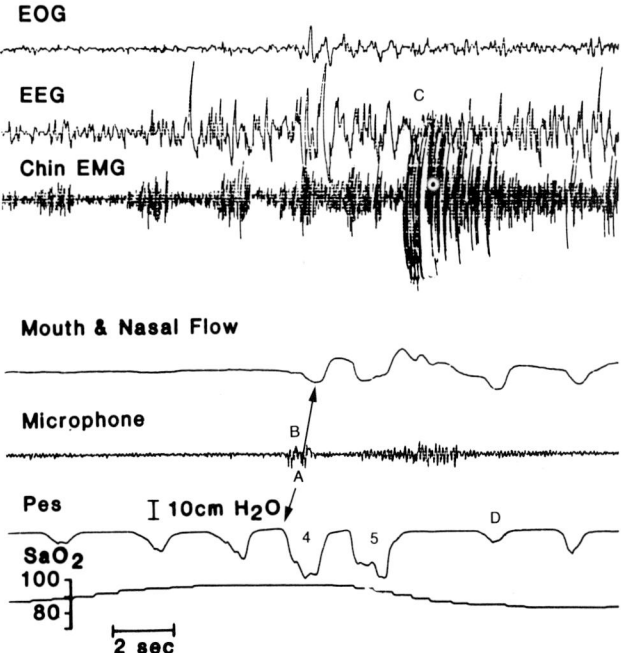

Fig. 2-5. Obstructive apnea. Inspiratory effort, as seen in the chin EMG and esophageal pressure tracings, increases over the first three breaths shown until the apnea is broken (A). During breaths four and five, large inspiratory efforts cause snoring (B) (microphone tracing) and some inspiratory flow. Following breath four, arousal occurs (C) and inspiratory resistance decreases as evidenced by the lower inspiratory esophageal pressure swings (D). Because of circulation time from lung to finger, arterial oxygen desaturation follows the apneas by several seconds.

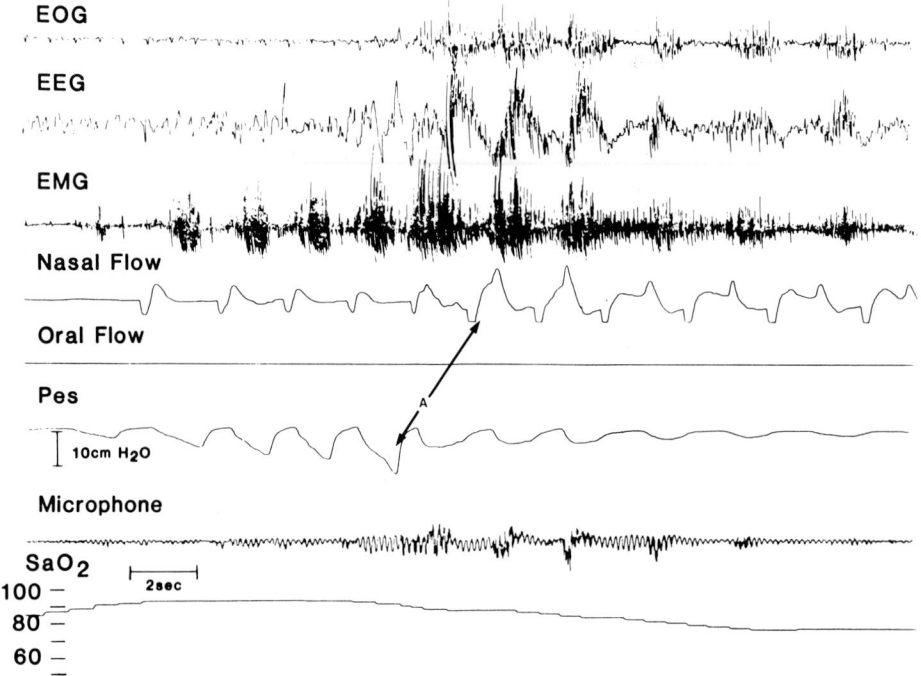

Fig. 2-6. Partial airway obstruction. Airflow and snoring are present as inspiratory efforts increase and moderate desaturation occurs. Airflow and snoring increase as the obstruction is relieved (A).

circulation time from lung to the finger but also because of a short machine delay. A partial airway obstruction is shown in Figure 2-6. During the event, some airflow persists but inspiratory pleural pressure swings increase and desaturation occurs. Snoring is present during inspiration of all breaths but amplifies when airflow increases. The pleural pressure swings are not as marked in the partial obstruction as in the totally obstructive apnea.

An example of a central apnea is presented in Figure 2-7. Both airflow and respiratory efforts cease. Minimal inspiratory EMG activity is seen during the apnea. With resumption of breathing, inspiratory upper airway muscle activity, as reflected by the submental EMG, increases dramatically. A mixed apnea is a combination of a central and obstructive apnea. Usually the central component appears first. There is a short central component at the beginning of the apnea in Figure 2-8.

Two other respiratory abnormalities can be observed especially in REM sleep, periodic and paradoxical breathing. Figure 2-9 demonstrates periodic breathing; a period of hyperpnea follows a period of hypopnea, which results in some arterial oxygen desaturation. With use of an inductance vest, paradoxical inward motion of the thorax can be seen during inspiratory outward motion of the abdomen, as shown in Figure 2-10. This pattern may be seen in REM sleep in patients with emphysema or chronic bronchitis.

Thus, with these relatively simple techniques the characteristics and severity of a particular type of apnea can be determined in a given patient. Whether observations made during one night in the sleep laboratory are truly representative of the usual pattern of the patient's ventilation during more "natural" conditions is un-

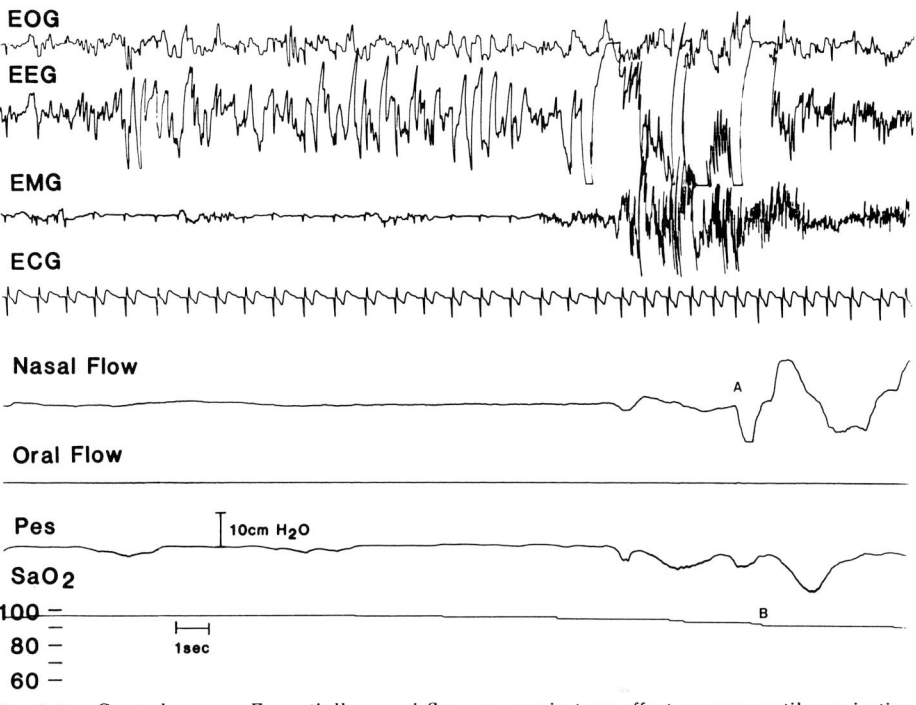

EOG

EEG

EMG

ECG

Nasal Flow

Oral Flow

Pes   10cm H$_2$O

SaO$_2$

100
80   1sec
60

Fig. 2-7. Central apnea. Essentially no airflow or respiratory effort occurs until respiration resumes (A). Mild desaturation occurs (B).

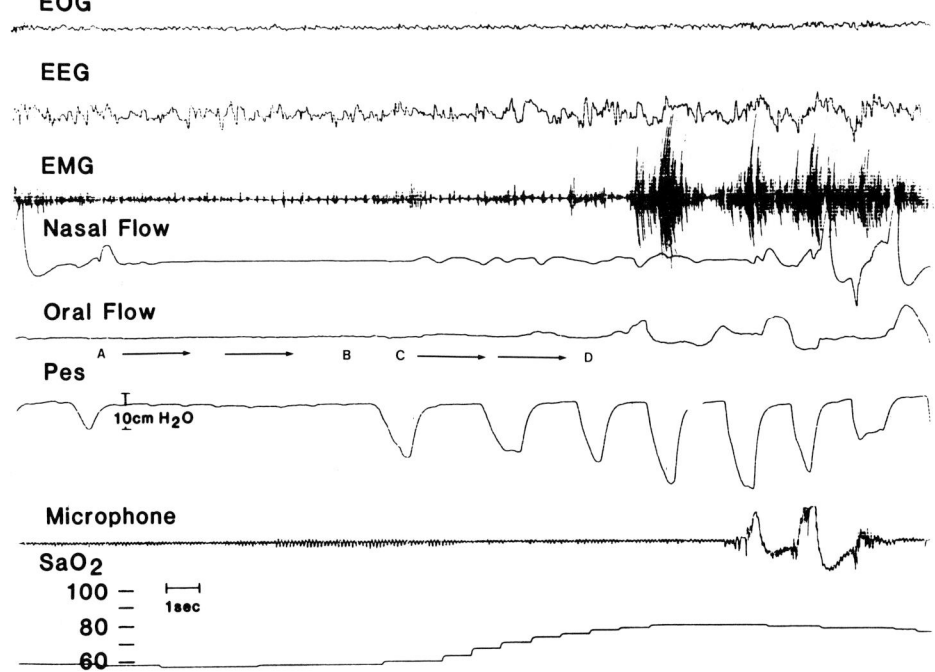

EOG

EEG

EMG

Nasal Flow

Oral Flow

Pes   10cm H$_2$O

Microphone

SaO$_2$

100   1sec
80
60

Fig. 2-8. Mixed apnea. An eight second central apnea (A → B), as evidenced by lack of inspiratory efforts in the chin EMG and esophageal pressure tracings, precedes a typical obstructive event (C → D).

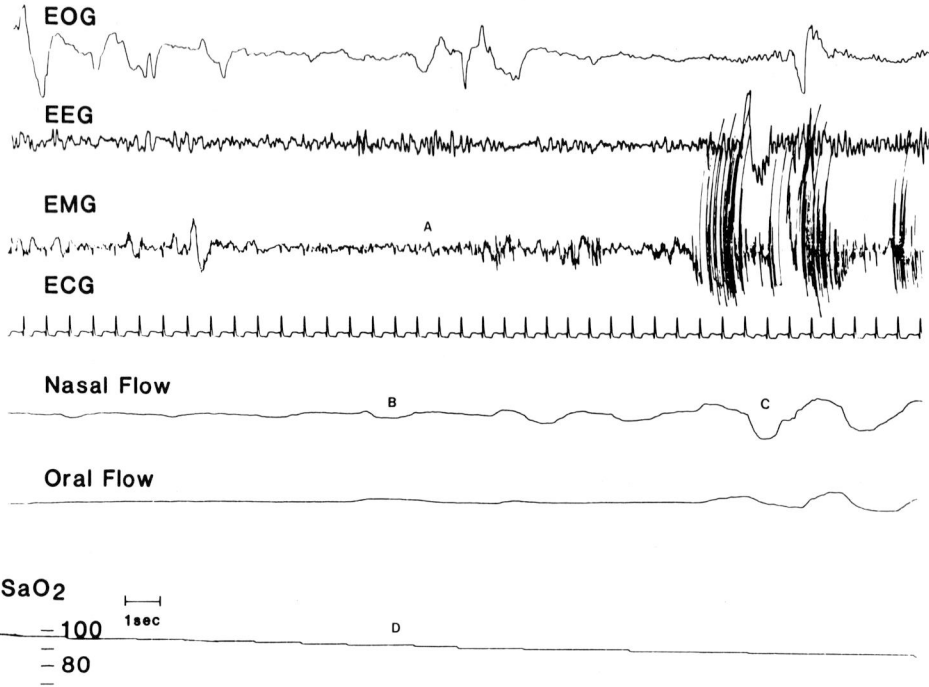

Fig. 2-9. Periodic breathing in REM sleep. Decreasing inspiratory EMG activity (A) and minimal airflow (B) alternate with periods of hyperpnea (C). Mild arterial oxygen desaturation (D) occurs secondary to the hypopneic breathing.

known. Obviously, some variability exists between nights but observations made on two nights in the laboratory are usually similar.

The technician in the laboratory must also make direct observations of the patient's breathing pattern, body position, restlessness, and characteristics of snoring. These observations help verify the recorded data and the bed partner history. It has become commonplace to count the number of apneic or hypopneic episodes lasting longer than ten seconds throughout the night and divide this number by the total sleep time to derive the "apnea index." Obviously, this variable is an oversimplification of the ventilatory variations and abnormalities that occur during sleep. Apneas or hypopneas that appear at sleep onset are normal, therefore, much less meaningful than apneas that occur in stage 2 or REM sleep. In addition, the apnea index ignores body position and ventilatory pattern or "context," in which these episodes occur. These important variables need to be assessed in addition to the apnea index.

It is not only important to use polysomnography for diagnosis but also to monitor therapy. The success rate of many forms of therapy for obstructive sleep apnea is in the neighborhood of 50 percent; therefore, response to a chosen therapeutic modality needs objective verification. Although tracheostomy and nasal continuous positive airway pressure (nasal CPAP) are usually successful therapies, a post-therapy evaluation of at least oximetry is needed to verify success.

Since a major indication for treatment of sleep apnea is daytime hypersomnolence, it is important to have followup evaluation of this problem. A successful

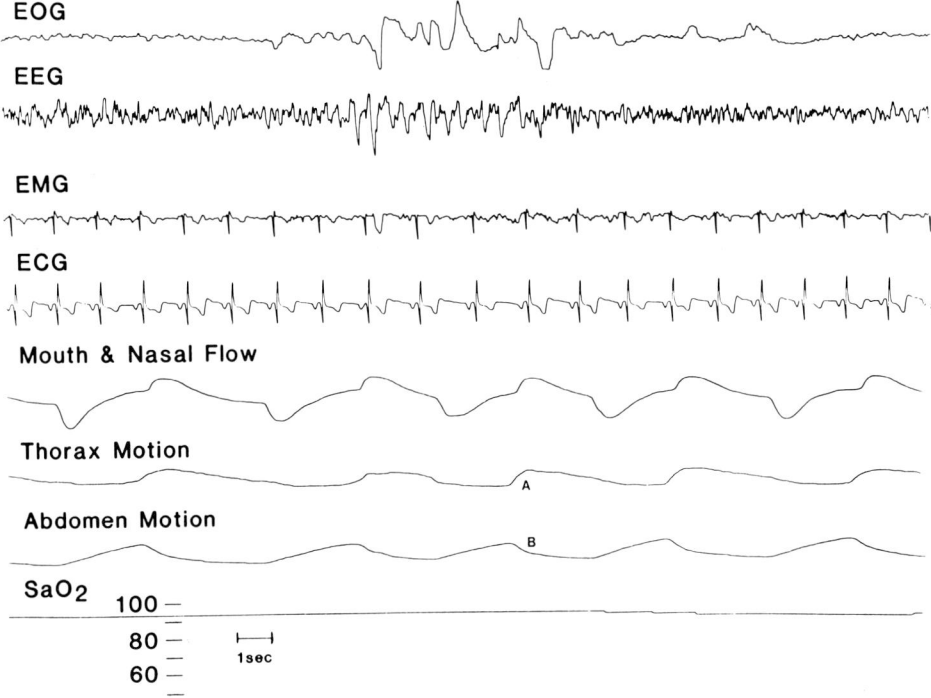

Fig. 2-10. Paradoxical breathing in REM sleep. An inductance vest is used to monitor thorax and abdomen motion. When abdominal inspiration [upward deflection (A)] is occurring the thorax is collapsing inward [downward deflection (B)].

therapy of obstructive apnea should produce dramatic improvement in the hypersomnolence, and the results are usually quite apparent to the patient and his family. However, two techniques are available that will quantitate sleep latency (time from lights out to sleep onset), a direct measurement of the degree of somnolence. Patients with severe somnolence will be asleep while the technician is putting the recording electrodes in place. Those patients with slightly less somnolence will fall asleep very soon after lights are turned out, usually within 1–3 minutes. Thus, some indication of the severity of somnolence can be made during routine nocturnal polysomnography. Another technique, the multiple sleep latency test,[9] was developed to quantitate level of daytime somnolence. With this technique the sleep latency is determined during each of four short naps over the course of a day. Thus a quantitation of the average sleep latency during the day can be accomplished. In most situations, assessment of sleepiness from the patient and family member histories and a bedtime sleep latency determination are usually an adequate guide to the degree of somnolence present.

SUMMARY

Within the past 10 years the medical community has become much more aware of the sleep apnea syndrome and its devastating complications. The *key* to proper diagnosis is the level of awareness of the primary health care provider of the symptoms and signs of sleep apnea. Family member's history often provides important clues to the diagnosis. Once a patient is suspected of having sleep apnea, screening oximetry and observation by a clinician during sleep is helpful. Referral to a sleep laboratory is ideal to verify the diagnosis and provide therapeutic recommendations and follow-up care. In the author's experience, the diagnosis of these entities is simple; it is the continued therapeutic efforts and modifications in therapy required that are difficult. Hypersomnolent patients are depressed and often do not follow through with advice. Therefore, physicians need to keep close tabs on these patients, since they may be peacefully sleeping away their lives, registering no complaints!

REFERENCES

1. Lugaresi E, Coccagna G, Cirignotta F: Snoring and its Clinical Implications, in Guilleminault C, Dement WC (eds): Sleep Apnea Syndromes, New York, Alan R. Liss, pp 13–21
2. Lugaresi E, Cirignotta F, Coccagna G, Baruzzi A: Snoring and the obstructive apnea syndrome, in Broughton RJ (ed): Henri Gastaut and the Marseilles School's Contribution to the Neurosciences (EEG Suppl No 35). Amsterdam, Elsevier Biomedical Press, 1982, pp 421–430
3. Lugaresi E, Coccagna G, Mantovani M: Hypersomnia with periodic apneas, in Weizman EH (ed): Advances in Sleep Research, Vol. 4. Jamaica, NY, Spectrum Publ.
4. Lavie P: Sleep disturbances in industry workers. Sleep Res 9:209–221, 1980
5. Block AJ, Boysen PG, Wynne JW, Hunt LW: Sleep apnea, hypopnea and oxygen desaturation in normal subjects: a strong male predominance. N Engl J Med 300:513–517, 1979
6. Block AJ, Wynne JW, Boysen PG, et al: Menopause, medroxyprogesterone, and breathing during sleep. Am J Med 70:506–510, 1981
7. Block AJ, Wynne JW, Boysen PG: Sleep-disordered breathing and nocturnal oxygen desaturation in postmenopausal women. Am J Med 69:75–79, 1980
8. Miller MM, Van den Hoed J, Carskadon MA, et al: REM sleep episodes during multiple sleep latency test in narcoleptic patients. Electroenceph Clin Neurophysiol 46:478–481, 1979
9. Reynolds CF III, Cobb PA, Kupfer DJ, Holzer BC: Application of the multiple sleep latency test in disorders of excessive sleepiness. Electroenceph & Clin Neurophysiol 53:443–452, 1982
10. Tilkian AG, Guilleminault C, Schroeder JS, et al: Hemodynamics in sleep-induced apnea. Studies during wakefulness and sleep. Ann Intern Med 85:714–719, 1976
11. Fletcher EC, DeBehnke RD, Lovoi MS, Gorin AB: Undiagnosed sleep apnea in patients with essential hypertension. Ann Int Med 103:190–195, 1985
12. Kales A, Bixler ED, Cadieux RJ, et al: Sleep apneas in a hypertensive population. Lancet 2:1005–1008, 1984
13. Bartall HZ, Tye K-H, Roper P, et al: Atrial flutter associated with obstructive apnea syndrome. A case report. Arch Int Med 140:121–122, 1980
14. Deedwania PC, Swiryn S, Dhingna RC, Rosen KM: Nocturnal atrioventricular block as a manifestation of sleep apnea syndrome. Chest 76:319–321, 1980
15. Tilkian AG, Guilleminault C, Schroeder JS, et al: Sleep-induced apnea syndrome. Prevalence of cardiac arrhythmias and their reversal after tracheostomy. Am J Med 63:348–358, 1977
16. Berrettini WH: Paranoid psychosis and sleep apnea syndrome. Am J Psychiatry 137:493–494, 1980
17. Brouillette RT, Fernbach SK, Hunt CE: Obstructive sleep apnea in infants and children. J Peds 100:31–40, 1982
18. Mandel EM, Reynolds CF III: Sleep disorders associated with upper airway obstruction in children. Symposium on pediatric otolaryngology. Pediatric Clinics of North America 28:897–903, 1981
19. Orr WC, Martin RJ: Obstructive sleep apnea associated with tonsillar hypertrophy in adults. Arch Intern Med 141:990–992, 1981
20. Mezon BJ, West P, Maclean JP, Kryger MH: Sleep apnea in acromegaly. Am J Med 69:615–618, 1980
21. Perks WH, Hovrocks PM, Cooper RA, et al: Sleep apnea in acromegaly. Brit Med J 280:894–897, 1980
22. Zorick F, Roth T, Kramer M, Flessa H: Exacer-

bation of upper-airway sleep apnea by lymphocytic lymphoma. Chest 77:689–690, 1980

23. Baker SR, Ross J: Sleep apnea syndrome and supraglottic edema. Acta Otolaryngol 106:486–491, 1980

24. Polnitsky CA, Sherter CB, Sugar JO: Irradiation-induced fibrosis of the neck and sleep apnea. Arch Otolaryngol 107:629–630, 1981

25. Davies SF: Obstructive sleep apnea associated with adult-acquired microagnathia from rheumatoid arthritis. Am Rev Respir Dis 127:245–247, 1983

26. Kravath RE, Pollak CP, Borowieck B, Weitzman ED: Obstructive sleep apnea and death associated with surgical correction of velopharyngeal incompetence. J Peds 96:645–648, 1980

27. Guilleminault C, Kurland G, Winkle R, Miles LE: Severe kyphoscoliosis, breathing and sleep. Chest 79:626–630, 1981

28. Hill R, Robbins AW, Arora NS: Sleep apnea syndrome after poliomyelitis. Am Rev Respir Dis 127:129–131, 1983

29. Frank Y, Kravath RE, Inovek, et al: Sleep apnea and hypoventilation syndrome associated with acquired nonprogressive dysautonomia. Ann Neurol 10:18–27, 1981

30. Hyland RH, Hutcheon MA, Perl A, et al: Upper airway occlusion induced by diaphragm pacing for primary alveolar hypoventilation. Am Rev Respir Dis 124:180–185, 1981

31. Mendelson WB, Ganett D, Gillin JC: Flurazepam-induced sleep apnea syndrome in a patient with insomnia and mild sleep-related respiratory changes. J Nervous & Mental Dis 169:261–264, 1981

32. Issa FG, Sullivan CE: Alcohol, snoring and sleep apnea. J Neurol, Neurosur & Psychiatry 45:353–359, 1982

33. Johnson MW, Anch AM, Remmers JE: Induction of the obstructive sleep apnea syndrome in a human by exogenous androgen administration. Am Rev Respir Dis 129:1023–1025, 1984

34. Wyler AR, Weymauller EA Jr: Epilepsy complicated by sleep apnea. Ann Neurol 9:403–404, 1981

35. White DP, Miller F, Erickson RW: Sleep apnea and nocturnal hypoventilation after western equine encephalitis. Am Rev Respir Dis 127:132–133, 1983

36. Sauerland SK, Harper RM: The human tongue during sleep: electromyographic activity of the genioglossus muscle. Exp Neurol 51:160–170, 1976

37. Hudgel DW, Martin RJ, Johnson B, Hill P: Mechanics of the respiratory system and breathing pattern during sleep in normal humans. J Appl Physiol: Respirat Environ Exercise Physiol 56:133–137, 1984

38. Rubin IG: Snoring. Proc Roy Soc Med 61:575–582, 1968

39. Cirignotta F, Lugaresi E: Some cineradiographic aspects of snoring and obstructive apneas. Sleep 3:225–226, 1980

40. Hudgel DW, Robertson DW: Nasal resistance during wakefulness and sleep in normal man. Acta Otolaryngol 98:130–135, 1984

41. Lavie P, Gertner R, Zomer J, Podoshin L: Breathing disorders in sleep associated with "microarousals" in patients with allergic rhinitis. Acta Otolaryngol 92:529–533, 1981

42. Sachner MA, Landa J, Forrest T, Greeneltch D: Periodic sleep apnea: chronic sleep deprivation related to intermittent upper airway obstruction and central nervous system disturbance. Chest 67:164–171, 1975

43. Orr WC, Martin RJ, Imes NK, et al: Hypersomnolent and nonhypersomnolent patients with upper airway obstruction during sleep. Chest 75:418–422, 1979

44. Cramer H, Warter J-M, Renaud B, et al: Cerebrospinal fluid adenosine $3',5'$-monophosphate, 5-hydroxy-indoleacetic acid and homovanillic acid in patients with sleep apnea syndrome. J Neurol, Neurosurg & Psychiatry 44:1165–1167, 1981

45. Santamaria J, Prior J, Fleetham JA: Hypothalamic-pituitary-testicular dysfunction in obstructive sleep apnea. Am Rev Resp Dis 131:A105, 1981

46. Mosko SS, Lewis E, Sassin JF: Impaired sexual maturation associated with sleep apnea syndrome during puberty. Sleep 3:13–22, 1980

47. Haponik EF, Bleecker ER, Allen RP, et al: Abnormal inspiratory flow-volume curves in patients with sleep-disordered breathing. Am Rev Respir Dis 124:571–574, 1981

48. Sanders MH, Martin RJ, Pennnock BE, Rogers RM: The detection of sleep apnea in the awake patient. JAMA 245:2414–2418, 1981

49. Rechtschaffen A, Kales A: A Manual of Standardized Terminology Techniques and Scoring System for Sleep Stages of Human Subjects. Washington DC, National Institute of Health, (Publ 204), 1968

50. Martin RJ, Block AJ, Cohn MA, Conway WA, Hudgel DW, Powles ACP, Sanders MH, Smith PL: Indications and standards for cardiopulmonary sleep studies. Sleep 8:371, 1985

John W. Shepard, Jr.

3

Hemodynamics in Obstructive Sleep Apnea

Following the vigorous activities of the day, sleep is welcomed and generally considered to be a period of physiological rest. In normal, quietly sleeping adults, the observed reductions in ventilation, heart rate, blood pressure, and metabolic rate lend credence to this point of view. In opposition to this perspective are the data of Smolensky et al[1] who observed an increase in human mortality rates between 0400 and 0700 when the rapid-eye-movement (REM) sleep state is more predominant. Morbidly stated, sleep is occasionally associated with permanent rather than recouperative rest. Dramatic advances in our knowledge and understanding of cardiopulmonary physiology and pathology during sleep have occurred over the past two decades. The purposes of this chapter will be to review briefly the hemodynamic changes that occur during normal sleep and more extensively discuss the hemodynamic changes and cardiac dysrhythmias that occur in patients with obstructive sleep apnea. While there is both humor and prophetic wisdom in Bedfellow's Rule, which states that "the one who snores will fall asleep first," somewhat more practical advice is contained in the First Law for Sleep Lab Referrals, which states that "the snorer who periodically pauses should be studied to determine what causes the purplish hue which ensues." Because no animal model of sleep apnea exists, it is from these sleep lab referrals, who have participated in clinical research, to whom we owe most of our current knowledge.

HEMODYNAMICS DURING SLEEP IN NORMALS

Using indirect methods to record blood pressure, early investigators found consistent but variable reductions in systemic blood pressure during sleep.[2-5] Subsequent studies, which included electrophysiological monitoring and staging of sleep, determined that part of this variability was related to changes in sleep state. During nonrapid-eye-movement (NREM) stages 1–2, mean arterial pressure decreased by an

ABNORMALITIES OF RESPIRATION DURING SLEEP   Copyright © 1986 by Grune & Stratton, Inc.
ISBN 0-8089-1812-5   All rights of reproduction in any form reserved.

average of 5 to 9 percent and by 8 to 14 percent during stages 3–4 compared to the awake resting state.[6,7] Although systemic blood pressure was found to be variable during REM sleep, it was generally four to six percent greater than the immediately preceding or succeeding NREM value.[7,8] Cyclical oscillations in systemic blood pressure (Mayer waves), which typically have an amplitude of 15 to 20 mmHg and periodicity of 20 to 30 seconds, have been reported in normal subjects.[9,10] These oscillations may occur in the absence of overt periodic breathing.

During NREM sleep, reductions in heart rate of five to eight percent have been observed.[7,8,11] During REM sleep, heart rate is characteristically variable with the mean rate approximating resting awake values. Cardiac output has been reported to decrease or remain unchanged during sleep in normal subjects.[7,11] There are insufficient data examining cardiac output as a function of sleep state in normals to reach any firm conclusions. The limited data on pulmonary artery pressures during sleep in normal subjects suggest that there are no major changes.[12] Cyclical oscillations in pulmonary artery pressure with an amplitude of 2 to 4 mmHg and periodicity of 20 to 30 seconds have also been reported in normal subjects and may occur during periods of regular breathing.[10]

In heavy snorers, Lugaresi et al[12,13] have reported increased systemic and pulmonary artery pressures both while awake and asleep compared to nonsnoring controls. While the snorers showed moderate increases in systemic systolic but not diastolic blood pressure during NREM sleep, the greatest increases in systolic pressure occurred during REM sleep when arterial oxygen tensions (PaO_2) were the lowest and arterial carbon dioxide tensions ($PaCO_2$) the highest.

ACUTE HEMODYNAMIC EFFECTS OF APNEAS

Systemic Blood Pressure

Figure 3-1 shows the characteristic systemic blood pressure response to repetitive episodes of arterial oxyhemoglobin desaturation associated with obstructive apneas following the onset of NREM sleep. Apneas are documented by the absence of thermistor deflection in the tracing labeled airflow and their obstructive nature is indicated by the detection of chest wall movement. The phasic inspiratory decreases in systemic blood pressure also confirm the presence of respiratory effort. The peak elevations in systolic and diastolic blood pressure, which closely coincide with the nadirs of the oximeter tracing, can be seen to be proportional to the magnitude of the oxyhemoglobin desaturation. The minimum values for arterial oxyhemoglobin saturation (SaO_2) are registered 6 to 10 seconds following apnea termination due to the circulation time from the capillary bed of the lung to the ear plus instrumental delay time. Shortly after SaO_2 returns to baseline, minimum values for systemic pressure are reached. Subsequently, there is a progressive rise in both systolic and diastolic pressures until apnea termination. At that time, an incremental rise in systemic pressure usually occurs coinciding with arousal and the resumption of ventilation.

In 10 subjects with obstructive sleep apnea, Shepard et al[14] have reported that systolic blood pressure (SBP) increased by an average of 33 mmHg from 126 to 159 mmHg while diastolic blood pressure (DBP) increased by an average of 18 mmHg from 65 to 83 mmHg. This occurred in response to a mean fall in SaO_2 of 18 percent from a mean high SaO_2 of 93 percent to a mean low SaO_2 of 75 percent. Although the

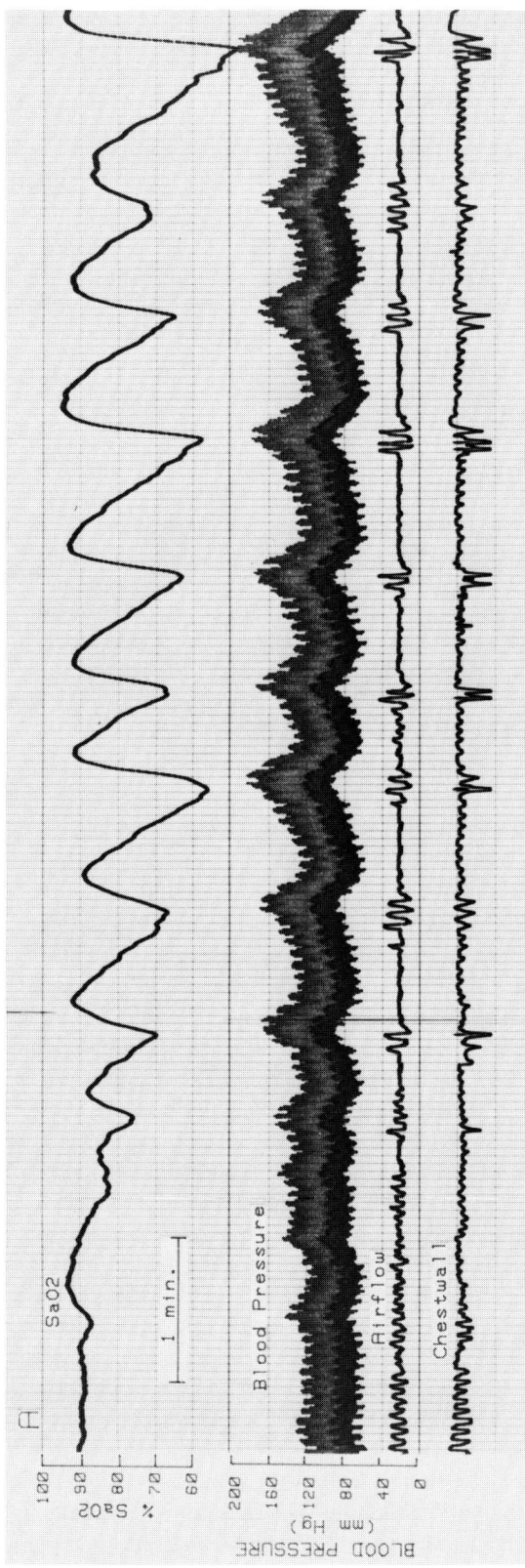

Fig. 3-1. Segment of a sleep record showing the onset of NREM sleep in a patient with obstructive sleep apnea. Note that the elevations in systemic blood pressure are proportional to the magnitude of the fall in arterial oxyhemoglobin saturation (SaO_2). (From Shepard JW Jr: Gas exchange and hemodynamics during sleep. Medical Clinics of North America 69:1243–1263, 1985. With permission.)

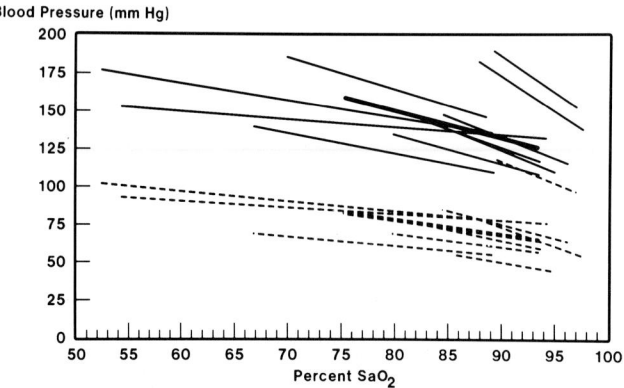

Fig. 3-2. Changes in systolic (solid lines) and diastolic (dashed lines) systemic blood pressures with episodes of oxyhemoglobin desaturation in 10 patients with obstructive sleep apnea. The heavy lines represent the mean data for the group. Note the marked differences in the slopes of the systemic pressor response to arterial hypoxemia that exists between individuals. (From Shepard JW Jr: Gas exchange and hemodynamics during sleep. Medical Clinics of North America 69:1243–1263, 1985. With permission.)

absolute magnitude of the increase in SBP was nearly double the rise in DBP, when expressed on a percentage basis, the 25 percent increase in SBP was virtually identical to the 27 percent increase in DBP. Figure 3-2 shows these group mean data as well as the mean data for each of the subjects. While the percent increases in SBP and DBP were quite uniform between patients, the magnitude of the oxyhemoglobin desaturation varied greatly. As a result, the systolic pressure response to oxyhemoglobin desaturation ($\Delta SBP/\Delta SaO_2$) ranged from 0.6 to 4.4 mmHg/percent with a mean of 2.4 ± 1.3 mmHg/percent. The diastolic pressure response ($\Delta DBP/\Delta SaO_2$) ranged from 0.4 to 2.8 mmHg/percent with a mean of 1.4 ± 0.8 mmHg/percent.

The slopes of the systemic pressure responses to oxyhemoglobin desaturation were found to be negatively correlated with the cardiothoracic ratios in the 10 subjects studied (Fig. 3-3). This interesting finding remains to be confirmed, correlated with variables of cardiac function, and the cause and effect relationships dissected. Although previous investigators[15,16] have reported systemic blood pressure elevations with apneas, Schroeder et al[17] specifically called attention to the progressive rise in peak systolic and diastolic pressures associated with increasingly severe oxyhemoglobin desaturations within individual subjects. While peak pressures frequently demonstrate this incremental pattern, systemic pressures usually return to a constant baseline provided SaO_2 returns to control (Fig. 3-1). Because of these observations, Shepard et al[14] further analyzed the relationship between the incremental increases in systolic (ΔSBP) and diastolic (ΔDBP) blood pressures and the decremental decreases in oxyhemoglobin saturation (ΔSaO_2) within each subject studied. In 9 of their 10 subjects, significant correlations were obtained. Figure 3-4 shows this relationship for one subject. Although the correlation was highly significant, $p < 0.001$, the correlation coefficient of 0.56 indicates that ΔSaO_2 would account for only 31 percent of the total variance reflecting the importance of other variables in determining the systemic pressure response.

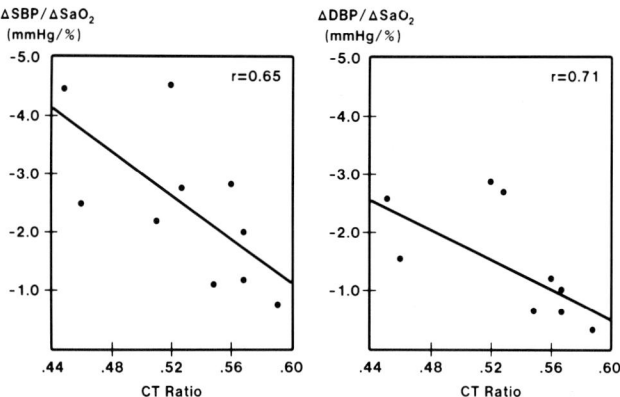

Fig. 3-3. Relationship between the slopes of the systolic and diastolic pressor responses to oxyhemoglobin desaturation and cardiothoracic ratios in 10 patients with obstructive sleep apnea. (From Shepard JW Jr: Gas exchange and hemodynamics during sleep. Medical Clinics of North America 69:1243–1263, 1985. With permission.)

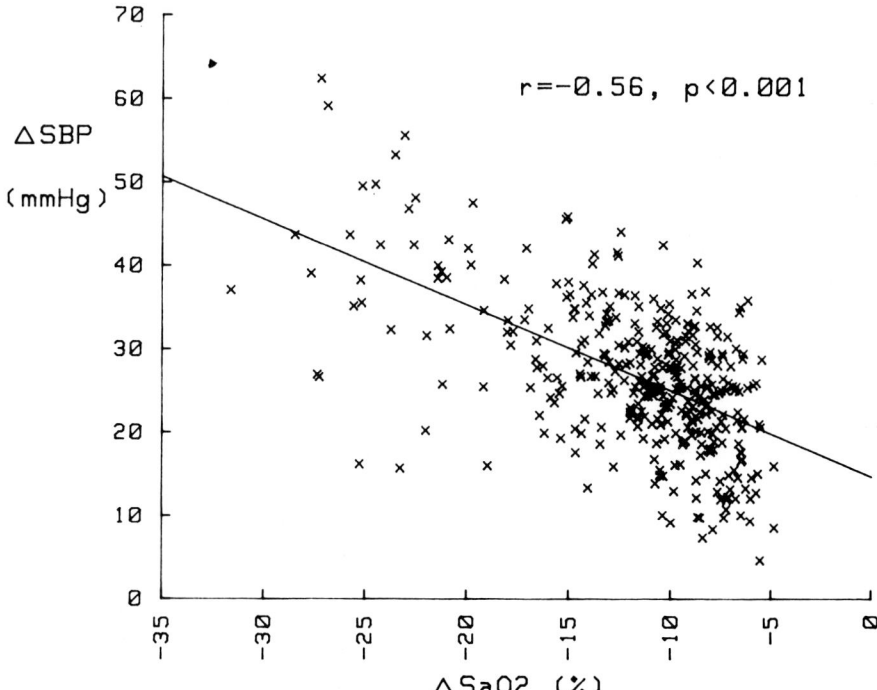

Fig. 3-4. Relationship between the increase in systolic blood pressure (ΔSBP) and decrease in SaO$_2$ (ΔSaO$_2$) in a patient with obstructive sleep apnea. While the rise in SBP is significantly related to the fall in SaO$_2$, p < 0.001, other variables are involved as indicated by the considerable scatter around the regression line.

Careful inspection of Figure 3-1 reveals that there are two components to the rise in systemic pressure. The first component is the progressive rise in systemic pressure, which occurs throughout the apnea and is correlated with the severity of oxyhemoglobin desaturation. The second component is the acute incremental rise in pressure, which occurs following apnea termination. The linear regression line in Figure 3-4 is given by the equation: $\Delta SBP = 15 - 1.0\ (\Delta SaO_2)$. In this equation, the constant term or y-axis intercept for $\Delta SaO_2 = 0$ percent is considered to represent the second component of pressure elevation, which is associated with arousal and the resumption of ventilation. The slope reflects the component of pressure elevation related to oxyhemoglobin desaturation. For ΔSBP, the values for the y-axis intercepts ranged from 14 to 27 mmHg with a mean of 21 mmHg for the 9 patients studied. The corresponding values for ΔDBP ranged from 7 to 15 mmHg with a mean of 11 mmHg. The slope of -1.0 mmHg/percent indicated that SBP increased by 1 mmHg for every 1 percent fall in SaO_2 in the depicted subject. For the group as a whole, the mean slope was -0.9 mmHg/percent for SBP (range -0.2 to -2.5 mmHg/percent) and -0.5 mmHg/percent for DBP (range 0 to -1.4 mmHg/percent).

While the inter-individual variability in the systemic pressure response to apnea related hypoxemia may have an underlying genetic basis similar to the differences in hypoxic ventilatory drive ($\Delta Ve/\Delta SaO_2$) that exist between individuals, alterations in cardiac function over time are likely to play a significant role in determining the systemic pressor response. Figure 3-5 shows a segment of the sleep data from the one subject to whom the rise in systemic pressures did not correlate with the fall in SaO_2. In this subject with cardiomegaly and overt left ventricular dysfunction, the elevations in systemic blood pressure occurred predominantly in the post-apneic period. Consequently, the total systemic pressure response to apneas can be viewed as being equal to the sum of the components related to apnea termination plus the rise related to oxyhemoglobin desaturation.

Pulmonary Artery Pressure

In an early study of pulmonary artery pressure (Ppa) during sleep in patients with obstructive sleep apnea, Ppa was found to increase progressively as subjects went from wakefulness through stages 1, 2, and 3–4 of NREM sleep with the highest values being recorded during REM sleep.[15] The elevations in Ppa paralleled the severity of the hypoxemia and hypercapnia, which were concomitantly observed. The maximum values for Ppa during sleep were double the awake resting values with the pattern of elevation being similar to the pattern observed for the systemic circulation. The increases in pulmonary systolic pressures were again greater than the elevations in diastolic pressures indicating widening of the pulse pressure. In subsequent reports from the Stanford group,[17,18] 59 percent of 22 patients had awake resting pulmonary hypertension defined as a mean Ppa of greater than 20 mmHg. In this group of patients, Ppa (systolic/diastolic) increased from 30/17 mmHg during wakefulness to 56/33 mmHg during sleep. Pulmonary artery wedge pressures were reported to be modestly elevated between 18 and 20 mmHg in three subjects in whom they were successfully recorded.[18]

In four patients with predominantly central sleep apnea Ppa increased from 26/16 mmHg while awake to maximum values of 41/26 mmHg during sleep.[17] The lesser degree of pressure elevation in these central apneics was likely due to the less severe

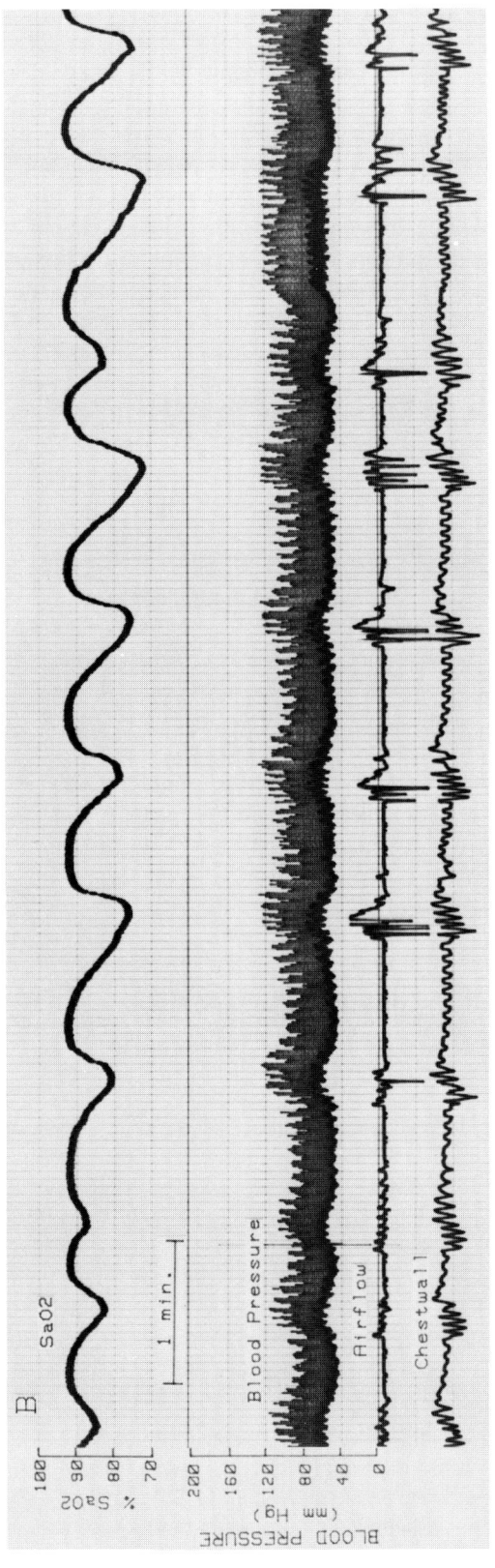

Fig. 3-5. Segment of the sleep record of a patient with obstructive sleep apnea and a left ventricular ejection fraction of 14 percent. With severe left ventricular dysfunction there was little systemic pressor response to hypoxemia during the apneic period. Following apnea termination a relatively consistent rise in pressure was observed. (From Shepard JW Jr: Gas exchange and hemodynamics during sleep. Medical Clinics of North America 69:1243–1263, 1985. With permission.)

45

oxyhemoglobin desaturation that was observed. Incremental elevations in pulmonary artery pressures have been observed following apnea termination similar to the pattern accompanying obstructive apneas.[17,19]

Figure 3-6 shows the typical changes that occur in Ppa during obstructive apneas. As illustrated, Ppa intermittently decreases to values less than atmospheric (Ppa < 0 mmHg) in association with the negative intrathoracic pressures generated by respiratory efforts in the presence of upper airway obstruction. While this effect complicates the analysis of pulmonary hemodynamics, examination of the Ppa trac-

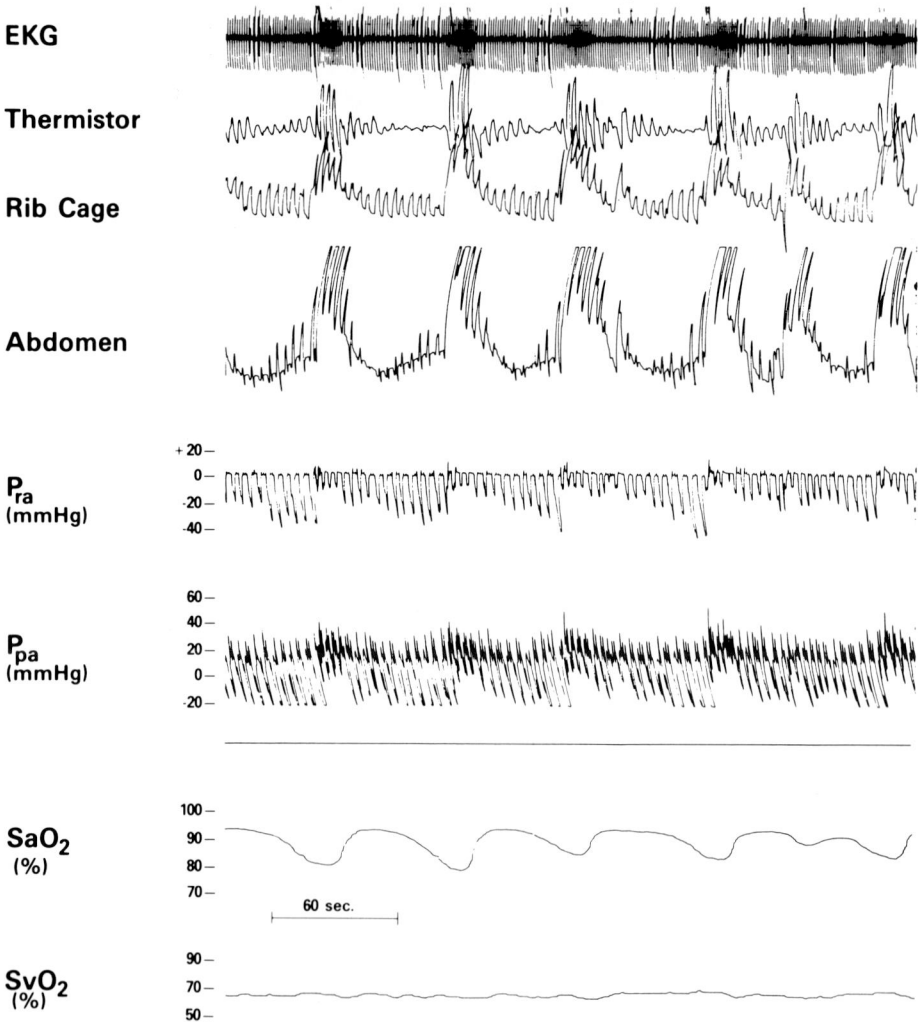

Fig. 3-6. Changes in pulmonary artery (P_{pa}) and right atrial (P_{ra}) pressures with sequential obstructive apneas. Note the negative intrathoracic pressures associated with inspiratory efforts against an obstructed upper airway as reflected by the decreases in Pra with corresponding reductions in Ppa. During expiration, Ppa can be observed to increase toward the end of the apneas and undergo an incremental rise following apnea termination. Small reductions in mixed venous oxyhemoglobin saturation (SvO_2) accompany the relatively mild decreases in SaO_2. Figure courtesy of Dr. E. Fletcher.

ing during expiration reveals a pattern similar to the one observed for systemic pressure. Cyclical elevations in Ppa occur with peak pressures being reached shortly after apnea termination again coinciding with the nadirs of the oximeter recording.

In order to obtain a true estimate of right ventricular afterload, pleural pressure (Ppl) should be subtracted from Ppa. The resulting value (Ppa − Ppl) represents the actual transmural pressure gradient against which the right ventricle must work. Although data on right ventricular transmural pressures (afterload) during obstructive apneas have not been published, the cardiac effects of negative intrathoracic pressure associated with the Mueller maneuver have been studied.[20–22] The increased venous return and right ventricular afterload associated with negative intrathoracic pressures combine to increase the dimensions of the compliant right ventricle. In addition, substantially negative intrathoracic pressures have also been documented to increase left ventricular transmural pressures and volumes despite reductions in systemic pressures recorded peripherally. Direct cinefluoroscopic evidence that heart size increases during obstructive apneas has been published.[23]

Heart Rate

The changes in heart rate during both apneas and voluntary breath holding have been extensively analyzed. Reductions in heart rate have been observed with central, obstructive, and mixed apneas with the extent of cardiac slowing being proportional to the severity of the oxyhemoglobin desaturation.[24] Both the cessation of ventilation and hypoxemia are important stimuli that contribute to the development of bradycardia during breath holds and apneas.[24,25] The inhalation of supplemental oxygen, which prevents hypoxemia, consistently ameliorates the bradycardia, which occurs during breath holding and apneas. Conversely, the degree of bradycardia is also reduced in rebreathing experiments that allow hypoxemia and hypercapnia to develop in the presence of continued chest wall movement and volume excursion of the lung. In contrast, hypoxemia resulting from the inhalation of hypoxic gas mixtures produces cardio-acceleration in association with increased ventilation and decreases in $PaCO_2$. The bradycardia that occurs during apneas is known to be mediated by an increase in vagal efferent activity as atropine markedly reduces or abolishes the bradycardia.[17,26,27]

Cardiac Output

Using the thermodilution technique, several studies have reported that there are no systematic changes in cardiac output during apneas.[17,18] Fletcher has obtained similar results with the exception that cardiac output fell substantially in one subject with marked apnea-associated bradycardia.* Because of the short duration of most apneic events, the difficulty in timing injections, and the fact that the thermodilution technique measures cardiac output over several cardiac cycles, future studies need to utilize techniques that are more responsive to the detection of transient changes in cardiac output and stroke volume.

Using impedance cardiography, an indirect but responsive technique of monitoring hemodynamic changes, Lin et al observed a decrease in cardiac output during

---

* Eugene C. Fletcher (personal communication, August, 1985).

90 second breath holds in normal subjects.[28] The maximal reduction in cardiac output, which occurred 30 seconds into the breath holds, was related to a 30 percent decrease in heart rate with stroke volume remaining unchanged. With increasing breath hold duration, heart rate remained reduced while stroke volume progressively increased returning cardiac output toward control. When hypercapnia was prevented during rebreathing experiments by passing expired gas through a carbon dioxide absorber, the rise in stroke volume was prevented and cardiac output remained reduced. Consequently, hypercapnia acts to increase stroke volume and maintain cardiac output despite reductions in heart rate.

In the breath holding literature cardiac output has been reported to show small increases, decreases, or to remain unchanged during breath holds.[29–31] In the absence of major changes in cardiac output, significant reductions in heart rate with increased systemic and pulmonary arterial pulse pressures during apneas strongly suggests that stroke volume is increased. Furthermore, increases in systemic and pulmonary arterial pressures with a relatively constant cardiac output directly imply increased systemic and pulmonary vascular resistances. Following apnea termination, the sudden increases in heart rate and maximal pulse pressures that are observed suggest that cardiac output is transiently increased. An increase in cardiac output in the presence of increased pulmonary and systemic vascular resistances in the immediate post apneic period is probably a significant factor contributing to the elevations in pulmonary and systemic pressures observed at this point in time.

Myocardial Oxygen Balance

Oxyhemoglobin desaturation during sleep in patients with chronic obstructive pulmonary disease has been shown by indirect methods to stress the flow reserves of the coronary circulation in order to provide adequate myocardial oxygen delivery to meet existing demands.[32] Applying this methodology, which utilizes the heart rate-systolic blood pressure product as an index of myocardial oxygen consumption (MVO_2) and the Fick equation to estimate myocardial blood flow (MBF), apneas associated with significant oxyhemoglobin desaturation have been found to produce intermittently high demands for MBF.[14]

The time course of the relationships between SaO_2 (corrected for a 5-second delay), heart rate, SBP, MVO_2 and MBF are illustrated in Figure 3-7 for a sequence of four obstructive apneas. In the early- to mid-portion of most apneas, MVO_2 estimated from the double product was found to decrease to its nadir. Because the arterial blood is well oxygenated and myocardial oxygen demands are low at this time, the level of MBF required to provide adequate oxygen delivery is also low. By the mid-portion of most apneas, SBP begins to rise in proportion to the reductions in SaO_2. Heart rate remains reduced, thereby limiting the rise in MVO_2 related to increasing SBP. As a result, bradycardia can be viewed as serving an important cardioprotective function by limiting myocardial oxygen demands when the oxygen content of arterial blood is reduced. Upon apnea termination, a rapid increase in heart rate occurs along with an accentuated increase in SBP. This combination of events produces near maximal myocardial oxygen demands at a time when SaO_2 is near its nadir and just beginning to increase. Consequently, transiently high demands for MBF are computed to be necessary to maintain adequate oxygen delivery to meet the concurrently elevated demands of the myocardium for oxygen.

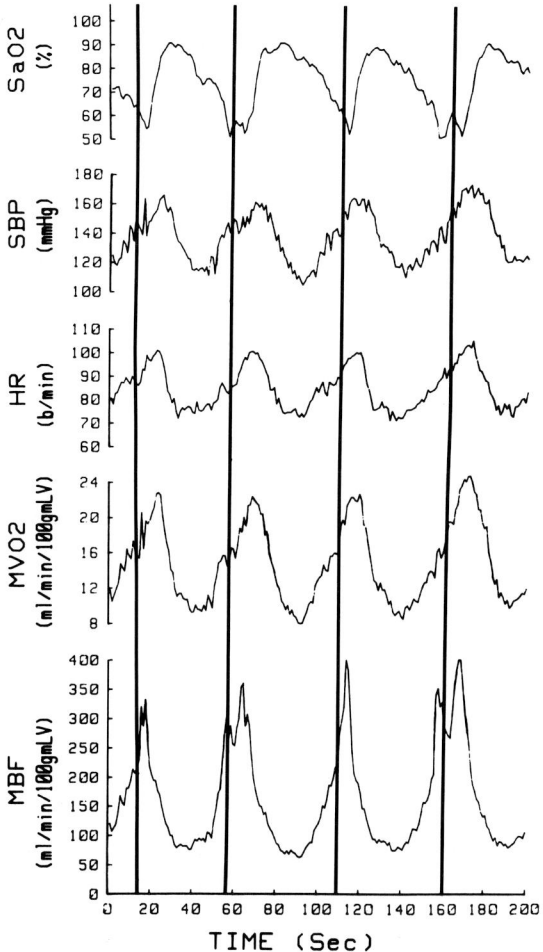

Fig. 3-7.   Sequential changes in SaO₂, systolic blood pressure (SBP), heart rate (HR), and myocardial oxygen consumption (MVO₂) estimated from the double product and myocardial blood flow (MBF) computed using the Fick equation with sequential obstructive apneas in one subject. The SaO₂ tracing has been corrected for an estimated 5 second delay in transit time from the heart to the ear. The vertical lines indicate apnea termination.

It is important to note that the oxyhemoglobin saturation of coronary sinus blood ($ScsO_2$) was assumed to remain constant at a normal level of 30 percent in the Fick equation used to calculate MBF. While this corresponds to a partial pressure of only 19 mmHg for oxygen in the coronary sinus blood, it is certainly possible that $ScsO_2$ falls during severe apneas with increased myocardial oxygen extraction contributing to oxygen delivery. Direct measurements of $ScsO_2$ will be required to resolve this issue. Figure 3-8 shows the percentages of NREM and REM sleep time that 10 patients with obstructive sleep apnea were calculated to have spent in each of 4 categorical levels of MBF. Normal values for MBF at rest range from 60 to

Percent of Total Sleep Time

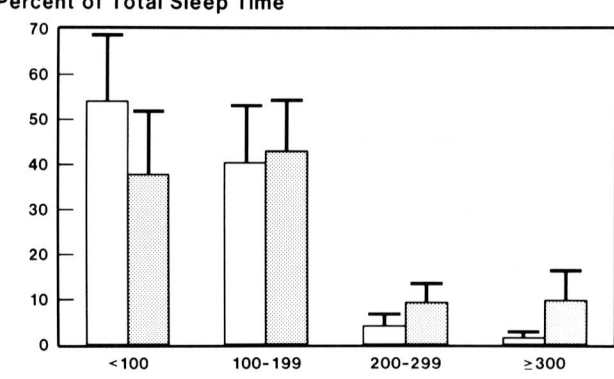

Level of MBF (ml/min/100gm LV)

Fig. 3-8. Percent of NREM (open bars) and REM (stippled bars) sleep calculated to have been spent in four categoric levels of myocardial blood flow (MBF). Data are means ±1 standard deviation for 10 subjects with obstructive sleep apnea.

100 ml/min/100 g LV and values exceeding 300 ml/min/100 g LV are associated with maximal exercise.

Mechanisms and Overview of the Hemodynamic Changes

The circulatory response to apneas involves the complex central integration of both the direct actions and cardiovascular reflexes to the stimuli of hypoxia, hypercapnia, acidosis, and ventilatory cessation that occur. Alveolar hypoxia and hypercapnic acidosis are potent stimuli known to produce vasoconstriction of the pulmonary vascular bed. The mechanism(s) by which hypoxia induces contraction of pulmonary vascular smooth muscle has been extensively studied and reviewed.[33–35] Recent studies have implicated products of arachidonic acid metabolism and calcium influx as important mediators of the local vasoconstrictory response to hypoxia.[36,37] While increased hydrogen ion concentrations have been shown to potentiate hypoxic pulmonary vasoconstriction[38–41] as well as to cause pulmonary vasoconstriction during normoxia,[42,43] the mechanism by which acidosis induces pulmonary vasoconstriction is not known. However, vasoconstriction secondary to hypercapnic acidosis is known to be related to the increase in hydrogen ion concentration as the direct effect of carbon dioxide on the pulmonary circulation is vasodilation.[44,45] Provided cardiac output does not fall, hypoxia and hypercapnic acidosis act in concert to produce pulmonary hypertension during apneas.

In contrast to their vasoconstrictory actions on the pulmonary circulation, the direct effects of hypoxia and acidosis on the systemic circulation are vasodilatory. These direct effects would produce a fall in systemic blood pressure were it not for the cardiovascular reflexes associated with arterial hypoxemia, hypercapnia, and the cessation of ventilation. It is important to note that the systemic hemodynamic response to hypoxia is substantially different when ventilation ceases (apneic-hypoxia) compared to when ventilation is increased (ventilated-hypoxia). Therefore, repetitively occurring apneas provide alternating exposure to hypoxia under conditions of apnea and increased ventilation during the post apneic period.

While apneic-hypoxia is associated with systemic hypertension, peripheral vasoconstriction and bradycardia with little change in cardiac output, hypoxia associated with increased ventilation results in elevations in heart rate, ventricular contractility, and cardiac output.[46–48] This increase in cardiac activity combined with selective redistribution of systemic blood flow functions to maintain systemic blood pressure despite the direct vasodilatory effects of hypoxia.[49–51] Hypocapnia and stimulation of pulmonary stretch receptors resulting from increased ventilation are considered to play a significant role contributing to the increase in heart rate based on the results of experimental work conducted in dogs.[52–54] In addition, heart rate is increased secondary to the direct effect of hypoxia on the central nervous system, which augments sympathetic efferent activity and catecholamine release.[55,56]

The carotid chemoreceptors have been shown to play an important role in mediating the bradycardic response to breath holding in both animals and man.[52,53,57] While breath holding with room air usually produces bradycardia in normal subjects, Gross et al observed a tachycardic response in each of five subjects who had undergone bilateral carotid body resections.[57] The rise in heart rate was directly related to the severity of the fall in oxygen tension indicating the central stimulatory effect of hypoxia on heart rate. In addition, systemic pressures in the carotid body resected group rose linearly with breath hold duration to levels 15 to 20 percent over control. Hypoxia mediated increases in sympathetic efferent activity likely contribute to the systemic hypertension during apneas as patients with the Shy-Drager syndrome who are sympathetically denervated do not elevate systemic pressure with apneas.[17,58]

While the complexity of analyzing the hemodynamic response to apneas should be evident from the preceding brief discussion, it should be further recognized that the circulatory responses to obstructive apneas are also influenced by fluctuations between wakefulness and sleep as well as the oscillations in intrathoracic pressures that alter ventricular preload and afterload. Part of the elevations in pulmonary and systemic arterial pressures with apnea termination may therefore be related to arousal as well as the cardiostimulatory effects of hypoxia associated with increased ventilation. Although the complexity of the centrally integrated response is great, what should be stressed is the fact that the hemodynamic response to apneas appears to be appropriate for survival.

With the onset of apnea, vasoconstriction of less essential peripheral vascular beds shifts blood centrally. This increases preload to maintain stroke volume and prevent precipitous declines in cardiac output with reductions in heart rate. Bradycardia beneficially reduces myocardial oxygen consumption and increases diastolic filling time, which acts to improve both coronary perfusion and ventricular filling. While the elevations in systemic pressure facilitate coronary and cerebral perfusion, they adversely increase myocardial oxygen consumption. In comparison, most diving mammals reduce heart rate and cardiac output to a greater extent than man with the balance between reduced cardiac output and elevated systemic vascular resistance leaving mean arterial pressure relatively unchanged. In highly conditioned humans, however, heart rate intervals in excess of 6 seconds have been reported during submersion.[59] These subjects may reflect the actual capacity of humans to limit myocardial oxygen consumption and thereby conserve oxygen during breath holding. The importance of apneic-bradycardia to conserving body oxygen stores and prolonging survival underwater has been well documented in both seals and ducks.[60,61]

While peripheral vasoconstriction, bradycardia and decreased cardiac output are beneficial during apneas, the converse is true following apnea termination. With the resumption of ventilation, repletion of the body's oxygen stores is best achieved by reducing systemic vascular resistance and increasing cardiac output to facilitate oxygen delivery to the peripheral tissues. Increasing heart rate, stroke volume, and cardiac output becomes a physiologically rational response as soon as oxygen can be transferred from the atmosphere to the blood at a rate that exceeds the metabolic cost of maintaining the increased cardiac output. While it remains to be experimentally documented that cardiac output increases following apnea termination, the sudden increase in heart rate and widening of the pulse pressures make it highly probable.

CARDIAC DYSRHYTHMIAS DURING SLEEP

Normal Subjects

Multiple studies using Holter monitoring have been conducted in young, middle-aged, and elderly normal subjects to determine the prevalence of cardiac dysrhythmias. These studies have indicated that ventricular ectopic activity decreases during sleep in association with reductions in heart rate.[62–66] However, despite reductions in nocturnal ectopic frequency, ventricular ectopy still occurred in 48 to 73 percent of normal subjects during the night. Ventricular ectopy was complex (multifocal, repetitive, or both) in 14 to 17 percent of the subjects with ventricular tachycardia being detected in 0 to 4 percent of the various study populations. Sinus arrhythmia was the most prominent nocturnal dysrhythmia occurring in 50 percent of young males. Almost one third had sinus pauses of 1.8 to 2.0 seconds duration and six percent demonstrated second degree (Mobitz type II) atrioventricular block.[62] Both the magnitude of sinus arrhythmia and prevalence of nocturnal bradyarrhythmias have been found to decrease with age.[64,67]

Although bradyarrhythmias have generally been considered to be benign in the younger population, Guilleminault et al[68] have questioned this assumption after observing 42 episodes of sinus arrest lasting from 2 to 9 seconds in 4 apparently healthy young adults. These prolonged episodes of asystole all occurred during REM sleep and none were associated with oxygen desaturation or significant apneas.

Lown et al[69] reported the case of a middle-aged male without organic heart disease who demonstrated increased ventricular ectopy during REM sleep and who survived a nocturnal episode of ventricular fibrillation. Because beta-adrenergic blockade effectively controlled this subjects ventricular ectopy, increased sympathetic neural activity, possibly linked to dream content, was implicated in the genesis of his ventricular arrhythmias.

Patients with Obstructive Sleep Apnea

Marked sinus arrhythmia, defined as a greater than 30 beat per minute variation in heart rate, is the most common dysrhythmia observed in patients with obstructive sleep apnea. It has been reported to occur in 78 to 100 percent of patients.[70–72] While

Table 3-1

Cardiac Dysrhythmias During Sleep in Patients
With Sleep Apnea

	Miller[71]	Guilleminault et al[75]	Shepard et al[74]
Patients (no.)	23	400	31
Sinus Bradycardia (<30 beats/min)	9%	7%	10%
Sinus Pauses (2–13 seconds)	9%	11%	10%
Second Degree Atrioventricular Block	4%	8%	6%
Ventricular Ectopy			
Any	57%	—	74%
Complex	9%	—	55%
Ventricular Tachycardia	0%	3%	3%

sinus arrhythmia is greatest for apneas associated with severe oxyhemoglobin desaturation, periodic breathing with only minimal oxyhemoglobin desaturation has also been observed to accentuate sinus arrhythmia. Large fluctuations in tidal volumes have been shown to increase sinus arrhythmia in man.[73] Table 3-1 presents the prevalence data for the more significant brady and tachyarrhythmias that have been reported in patients with sleep apnea. The results are consistent except for the higher prevalence of complex ventricular ectopy in the more severe apneics studied by Shepard et al.[74] Because Miller[71] found no difference in ventricular ectopic frequency between wakefulness and sleep, he concluded that ventricular ectopy was not related to the sleep apneic state. While this was also true for the majority of patients in the series reported by Guilleminault et al,[75] they observed a sleep related increase in ventricular ectopy in 55 or 14 percent of their 400 patients with sleep apnea. Furthermore, episodes of unsustained ventricular tachycardia were observed in eight patients in association with apnea-induced oxyhemoglobin desaturations to less than 65 percent.

The relationship between premature ventricular complex (PVC) frequency and SaO_2 has been recently reported for a group of 31 patients with moderate to severe sleep apnea.[74] When SaO_2 remained greater than 60 percent, no significant increase in PVC frequency was detected. However, in patients desaturating below 60 percent, PVC frequency increased nearly threefold when SaO_2 was less than 60 percent compared to when SaO_2 was greater than 90 percent (Fig. 3-9). Ventricular bigeminy occurred with desaturation below 60 percent in three patients. These results along with those of Guilleminault et al,[75] indicate that patients with sleep apnea are at increased risk of developing significant ventricular arrhythmias when SaO_2 decreases below 60 percent.

Figure 3-10 shows multiple PVCs coinciding with the nadirs of the oximeter tracing that has not been corrected for circulatory and instrumental delay. Careful inspection of the data reveals that the ventricular ectopy occurs during the period of cardio-acceleration immediately following the resumption of ventilation. This is a frequent point in time for ventricular ectopy to be observed. It is likely that the shift from parasympathetic predominant to sympathetic dominant neural activity follow-

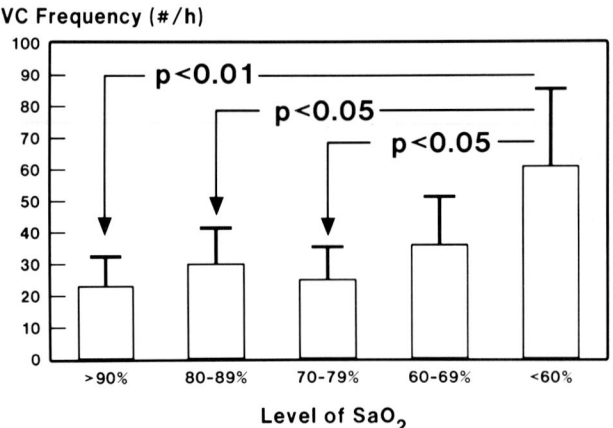

PVC Frequency (#/h)

Level of SaO$_2$

Fig. 3-9. Frequencies of PVCs in five categoric levels of SaO$_2$ for 16 patients with obstructive sleep apnea and desaturation below 60 percent. Data are means ±1 standard error of the mean. (From Shepard JW Jr, Garrison MW, Grither DA, et al: Chest 88:335–340, 1985. With permission.)

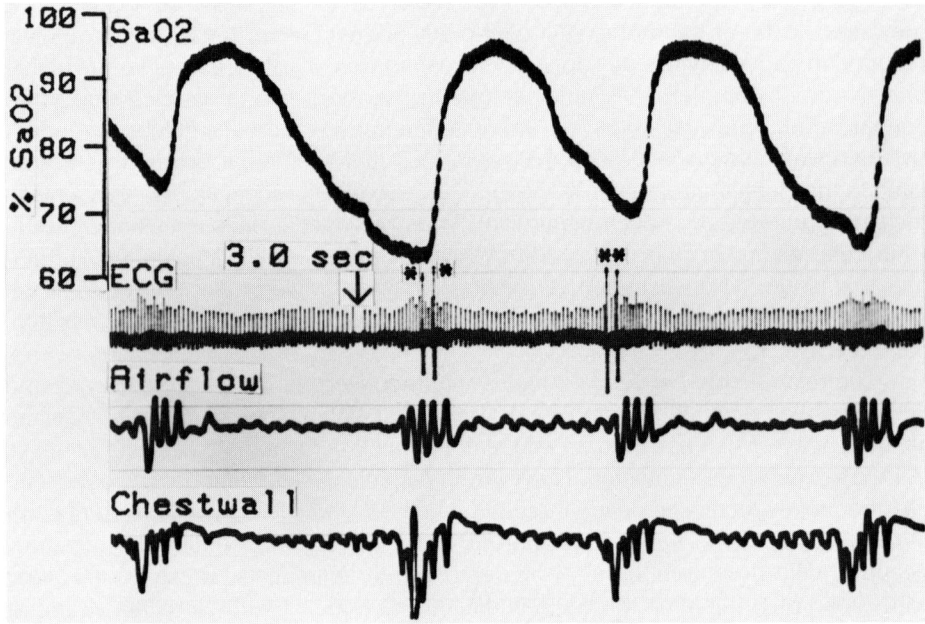

Fig. 3-10. Segment of a patient's sleep record showing the characteristic sinus arrhythmia associated with obstructive apneas along with a 3.0 second sinus pause. Note premature ventricular ectopic complexes indicated by the asterisks coinciding with cardio-acceleration immediately following apnea termination.

ing apnea termination acts to lower the ectopic threshold of the myocardium. Fluctuations in sympathetic-parasympathetic neural activity have been implicated in the pathogenesis of both supraventricular and ventricular arrhythmias by several authors.[76–78] In addition, mechanical stresses or biochemical changes associated with the reoxygenation of hypoxic myocardium may be involved in the generation of the ventricular ectopy.

CHRONIC HEMODYNAMIC EFFECTS OF APNEAS

While there is uniform agreement that apneas produce cyclical elevations in blood pressures, the relationship of sleep apnea to sustained systemic and pulmonary hypertension is a more complicated issue. Multiple variables, which include apnea severity, the degree of obesity, and the co-existence of cardiac or pulmonary disorders are all involved. Diurnal systemic hypertension has been reported to occur in 48 to 96 percent of patients with obstructive sleep apnea.[74,79–81] While obesity certainly contributes to this high incidence of systemic hypertension, Lugaresi and colleagues[12,23] consider apnea severity to be an important determinant of systemic hypertension based on data showing progressively greater pressures in hypersomnolent apneics compared to heavy snorers and non-snoring controls. Evidence that tracheostomy decreases the severity of diurnal hypertension in apneics further supports a contributory role for sleep apnea in the pathogenesis of systemic hypertension. In addition, urinary norepinephrine and normetanephrine have been reported to decrease following tracheostomy for obstructive sleep apnea.[82]

Because of the frequent occurrence of hypertension in sleep apneics and the fact that clinical symptoms are often not present in mild to moderate apneics, three groups have prospectively studied hypertensive patient populations to ascertain the underlying prevalence of sleep apnea in essential hypertension. Using a definition of greater than 30 apneas per night to diagnose sleep apnea, Kales et al[83] detected sleep apnea in 30 percent of 50 hypertensive patients and none of 50 age and sex matched controls. Using a diagnostic criteria of greater than 10 apneas per hour, Lavie et al[84] confirmed the presence of sleep apnea in 22 percent of 50 subjects with essential hypertension. Employing this same diagnostic criteria, Fletcher et al[85] detected sleep apnea in 30 percent of 46 men with essential hypertension. Sleep apnea was detected in nine percent of their age, sex, and weight matched nonhypertensive control population.

The pathogenesis of essential hypertension is a multifactorial process involving dietary, hormonal, neurogenic, vascular, and hemodynamic factors.[86] While the male sex and caloric excess are important common denominators in both sleep apnea and systemic hypertension, recurrent oxyhemoglobin desaturation leading to chronic stimulation of the sympathetic nervous system and catecholamine excretion has been postulated to play an significant role in the development of diurnal hypertension. Clark et al[87] reported that plasma and urinary catecholamine levels were increased by 47 and 67 percent respectively in patients with sleep apnea compared to controls. Fletcher et al[82] measured urinary free epinephrine, free norepinephrine, and their respective metabolic products metanephrine and normetanephrine in six patients with sleep apnea before and after tracheostomy. These subjects failed to show the normal pattern of nocturnal reductions in norepinephrine and normetanephrine excretion consistent with increased sympathetic neural activity during sleep. Levels of norepinephrine and normetanephrine (sympathetic neurotransmitters) were high before tracheostomy and returned to control values after tracheostomy. Consequently, these studies provide direct evidence for hyperactivity of the sympathetic nervous system that may contribute to either the development of diurnal hypertension, increased ventricular ectopy or both.

The deleterious effects of obesity and systemic hypertension on the heart are widely recognized. While obesity tends to produce left ventricular dilatation and hypertrophy (eccentric hypertrophy), hypertension results in concentric hypertrophy and both contribute to long term elevations in left ventricular stroke work, which increase the risk of congestive heart failure.[88] Although excessive exposure of the cardiovascular system to catecholamines results in hypertension as well as cardiomyopathic changes, the catecholamine elevations in sleep apnea are not impressive when compared to those observed with pheochromocytomas. An interesting question that has not been raised is whether or not repetitive pressure elevations related to apneas have more deleterious cardiovascular effects than constantly maintained increases in pressure. While stop and go driving in traffic clearly has a negative impact on mechanical longevity in automobiles, it is not known whether repetitive accelerations and decelerations in heart rate and blood pressure with associated shear stresses have an adverse effect on the longevity of the cardiovascular system.

The prevalence of pulmonary hypertension in sleep apnea is not well established because patients without clinical evidence of right ventricular dysfunction are seldom exposed to the risks of hemodynamic monitoring. Recently, Bradley et al[89] reported that 12 percent of 50 consecutively studied patients with obstructive sleep apnea had clinically evident right heart failure. Because the patients with right heart failure were hyperinflated, had substantial expiratory airflow obstruction, and were considerably more hypoxemic (PaO_2 = 52 versus 75 mmHg) and hypercapnic ($PaCO_2$ = 51 versus 36 mmHg) than those without right heart failure, they concluded that concomitant obstructive airways disease, which produced diurnal as well as nocturnal hypoxemia, played a major role in the development of cor pulmonale. The fact that no differences in apnea plus hypopnea frequency, apnea duration, or total apnea time per hour of sleep were detected between patients with and without right heart failure further suggested that differences in apnea severity were not a primary determinant of right heart failure. Although the role of obesity was de-emphasized, the subjects with right heart failure were massively obese weighing 186 percent of their ideal body weight. In the absence of obesity, the degree of obstructive airways disease reported would not likely have produced the severe impairments in gas exchange that were observed. Although the results of this study suggest that clinically apparent right heart failure is unlikely to develop in the absence of diurnal hypoxemia, milder degrees of pulmonary hypertension and right ventricular dysfunction may be present in a significant number of patients with sleep apnea alone.

It is surprising that none of the obese hypercapnic and hypoxemic subjects with right heart failure in Bradley's study were found to have a restrictive pattern without airflow obstruction on pulmonary function testing. Clearly, there are considerable numbers of obese patients without obstructive airways disease who are diurnally hypercapnic, hypoxemic, and develop clinically evident right heart failure.[90] Whether these patients, who are diagnostically classified as having the obesity-hypoventilation (Pickwickian) syndrome are more frequently encountered than obese apneics with obstructive airways disease (blue bloaters) remains to be determined. Certainly, the greater the severity and duration of alveolar hypoxia, the greater the pulmonary hypertension and incidence of right heart failure. At the present time, it appears unlikely that intermittent episodes of nocturnal oxyhemoglobin desaturation alone are sufficient to induce substantial pulmonary hypertension in the absence of diurnal alveolar hypoxia.

EFFECTS OF TREATMENT ON HEMODYNAMICS AND CARDIAC DYSRHYTHMIAS

Effective treatment of obstructive sleep apnea by tracheostomy has been documented both to eliminate nocturnal elevations in systemic pressures as well as to decrease the severity of diurnal hypertension.[15,17,70,81,91,92] Coccagna et al[15] reported reductions in systemic pressures from 170/97 mmHg to 133/66 mmHg following tracheostomy in five patients with sleep apnea. Burack et al[81] confirmed this hemodynamically beneficial effect observing reductions in systemic pressures from 157/100 mmHg pre-surgery to 124/74 mmHg in 10 patients 1 week post-tracheostomy. In the eight patients reported by the Stanford group, systolic and diastolic blood pressures decreased by 18 and 15 mmHg, respectively, following tracheostomy.[17,70,91] However, it should be noted that weight loss associated with tracheostomy, which averaged 15 kg in one series,[70] may account for some of the improvement.

Tracheostomy has been found to abolish nocturnal increases in pulmonary artery pressures in the limited number of patients who have been studied before and after surgery.[15,17,91] Pressure recordings during wakefulness have documented reductions in pulmonary hypertension toward normal in three cases.[93,94] However, six subjects with borderline pulmonary hypertension before surgery showed no significant changes in pressure post-tracheostomy.[17,91]

Tracheostomy effectively eliminates the occurrence of the cardiac dysrhythmias, which are specifically related to obstructive apneas. Consequently, sinus bradycardia, sinus pauses, and atrioventricular block are greatly reduced following surgery.[15,27,70,72,92] However, Tilkian et al[95] have pointed out that these bradyarrhythmias may persist in association with central apneas. Atrial fibrillation and flutter have also been reported to resolve in several cases after tracheostomy possibly due to reductions in ventricular afterload and atrial distension.[15,27] Ventricular tachycardia specifically related to episodes of oxyhemoglobin desaturation has been reported to resolve following tracheostomy and ventricular ectopy in general has been considered to decrease.[70,75,92,95]

Although tracheostomy has been documented to have beneficial effects on systemic and pulmonary hemodynamics as well as cardiac dysrhythmias, it is associated with both short and long term complications.[92] In addition, Fletcher et al[96] have recently demonstrated that tracheostomy for obstructive sleep apnea may not always produce resolution of nocturnal hypoxemia and yield improvement in cardiovascular status if concomitant cardiopulmonary disorders are present. In the future, the therapeutic benefit to risk ratios for the newer forms of therapy will need to be compared with classical management by tracheostomy.

ACKNOWLEDGMENTS

This work was supported by the Veterans Administration.

REFERENCES

1. Smolensky M, Holberg F, Sargent F: II. Chronobiology of the life sequence, in Itoh S, Ogata K, Yoshimura H (eds): Advances in Climatic Physiology. Tokyo, Igaku Shoin Ltd., 1972, pp 281–318

2. Brooks H, Carrol JH: A clinical study of the effects of sleep and rest on blood pressure. Arch Intern Med 10:97–102, 1912

3. Littler WA, Honour AJ, Carter RD, et al: Sleep and blood pressure. Br Med J 3:346–348, 1975

4. MacWilliams JA: Blood pressure and heart action in sleep and dreams: Their relation to hemorrhages, angina and sudden death. Br Med J 22:1196–1200, 1923

5. Richardson DW, Honour AJ, Fenton GW, et al: Variation in arterial pressure throughout the day and night. Clin Sci 26:445–460, 1964

6. Coccagna G, Mantovani M, Brignani F, et al: Arterial pressure changes during spontaneous sleep in man. Electroenceph Clin Neurophysiol 31:277–281, 1971

7. Khatri IM, Freis ED: Hemodynamic changes during sleep. J Appl Physiol 22:867–873, 1967

8. Snyder F, Hobson JA, Morrison DF, et al: Changes in respiration, heart rate, and systolic blood pressure in human sleep. J Appl Physiol 19:417–422, 1964

9. Andersson B, Kenney RA, Neil E: The role of the chemoreceptors of the carotid and aortic regions in the production of Mayer waves. Acta Physiol Scand 20:203–220, 1950

10. Lugaresi E, Coccagna G, Mantovani M, et al: Some periodic phenomena arising during drowsiness and sleep in man. Electroenceph Clin Neurophysiol 32:701–705, 1972

11. Bristow JD, Honour AJ, Pickering TG, et al: Cardiovascular and respiratory changes during sleep in normal and hypertensive subjects. Cardiovasc Res 3:476–485, 1969

12. Lugaresi E, Coccagna G, Cirignotta F: Snoring and its clinical implications, in Guilleminault C, Dement WC (eds): Sleep Apnea Syndromes. New York, Alan R. Liss, Inc., 1978, pp 13–21

13. Lugaresi E, Coccagna G, Farneti P, et al: Snoring. Electroenceph Clin Neurophysiol 39:59–64, 1975

14. Shepard JW Jr, Garrison M, Grither D, et al: Hemodynamic responses to O_2 desaturation in obstructive sleep apnea. Am Rev Respir Dis 131:A106, 1985

15. Coccagna G, Mantovani M, Brignani F, et al: Continuous recording of the pulmonary and systemic arterial pressure during sleep in syndromes of hypersomnia with periodic breathing. Bull Physiopathol Respir 8:1159–1172, 1972

16. Lonsdorfer J, Meunier-Carus J, Lampert-Benignus E, et al: Haemodynamic and respiratory aspects of the Pickwickian syndrome. Bull Physiopathol Respir 8:1181–1192, 1972

17. Schroeder JS, Motta J, Guilleminault C: Hemodynamic studies in sleep apnea, in Guilleminault C, Dement WC (eds): Sleep Apnea Syndromes. New York, Alan R. Liss, Inc., 1978, pp 177–196

18. Tilkian AG, Guilleminault C, Schroeder JS, et al: Hemodynamics in sleep-induced apnea. Studies during wakefulness and sleep. Ann Int Med 85:714–719, 1976

19. Shepard JW Jr: Gas exchange and hemodynamics during sleep. Med Clinics of North Amer 69:1243–1263, 1985

20. Buda AJ, Pinsky MR, Ingels NB Jr, et al: Effect of intrathoracic pressure on left ventricular performance. N Engl J Med 301:453–459, 1979

21. Scharf SM, Brown R, Tow DE, et al: Cardiac effects of increased lung volume and decreased pleural pressure in man. J Appl Physiol 47:257–262, 1979

22. Scharf SM: Influence of sleep state and breathing on cardiovascular function, in Saunders NA, Sullivan CE (eds): Sleep and Breathing. New York, Marcel Dekker, Inc., 1984, pp 221–240

23. Lugaresi E, Cirignotta F, Coccagna G, et al: Clinical significance of snoring, in Saunders NA, Sullivan CE (eds): Sleep and Breathing. New York, Marcel Dekker, Inc., 1984, pp 283–298

24. Zwillich C, Devlin T, White D, et al: Bradycardia during sleep apnea: Characteristics and mechanism. J Clin Invest 69:1286–1292, 1982

25. Lin YC, Shida KK, Hong SK: Effects of hypercapnia, hypoxia, and rebreathing on heart rate response during apnea. J Appl Physiol 54:166–171, 1983

26. Imaizumi T: Arrhythmias in sleep apnea. Am Heart J 100:513–516, 1980

27. Kryger M, Quesney LF, Holder D, et al: The sleep deprivation syndrome of the obese patient. A problem of periodic nocturnal upper airway obstruction. Am J Med 56:531–539, 1974

28. Lin YC, Shida KK, Hong SK: Effects of hypercapnia, hypoxia, and rebreathing on circulatory responses to apnea. J Appl Physiol 54:172–177, 1983

29. Hong SK, Lin YC, Lally DA, et al: Alveolar gas exchanges and cardiovascular functions during breath holding with air. J Appl Physiol 30:540–547, 1971

30. Kawakami Y, Natelson BH, DuBois AB: Cardiovascular effects of face immersion and factors affecting diving reflex in man. J Appl Physiol 23:964–970, 1967

31. Paulev PE, Wettergvist H: Cardiac output during breath-holding in man. Scand J Clin Lab Invest 22:115–123, 1968

32. Shepard JW Jr, Schweitzer PK, Keller CA, et al: Myocardial stress: Exercise versus sleep in patients with COPD. Chest 86:366–374, 1984

33. Grover RF, Wagner WW, McMurtry IF, et al: Pulmonary circulation, in Shepherd JT, Abboud FM (eds): Handbook of Physiology. Bethesda, American Physiological Society, 1983, pp 103–136

34. Fishman AP: Hypoxia on the pulmonary circulation: how and where it acts. Circ Res 38:221–231, 1976

35. Weir EK: Acute hypoxic pulmonary hypertension, in Weir EK, Reeves JT (eds): Pulmonary Hypertension. Mount Kisco, Futura Publishing Co, 1984, pp 251–290

36. Morganroth ML, Reeves JT, Murphy RC, et al: Leukotriene synthesis and receptor blockers block hypoxic pulmonary vasoconstriction. J Appl Physiol 56:1340–1346, 1984

37. Stanbrook HS, Morris KG, McMurtry IF: Prevention and reversal of hypoxic pulmonary hypertension by calcium antagonists. Am Rev Respir Dis 130:81–85, 1984

38. Enson YC, Giuntini ML, Lewis TQ, et al: The influence of hydrogen ion concentration and hypoxia on the pulmonary circulation. J Clin Invest 43:1146–1162, 1964

39. Harvey RM, Enson Y, Betti R, et al: Further observations on the effect of hydrogen ion on the pulmonary circulation. Circulation 35:1019–1027, 1967

40. Rudolph AM, Yuan S: Response of the pulmonary vasculature to hypoxia and H^+ ion concentration changes. J Clin Invest 45:399–411, 1966

41. Vogel JHK, Blount SG Jr: The role of hydrogen ion concentration in the regulation of pulmonary arterial pressure. Circulation 32:788–796, 1965

42. Nisell OI: The action of oxygen and carbon dioxide on the bronchioles and vessels of the isolated perfused lungs. Acta Physiol Scand Suppl 73:7–62, 1950

43. VonEuler US, Liljestrand G: Observations on the pulmonary arterial blood pressure in the cat. Acta Physiol Scand 12:301–320, 1946

44. Emery CJ, Sloan PJM, Mohammed FH, et al: The action of hypercapnia during hypoxia on pulmonary vessels. Bull Eur Physiopathol Respir 13:763–776, 1977

45. Viles PH, Shepherd JT: Evidence for a dilator action of carbon dioxide on the pulmonary vessels of the cat. Circ Res 22:325–332, 1968

46. Kontos HA, Levasseur JE, Richardson DW, et al: Comparative circulatory responses to systemic hypoxia in man and in unanesthetized dog. J Appl Physiol 23:381–386, 1967

47. Slutsky AS, Rebuck AS: Heart rate response to isocapnic hypoxia in conscious man. Am J Physiol 234:H129–H132, 1978

48. Kahler RL, Goldblatt A, Braunwald E: The effects of acute hypoxia on the systemic venous and arterial system and myocardial contractile force. J Clin Invest 41:1553–1563, 1962

49. Adachi H, Strauss HW, Ochi H, et al: The effect of hypoxia on the regional distribution of cardiac output in the dog. Circ Res 39:314–319, 1976

50. Pelletier CL: Circulatory responses to graded stimulation of the carotid chemoreceptors in the dog. Circ Res 31:431–443, 1972

51. Krasney JA, Magno MG, Levitzky MG, et al: Cardiovascular responses to arterial hypoxia in awake sinoaortic-denervated dogs. J Appl Physiol 35:733–738, 1973

52. Daly M deB, Scott MJ: The effects of stimulation of the carotid body chemoreceptors on heart rate in the dog. J Physiol 144:148–166, 1958

53. Daly M deB, Scott MJ: An analysis of the primary cardiovascular reflex effects of stimulation of the carotid body chemoreceptors in the dog. J Physiol 162:555–573, 1962

54. Daly M deB, Hazzledine JL: The effects of artificially induced hyperventilation on the primary cardiac reflex response to stimulation of the carotid bodies in the dog. J Physiol 168:872–889, 1963

55. DeGeest H, Levy MN, Zieske H: Reflex effects of cephalic hypoxia, hypercapnia, and ischemia upon ventricular contractility. Circ Res 17:349–357, 1965

56. Downing SE, Mitchell JH, Wallace AG: Cardiovascular responses to ischemia, hypoxia, and hypercapnia of the central nervous system. Am J Physiol 204:881–887, 1963

57. Gross PM, Whipp B, Davidson JT, et al: Role of the carotid bodies in the heart rate response to breath holding in man. J Appl Physiol 41:336–340, 1976

58. Briskin JB, Lehrman KL, Guilleminault C: Shy-Drager syndrome and sleep apnea, in Guilleminault C, Dement WC (eds): Sleep Apnea Syndrome. New York, Alan R. Liss, 1978, pp 317–322

59. Stromme SB, Kerem D, Elsner R: Diving bradycardia during rest and exercise and its relation to physical fitness. J Appl Physiol 28:614–621, 1970

60. Murdaugh HV Jr, Seabury JC, Mitchell WL: Electrocardiogram of the diving seal. Circ Res 9:358–361, 1961

61. Jones DR, Purves MJ: The carotid body in the duck and the consequences of its denervation upon the cardiac responses to immersion. J Physiol 211:279–294, 1970

62. Brodsky M, Wu D, Denes P, et al: Arrhythmias documented by 24 hour continuous electrocardiographic monitoring in 50 male medical students without apparent heart disease. Am J Cardiol 39:390–395, 1977

63. Clarke JM, Shelton JR, Hamer J, et al: The rhythm of the normal human heart. Lancet ii:508–512, 1976

64. Fleg JL, Kennedy HL: Cardiac arrhythmias in a healthy elderly population. Chest 81:302–307, 1982

65. Pickering TG, Johnston J, Honour AJ: Comparison of the effects of sleep, exercise and autonomic drugs on ventricular extrasystoles, using ambulatory monitoring of electrocardiogram and electroencephalogram. Am J Med 65:575–583, 1978

66. Winkle RA: The relationship between ventricular ectopic beat frequency and heart rate. Circulation 66:439–446, 1982

67. Camm AJ, Evans KE, Ward DE, et al: The rhythm of the heart in active elderly subjects. Am Heart J 99:598–603, 1980

68. Guilleminault C, Pool P, Motta J, et al: Sinus arrest during REM sleep in young adults. N Engl J Med 311:1006–1010, 1984

69. Lown B, Temte JV, Reich P, et al: Basis for recurring ventricular fibrillation in the absence of coronary heart disease and its management. N Engl J Med 294:623–629, 1976

70. Guilleminault C, Simmons FB, Motta J, et al: Obstructive sleep apnea syndrome and tracheostomy. Arch Intern Med 141:985–988, 1981

71. Miller WP: Cardiac arrhythmias and conduction disturbances in the sleep apnea syndrome. Am J Med 73:317–321, 1982

72. Tilkian AG, Guilleminault C, Schroeder JS, et al: Sleep-induced apnea syndrome. Am J Med 63:348–358, 1977

73. Eckberg DL: Human sinus arrhythmia as an index of vagal cardiac outflow. J Appl Physiol 54:961–966, 1983

74. Shepard JW Jr, Garrison MW, Grither DA, et al: Relationship of ventricular ectopy to nocturnal O2 desaturation in patients with obstructive sleep apnea. Chest 88:335–340, 1985

75. Guilleminault C, Connolly SJ, Winkle RA: Cardiac arrhythmia and conduction disturbances during sleep in 400 patients with sleep apnea syndrome. Am J Cardiol 52:490–494, 1983

76. Findley LJ, Ries AL, Tisi GM, et al: Case report: Apneas and oscillation of cardiac ectopy in Cheyne-Stokes breathing during sleep. Am Rev Respir Dis 130:937–939, 1984

77. Lown B, Tykocinski M, Garfein A, et al: Sleep and ventricular premature beats. Circulation 48:691–701, 1973

78. Rosenblatt G, Hartmann E, Zwilling GR: Cardiac irritability during sleep and dreaming. J Psychosom Res 17:129–134, 1973

79. Guilleminault C, van den Hoed J, Mitler MM: Clinical overview of the sleep apnea syndromes, in Guilleminault C, Dement WC (eds): Sleep Apnea Syndromes. New York, Alan R. Liss, 1978, pp 1–12

80. Guilleminault C, Tilkian A, Dement WC: The sleep apnea syndromes. Ann Rev Med 27:465–484, 1976

81. Burack B, Pollak C, Borowiecki B, et al: The hypersomnia-sleep apnea syndrome (HSA): a reversible major cardiovascular hazard. Circulation 56:177, 1977

82. Fletcher E, Miller J, Schaaf J, et al: Urinary catecholamines before and after tracheostomy in obstructive sleep apnea. Sleep Research 114:154, 1985

83. Kales A, Bixler EO, Cadieux RJ, et al: Sleep apnoea in a hypertensive population. Lancet ii:1005–1008, 1984

84. Lavie P, Ben-Yosef R, Rubin AE: Prevalence of sleep apnea syndrome among patients with essential hypertension. Am Heart J 108:373–376, 1984

85. Fletcher EC, DeBehnke RD, Lovoi MS, et al: Undiagnosed sleep apnea among patients with essential hypertension. Ann Int Med 103:190–194, 1985

86. Kaplan NM: Clinical Hypertension (ed 3). Baltimore, Williams and Wilkins, 1982, pp 1–41

87. Clark RW, Boudoulas H, Schaal SF, et al: Adrenergic hyperactivity and cardiac abnormal-

ity in primary disorders of sleep. Neurology 30:113–119, 1980

88. Messerli FH, Sundgaard-Riise K, Reisin ED, et al: Dimorphic cardiac adaptation to obesity and arterial hypertension. Ann Int Med 99:757–761, 1983

89. Bradley TD, Rutherford R, Grossman RF, et al: Role of daytime hypoxemia in the pathogenesis of right heart failure in the obstructive sleep apnea syndrome. Am Rev Respir Dis 131:835–839, 1985

90. Jones JB, Wilhoit SC, Findley LJ, et al: Oxyhemoglobin saturation during sleep in subjects with and without the obesity-hypoventilation syndrome. Chest 88:9–15, 1985

91. Motta J, Guilleminault C, Schroeder JS, et al: Tracheostomy and hemodynamic changes in sleep-induced apnea. Ann Int Med 89:454–458, 1978

92. Conway WA, Victor LD, Magilligan DJ, et al: Adverse effects of tracheostomy for sleep apnea. JAMA 246:347–350, 1981

93. Lugaresi E, Coccagna G, Mantovani M, et al: Effects of tracheostomy in two cases of hypersomnia with periodic breathing. J Neurol Neurosurg Psych 36:15–26, 1973

94. Aubert-Tulkens G, Willems B, Veriter C, et al: Increase in ventilatory response to CO_2 following tracheostomy in obstructive sleep apnea. Bull Eur Physiopathol Respir 16:587–593, 1980

95. Tilkian AG, Motta J, Guilleminault C: Cardiac arrhythmias in sleep apnea, in Guilleminault C, Dement WC (eds): Sleep Apnea Syndromes. New York, Alan R. Liss, Inc., 1978, pp 197–210

96. Fletcher EC, Brown DL: Nocturnal oxyhemoglobin desaturation following tracheostomy for obstructive sleep apnea. Am J Med 79:35–42, 1985

Samuel T. Kuna
John E. Remmers

4
Pathophysiology and Mechanisms of Sleep Apnea

The upper airway serves as a common pathway for the respiratory, digestive, and phonatory tracts. Its anatomy has been dictated by the multiplicity of its functions. Patency of the upper airway is required for the normal function of respiration. But, as a part of the digestive tract, the upper airway must be able to close in order to initiate swallowing. As a phonatory tract, the upper airway is interrupted by a series of valves: the larynx, the velopharynx, and the lips. The opening and closing of these valves creates vibrations in the air column producing speech. The specific anatomic requirements that make swallowing and verbal communication possible compromise the upper airway as a continuous conduit of air. Throughout most of the proximal respiratory tract, the patency of the air column is protected by walls reinforced with cartilage and/or bone. The trachea and proximal bronchi are supported by rings or plates of cartilage. The larynx is also furnished with cartilagenous rings, and the nasal passages are enveloped by bone and cartilage. By contrast, a long segment of the upper airway, the pharynx, is potentially collapsible. Despite this compromise, an intricate anatomic and physiologic integration allows the upper airway to function as a respiratory as well as a digestive and phonatory tract. Normally the upper airway closes momentarily during such actions as swallowing, regurgitation, eructation, and speech, but otherwise it remains open.[1] This almost continuous patency of the upper airway during wakefulness and sleep is in large part due to the upper airway's morphologic design. In addition, physiologic mechanisms safeguard against airway closure and restore patency of a collapsed airway. Pathologic conditions can disrupt this intricate balance between structure and function leading to collapse of the upper airway during sleep with potential asphyxiation. Such pathologic conditions may arise from gross anatomic abnormalities and/or an abnormal alteration of the physiologic defense mechanisms.

ABNORMALITIES OF RESPIRATION DURING SLEEP
ISBN 0-8089-1812-5
Copyright © 1986 by Grune & Stratton, Inc.
All rights of reproduction in any form reserved.

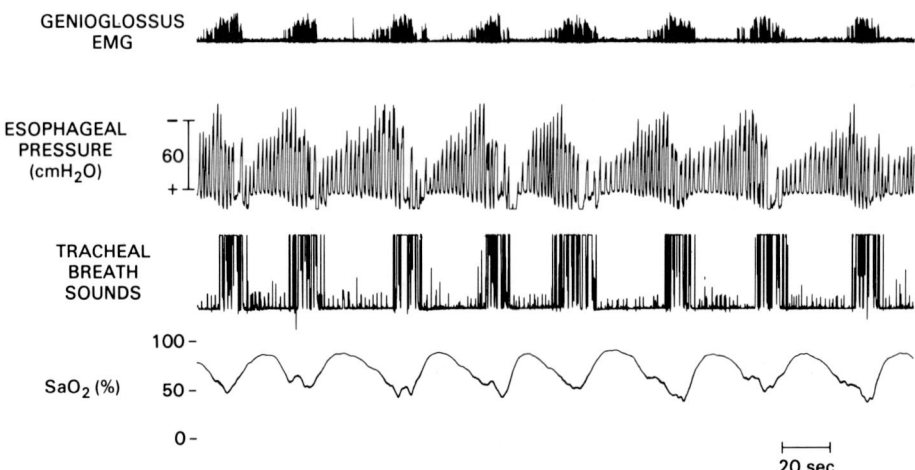

GENIOGLOSSUS
EMG

ESOPHAGEAL
PRESSURE
(cmH₂O)

TRACHEAL
BREATH
SOUNDS

SaO₂ (%)

20 sec

Fig. 4-1. Recording obtained during sleep in a patient with obstructive sleep apnea. Tracings are from top to bottom: rectified genioglossus electromyogram (EMG), esophageal pressure in cm H₂O, tracheal breath sounds, and arterial oxygen saturation (SaO₂).

SEQUENTIAL EVENTS OF UPPER AIRWAY CLOSURE DURING SLEEP

A polygraphic recording from a sleeping patient who has multiple upper airway closures during sleep is shown in Figure 4-1. The tracheal breath sounds indicate the presence or absence of airflow and show repetitive intervals in which airflow is absent. During these so called apneic episodes, the subject is generating enormous respiratory efforts. Esophageal, i.e., intrathoracic, pressures near the end of each apneic episode reach −60 cm of the H_2O. The absence of airflow in the presence of respiratory efforts indicates a collapse of the upper airway. That the upper airway is indeed the site of closure is demonstrated by the ability to completely eliminate these apneic episodes by performing a tracheostomy.[2] During sleep, these obstructive apneas are terminated when the upper airway opens and airflow resumes. However, this is a transient state; after several breaths the upper airway again closes initiating the onset of another apneic episode. As is evident in this record, one of the dire consequences of intermittent upper airway closure during sleep is the marked arterial oxygen desaturation consequent to each apneic episode. During this five minute sleep recording, the subject had seven apneic episodes. During the course of the night, hundreds more were recorded, unequivocally establishing the diagnosis of obstructive sleep apnea (OSA).

SITE OF UPPER AIRWAY CLOSURE

Fluoroscopic and fiberoptic studies during sleep in patients with OSA indicate that the pharynx is the usual site of upper airway closure.[3–6] In general, pharyngeal airway collapse occurs with concentric closure of the pharyngeal lumen due to the apposition of the tongue to the lateral and posterior pharyngeal walls. Whether or not

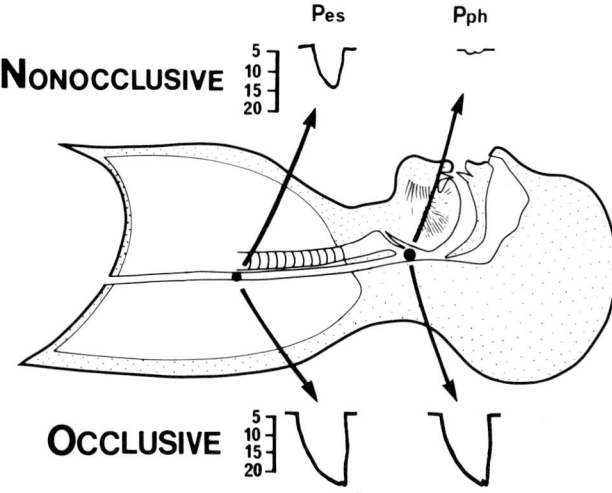

Fig. 4-2. Schematic diagram showing transmission of subatmospheric intrathoracic pressure into the hypopharynx. With a patent airway (upper tracing) only small pressure fluctuations occur in the upper airway during inspiration. Airway occlusion above the hypopharynx (lower tracing) results in an equalization of intrathoracic and upper airway pressure. (From Block AJ, Faulkner JA, Hughes RL, et al: Factors influencing upper airway closure. Chest 86:117, 1984. With permission.)

there is distal migration or extension of collapse into more caudal regions during successive respiratory efforts is unknown, but may be answered by somnofluroscopy. Physiologic measurements of upper airway pressure in OSA patients during sleep confirm these visual observations[7] (Fig. 4-2). When the airway is patent, normal tidal breathing creates relatively small fluctuations in pharyngeal pressure reflecting the resistance to airflow presented by the pharynx and nose (Fig. 4-2, upper tracing). During airway occlusion, however, intrathoracic and epiglottic pressures are equal, indicating that the site of closure is the collapsible portion of the pharynx (Fig. 4-2, lower tracing). Successful prevention of upper airway closure with a nasopharyngeal tube also implicates the pharynx as the site of closure. When inserted through the naris, the tip of this tube reaches the level of the hypopharynx.

MECHANISMS OF PHARYNGEAL OCCLUSION IN OSA

Based on their clinical observations in patients with OSA, Remmers et al proposed that the patency of the upper airway is determined by two counteracting forces[7,8] (Fig. 4-3). Subatmospheric intraluminal pressure during inspiration promotes narrowing of the collapsible upper airway segment. This inward narrowing force is counterbalanced by an outward dilating force created by the activation of skeletal muscles surrounding the upper airway. The net balance between these two forces will determine upper airway patency. Normally, during wakefulness and sleep, the net balance of forces favors airway patency. A disruption in the balance between

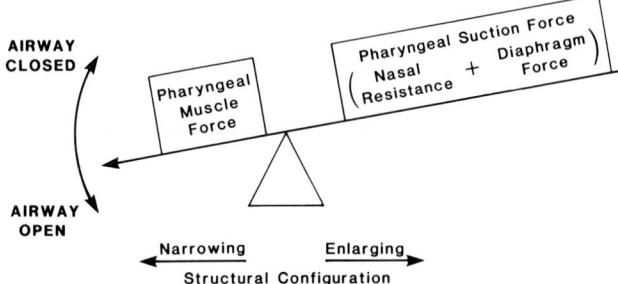

Fig. 4-3. Schematic model of pharyngeal airway maintenance, showing airway narrowing and dilating forces on either
side of a fulcrum. Change in airway configuration shifts the
position of the fulcrum. (From Block AJ, Faulkner JA, Hughes
RL, et al: Factors influencing upper airway closure. Chest
86:116, 1984. With permission.)

these opposing forces can result in upper airway closure. For example, upper airway
closure could result from excessive suppression of upper airway muscle activity or a
disproportionate increase in subatmospheric intraluminal pressure. Evidence suggests that both of these mechanisms play a role in the pathogenesis of upper airway
closure during sleep.

The cyclical change in genioglossus muscle activity in association with upper
airway closure, shown in Figure 4-1, suggests that upper airway muscle activity plays
a role in maintaining a patent upper airway. The genioglossus protrudes the tongue,
and its contraction increases the size of the pharyngeal lumen. The onset of the
airway occlusions corresponds to a nadir in genioglossal activity, while termination
of each apneic episode coincides with greatest activation of the genioglossus muscle. Electromyographic recordings of other upper airway muscles in patients with
OSA during sleep display cyclical variation similar to that of the genioglossus.[3,9,10]

The interaction between upper airway muscle activity and subatmospheric intraluminal pressure has been studied by comparing the pressure required to collapse
the upper airway in infant cadavers.[11] Subatmospheric pressure was applied to the
upper airway via a face mask. The closing pressure in dead infants was about +1.4
cm H_2O. Further support for the effect of subatmospheric intraluminal pressure on
upper airway configuration, independent of upper airway muscle activity, comes
from observations made during the clinical treatment of central, i.e., nonobstructive,
apneas with phrenic nerve stimulation.[12] During central apneas, there is a global loss
in respiratory-related neural activity. Stimulation of the phrenic nerve during these
apneas can precipitate and/or unmask upper airway closure. Diaphragmatic contraction by phrenic nerve pacing would not be accompanied by co-activation of upper
airway muscles, leaving unopposed the airway constricting effect of the subatmospheric intraluminal pressure.

Activation of upper airway muscles not only stabilizes but even dilates the upper
airway. Strohl and Fouke measured the change in pressure in an isolated, sealed
upper airway in spontaneously breathing tracheostomized dogs.[13] Pressure within
this upper airway compartment decreased during inspiration in association with
phasic activation of upper airway muscles, proving that with each inspiration these

muscles act to dilate the pharynx. Increased upper airway muscle activity changes airway configuration thereby altering airway resistance. In normal subjects, the hypercapnia induced increase in phasic inspiratory activity of the alae nasi muscles, which flare the nostrils, is associated with a significant drop in specific nasal airway resistance.[14,15] Conversely, phrenic nerve stimulation in the anesthetized dog, which would not be associated with co-activation of alae nasi muscles, leads to an increase in nasal resistance.[16]

MECHANICAL FACTORS INFLUENCING UPPER AIRWAY CLOSURE:

Compliance

Certain mechanical properties of the upper airway will also influence the effect of subatmospheric intraluminal pressure on upper airway configuration. These include: airway compliance, surface adhesive forces, and airway configuration itself. Fiberoptic studies of the upper airway in infant cadavers have shown that pressure reduction causes narrowing of the entire upper airway from the nasal choanae to the vocal cords.[17] The most compliant area, the oropharynx, has a mean closing pressure of -0.04 ± 1.5 (SE) cm H_2O. Greater negative pressures are required to achieve closure of the nasopharynx. Closing pressures in the hypopharynx are still lower and, at the vocal cords, closing pressures, when present, are lowest of all, ranging from -24 to -59 cm H_2O. In vivo, the degree of upper airway muscle activity will influence this regional airway compliance.

Surface Adhesive Forces

Clinical observations suggest that surface adhesive forces between the apposed membranes may help generate and/or perpetuate upper airway closure. Fiberoptic studies show that as the upper airway narrows, the mucous film lining the surface becomes thicker and further narrows the airway.[17,18] One may speculate that with diminishing airway size, the increase in surface tension forces may decrease airway stability. When using nasal airway positive pressure (NAPP) during sleep in OSA patients, higher pressures are needed to open an already closed airway than to prevent closure of a patent airway.[19] Similar findings have been reported in infant cadavers and sleeping infants.[11,20] These higher opening pressures may be required to overcome surface adhesive forces.

Airway Configuration

Although the relative importance of surface adhesive forces is unknown, another mechanical factor, upper airway configuration, appears to play a very important role in the maintenance of upper airway patency. Acoustic reflection studies reveal that changes in body position causes narrowing of the pharynx in awake normal human subjects.[21] Mean pharyngeal cross sectional area decreases 23 ± 8 (SEM) percent when adult subjects change from an upright to supine position. In contrast, area in the laryngeal and tracheal segments is unchanged. Decreases in pharyngeal cross sectional area have also been noted with neck flexion.[22] Changes in genioglossus and posterior cricoarytenoid muscle activity occur with changes in head position.[23] The postural changes in airway area cannot be solely due to reflex muscle activation, as similar results have been obtained with changing head position in curarized adults and dead infants.[11,24] However, decreased upper airway muscle activity is associated with states of unconsciousness, conditions predisposing to upper airway closure. Safar and colleagues studied the effect of head position on pharyngeal closure in anesthetized adults and found that all subjects developed an upper airway occlusion with neck flexion.[25] Appreciation of this problem in the unconscious patient has led to the incorporation of the neck extension/mandible protrusion technique for maintenance of upper airway patency during cardiopulmonary resuscitation. Stark and Thach extended this work by showing that sleeping infants also develop airway closure upon neck flexion.[26]

Upper Airway Resistance

As resistance to flow through a tube is inversely proportional to the fourth power of the radius, a relatively small decrease in the size of the pharyngeal airway results in relatively large increases in airway resistance. Anch et al studied the effect of body position on upper airway resistance in normal adults.[27] Resistance was calculated by measuring nasal airflow and pressure at the epiglottis referenced to atmospheric pressure. The relationship between pressure and flow, during normal tidal breathing in a patient with OSA, is shown in Figure 4-4. Resistance to airflow, the slope of a line

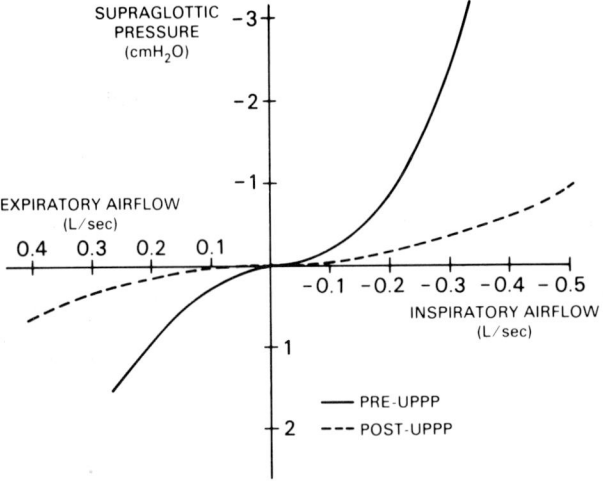

Fig. 4-4. Change in pressure across the upper airway during normal tidal breathing in a patient with OSA. Pressure transducer located at level of epiglottis. Nasal airflow measured by pneumotachograph attached to a nose mask. Solid line: before UPPP; dashed line: several months after UPPP. Although the operation resulted in a marked decrease in upper airway resistance, a followup sleep study revealed a persistence of upper airway closures.

connecting the origin with any point on the curve, varies throughout the respiratory cycle. The parabolic pressure-flow relationship can also be analyzed by fitting it to the Rohrer equation ($P = K_1V + K_2V^2$) where K_1 and K_2 are constants that describe the steepness of the curve. Using both of the above methods, Anch et al found that impedance to airflow presented by the supraglottic airway increased in all subjects when they went from a sitting to supine position. This impedance decreased significantly after topical application of a nasal decongestant indicating an important contribution from mucosal congestion. However, positional changes in upper airway resistance were apparent even after the use of nasal decongestant. The decrease in pharyngeal cross-sectional area may result from a realignment of soft tissue structures by gravity.

Increased upper airway resistance predisposes to upper airway closure. Two clinical studies have shown that upper airway closure during sleep can be induced in normal subjects by increasing their nasal resistance. Lavie et al studied subjects during and after an upper airway viral infection with associated nasal rhinitis.[28] They found an increased incidence in respiratory dysrhythmias during sleep in association with the nasal congestion. Other investigators have induced increased respiratory dysrhythmias during sleep by blocking the nasal passages in normal subjects.[29,30] Although the nasal passages are not felt to be the actual sites of closure, the resistance in this segment of the upper airway plays an important role in the pathogenesis of upper airway closure. Nasal airway resistance will help determine the upstream pressure acting on the collapsible segments of the upper airway.

UPPER AIRWAY MUSCLES

The upper airway is surrounded by muscles. The extrinsic and intrinsic muscles of the tongue exemplify the complex arrangement of these upper airway muscles (Figure 4-5). On each side, the extrinsic tongue muscles include the genioglossus, hypoglossus, styloglossus, and geniohyoid. Whereas activation of the genioglossus

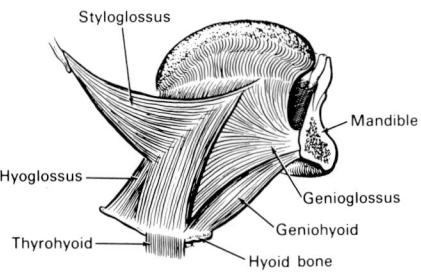

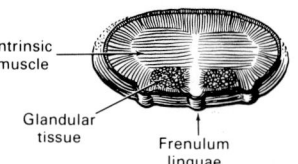

Fig. 4-5. Tongue musculature and its relationship with the mandible and hyoid bone. Upper drawing: lateral view; lower drawing: cross section.

protrudes the tongue, hypoglossal and styloglossal activation causes tongue retraction. The intrinsic muscle fibers enable rolling of the tongue. All of these muscles are innervated by cranial nerve XII carrying motoneurons from the hypoglossal nucleus in the medulla. In the cat, the motoneurons to these different muscles are myotopically arranged within the nucleus. Efferent discharge from this motoneuron pool activates these muscles and coordinates tone and movement of the tongue. Development of a detailed knowledge of the functional anatomy of upper airway muscles, required to understand their interaction, has been hampered by their complex anatomy. Twenty-three pairs of muscles envelop the pharyngeal airway alone. The inspiratory activity is commonly assumed to dilate the upper airway. While this may not be entirely correct, it certainly is valid for three well studied muscles, namely: (1) the genioglossi, (2) the alae nasi, which are innervated by the facial nerves, and (3) the posterior cricoarytenoids, which abduct the vocal cords and are innervated by the recurrent laryngeal nerves. Extrapolating the characteristics of these specific muscles to other upper airway muscles may seem useful, but will certainly lead to pitfalls if done indiscriminately.

Upper airway muscles can exhibit tonic and respiratory-related phasic activity, and the majority display a burst of activity during inspiration. Figure 4-6 compares the representative efferent discharge patterns of the recurrent laryngeal nerve and the medial branch of the hypoglossal nerve (innervating the genioglossus muscle) with phrenic efferent discharge. During the first inspiratory burst, the lung volume in-

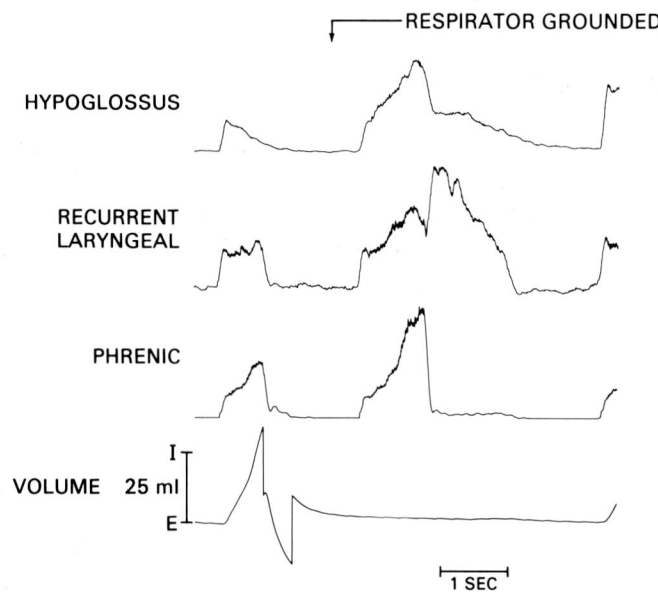

Fig. 4-6. Efferent discharge patterns of hypoglossal, recurrent laryngeal and phrenic nerves in a paralyzed decerebrate cat ventilated with a phrenic driven servo respirator. Two discharges for each nerve are shown. In the first, the phrenic discharge initiates and regulates the size of the tidal volume delivered. During expiration, the respirator is then grounded so that no increment in lung volume occurs with the second phrenic discharge.

creases normally during inspiration. Phrenic activity augments continuously. However, efferent upper airway motoneuron activity typically reaches a peak relatively early in inspiration followed by a gradual decrement or plateau. Characteristically, the onset of upper airway motoneuron phasic inspiratory activity precedes the onset of phrenic discharge by 50 to 100 msec.[9,31–33] Preactivation of upper airway muscles increases with increasing levels of chemical drive and in the presence of increased subatmospheric pressure in an isolated upper airway.[33,34] Under physiologic conditions, this preactivation of upper airway muscles may serve to stabilize the wall of the upper airway in anticipation of the constrictive action of subatmospheric intraluminal pressure.

FACTORS CONTROLLING UPPER AIRWAY MUSCLE ACTIVITY

Volume Feedback

Studies of the factors that influence upper airway muscle activity have helped elucidate the pathogenesis of upper airway closure during sleep. The second inspiratory burst in Figure 4-6 occurred when lung volume was held at FRC. In the absence of phasic volume feedback, all three nerves display a continuously augmenting pattern, indicative of input from central inspiratory activity. Comparing the first and second inspiratory efforts in Figure 4-6, i.e., one with and one without phasic volume feedback, reveals that in contrast to the phrenic, the activity of upper airway motoneurons is readily suppressed by incrementing lung volume. In addition, this phasic volume feedback exerts a differential effect on upper airway motoneuron activity; hypoglossal motoneurons are affected much more than recurrent laryngeal motoneurons.[35,36] Phasic volume feedback also inhibits the alae nasi, but not as prominently as the genioglossus.[36] The alterations in discharge patterns in the presence of phasic changes in lung volume appear to be mediated by vagal afferents from lung mechanoreceptors, since the changes are abolished by bilateral cervical vagotomy.[31,37,38]

Volume feedback plays an important role in the regulation of upper airway motoneuron activity in many animal preparations justifying a more detailed examination of this phenomenon. Hypoglossal motoneurons are much more sensitive than phrenic motoneurons to phasic volume feedback.[39] Figure 4-7 shows the increment in lung volume above end expiratory volume at a particular time after the onset of inspiration, which will cause an initial suppression of efferent motoneuron discharge. Suppression begins at much lower lung volumes and begins much earlier in inspiration for hypoglossal motoneurons then for phrenic motoneurons. Figure 4-7 also indicates that the mechanisms by which phasic volume feedback affects hypoglossal and phrenic activity markedly differ from one another. The steeply declining curve for the phrenic nerve indicates a dramatic decrease in volume threshold as a function of time. It requires a much larger lung volume to initiate suppression of phrenic activity early in inspiration. The hypoglossal system displays a flat volume-time relationship. The same increment in lung volume is required throughout inspiration to start suppressing hypoglossal activity. The volume threshold for suppression of hypoglossal activity does not change with time.

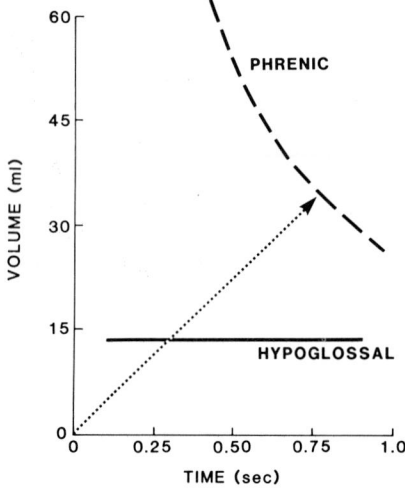

Fig. 4-7. Schematic diagram of effect of phasic volume feedback on suppression of phrenic (dashed line) and hypoglossal (solid line) nerve efferent activity. Increase in lung volume during inspiration (dotted line) would reach volume threshold for inhibition of hypoglossal activity earlier in inspiration.

In the barbiturate anesthetized cat, phasic volume feedback causes a graded suppression of phrenic activity[40] (Fig. 4-8A). Once volume threshold is reached, progressively smaller lung volume increments are needed to achieve further suppression of phrenic activity. Phasic volume feedback causes a graded suppression of hypoglossal activity. However, once volume threshold for suppression of hypoglossal activity is reached, it becomes progressively more difficult to suppress hypoglossal activity (Fig. 4-8B).

This effect of phasic volume feedback can explain the different discharge patterns of upper airway motoneurons as compared to phrenic motoneurons. Once volume threshold for suppression of phrenic activity is reached, smaller and smaller volume increments are needed to achieve further suppression. Consequently, termination of phrenic activity is relatively abrupt. Once volume threshold for suppression of hypoglossal activity is reached, larger and larger volume increments are needed to cause further suppression, resulting in a gradual decline in hypoglossal activity.

What is the functional significance of phasic volume feedback suppression on upper airway motoneuron activity? Normally the upper airway is patent. In the presence of phasic volume feedback, hypoglossal activity is suppressed early in inspira-

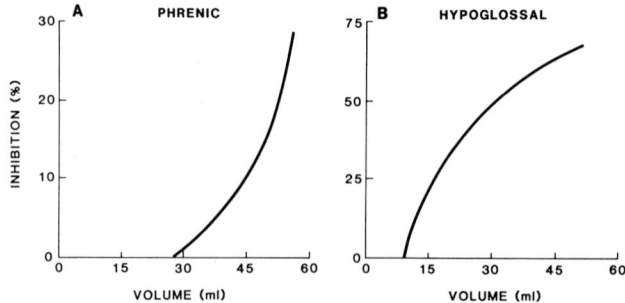

Fig. 4-8. Schematic diagram of effect of lung volume on the graded inhibition of hypoglossal (left panel) and phrenic (right panel) activity at a particular time in inspiration.

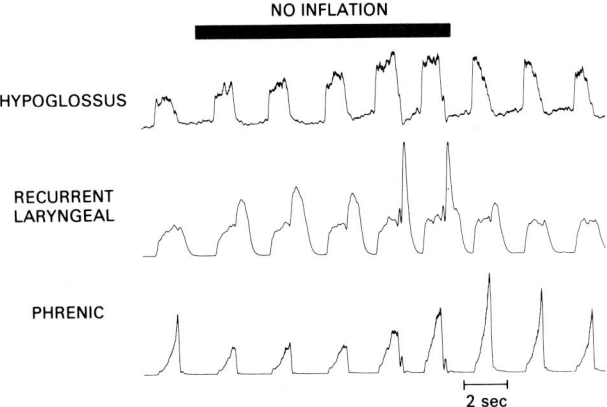

Fig. 4-9. Efferent discharge patterns of hypoglossal, recurrent laryngeal, and phrenic nerves in a paralyzed decerebrate cat on a phrenic driven servo respirator. During the period indicated by the solid bar, the respirator is grounded and no inflation occurs.

tion. In the absence of phasic volume feedback, the continuously augmenting pattern of hypoglossal activity results in a marked activation of the genioglossus muscle. With an inappropriately low increment in lung volume for a given respiratory effort, the volume threshold for suppression of hypoglossal activity will not be reached early in inspiration. Hypoglossal activation will continue to increase, further activating the genioglossus muscle. Genioglossal activation protrudes the tongue and increases the size of the pharyngeal lumen. This reflex response would help ensure that the absent or inappropriate increase in lung volume is not due to closure or narrowing of the upper airway. Although phasic volume feedback appears to play an important role in the activation of upper airway muscles and in the defense of upper airway patency in animals, its importance in man is unknown.

Figure 4-9 shows the effect of withdrawal of phasic volume feedback on phrenic, hypoglossal, and recurrent laryngeal nerve activity in a paralyzed cat on a phrenic driven servo-respirator. In this example, there is a marked decrease in phrenic discharge on the first no-inflation respiratory effort. There is a decrease in both the mean rate of rise and peak height of phrenic activity. This is in marked contrast to the classically described response to withdrawal of phasic volume feedback: a prolongation of the time of inspiration and expiration without a change in mean rate of rise in activity. The latter type response is evident in the simultaneous discharges of the hypoglossal and recurrent laryngeal nerves. The seemingly paradoxical response of the phrenic nerve has been described in a number of different animal preparations and is accounted for by an excitation of phrenic activity by phasic volume feedback.[41,42] This vagally mediated facilitation of phrenic activity may represent another defense mechanism protecting upper airway patency. With compromise of upper airway patency, an increase in phrenic discharge would further increase subatmospheric intraluminal pressure and might exaccerbate the problem. On the other hand, a differential decrease in phrenic discharge would decrease subatmospheric intraluminal pressure helping to shift the balance of forces acting on the upper airway in an outward direction.

Changes in Chemical Drive

Upper airway muscle activity increases when chemoreceptors are stimulated, and Figure 4-9 shows the effect of asphyxia on upper airway motoneuron activity. Inflation is withheld for five successive respiratory efforts. As described above, the changes in neural activity associated with the first no-inflation respiratory effort are due to withdrawal of phasic volume feedback. The crescendo increase in peak phasic inspiratory activity of all three nerves with subsequent respiratory efforts reflects their response to the ensuing progressive increase in chemical drive. Upper airway motoneuron activity increases with either hypercapnia and/or hypoxia.[37,43-49] Phasic activity, which may be absent under eucapnic conditions, will often appear at increased levels of chemical drive. The relationship between increasing levels of CO_2 and peak phasic activity has been described as being both linear and nonlinear[32,37,49] (Fig. 4-10). This apparent discrepancy may be due to differences in species, technique, or the starting location on the stimulus response curve. Similar controversy exists as to whether the relative activation of upper airway motoneurons under conditions of increased chemical drive is greater than that of the phrenic. A preferential activation of upper airway motoneurons could alter the balance of forces acting on the upper airway, shifting the net vector in an outward direction.

Upper airway and phrenic motoneurons also differ in their response to hypocapnia.[37,50] Upper airway motoneurons appear to have a higher CO_2 threshold for activation. With passive hyperventilation in an intubated, vagotomized anesthetized animal, phasic upper airway motoneuron activity disappears prior to phrenic activity. When the CO_2 is then allowed to rise, phasic activity first reappears in the phrenic. Thus cyclical changes in arterial CO_2 around the CO_2 threshold for activation of upper airway motoneuron activity could lead to an imbalance of forces acting on the upper airway.

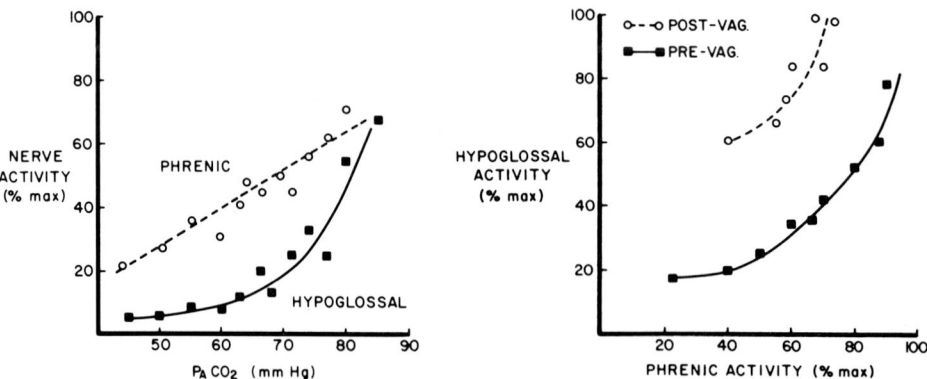

Fig. 4-10. Left panel: Effect of hypercapnea on peak hypoglossal (closed squares) and phrenic (open circles) nerve activity in a paralyzed anesthetized dog on a cycle controlled ventilator. Right panel: Relationship between hypoglossal and phrenic nerve activity during hypercapnia in the same animal preparation pre (closed squares) and post (open circles) bilateral cervical vagotomy. (From Weiner D, Mitra J, Salamone J, Cherniack NS: Effect of chemical stimuli on nerve supplying upper airway muscles. J Appl Physiol 52:532, 534, 1982. With permission.)

Tonic Activity

Changes in tonic, as well as phasic upper airway motoneuron activity, may help maintain upper airway patency. During airway occlusion, not only phasic but also tonic hypoglossal activity increases (Figs. 4-6 and 4-9). Greater tonic activity develops with increased chemical drive in spontaneously breathing animals, but these changes seem far less dramatic than those seen in the absence of phasic volume feedback.[37,43,45,49] This suggests that changes in lung volume may effect tonic as well as phasic upper airway motoneuron activity. Increased tonic activity would decrease the compliance of the upper airway or even cause dilatation of the upper airway lumen. The relative contributions of phasic versus tonic activity in the maintenance of upper airway patency remain unknown, but phasic inspiratory activity certainly plays an important role as it directly counteracts inspiratory subatmospheric intraluminal pressure.

RESPIRATORY-RELATED UPPER AIRWAY RECEPTORS

The upper airway is richly endowed by receptors. Sant'Ambrogio, Mathew, and colleagues have elegantly characterized the respiratory-related receptors of the larynx.[51–53] From single fiber recordings of superior laryngeal nerve afferents, three types of laryngeal receptors have been identified: pressure receptors, drive receptors,

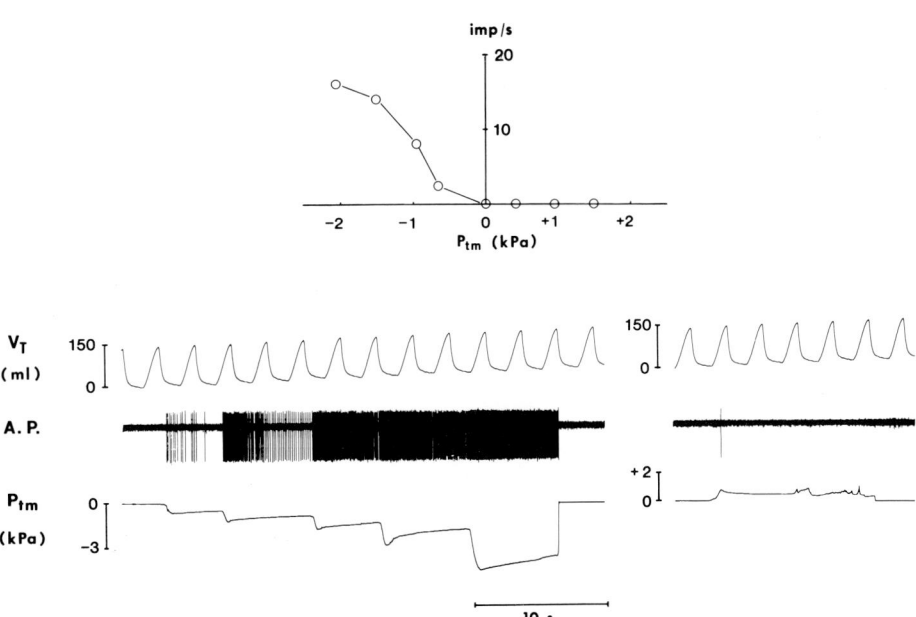

Fig. 4-11. Response of a negative pressure receptor to maintained negative and positive pressure in the upper airway of an anesthetized, paralyzed artificially ventilated dog. Vt = tidal volume, A.P. = action potentials, Ptm = transmural pressure in the upper airway. Top panel represent the static response (imp/sec) of the receptor to maintained transmural pressure. (From Mathew OP, Sant'Ambrogio G, Fisher JT, Sant'Ambrogio FB: Laryngeal pressure receptors. Respir Physiol 57:116, 1984. With permission.)

and flow or cold receptors. Compared to respiratory-related receptors in the tracheo-bronchial tree, these upper airway receptors have unique characteristics. Pressure receptors, the most common laryngeal receptors, are frequently active during sponta-neous tidal breathing. They fire during inspiration and/or expiration. Some are acti-vated by positive and others by negative transmural pressure. In these respects they resemble slowly adapting receptors of the tracheobronchial tree. However, unlike this potential counterpart, pressure receptors of the upper airway are rapidly adapt-ing. The pressure receptor in Figure 4-11 responds to negative transmural pressure and shows a characteristic progressive increase in firing rate with successive in-creases in negative transmural pressure. This particular receptor is silent when transmural pressure is zero or positive. Flow receptors also have no direct counter-part in the lower airway. These receptors usually fire on inspiration and are active during normal tidal breathing. They are not activated during respiratory efforts against a closed upper airway or tracheal occlusion. Flow receptors are actually temperature receptors stimulated by cold air, and they become silent when 37° C air is introduced into the upper airway.

The third type of receptor, the "drive" or motion receptor, is also active on inspiration during spontaneous tidal breathing. These receptors continue to fire in an acutely tracheostomized animal, but become silent during mechanical ventilation in a tracheostomized, paralyzed animal. These receptors appear to be activated by laryngeal movements induced by muscle contraction.

REFLEX ACTIVATION OF RESPIRATORY-RELATED MUSCLES BY UPPER AIRWAY RECEPTORS

Upper airway receptors exert a reflex effect on the activity of upper airway muscles. Diverting airflow from the nose to a tracheostomy in spontaneously breath-ing, anesthetized animals immediately decreases upper airway muscle activity.[54,55] Abu-Osba et al noted pharyngeal collapse in anesthetized rabbits after bypassing airflow from the upper airway to tracheostomy, and comparable observations have been described in tracheostomized sleeping infants.[34] A bypass of upper airway receptors resulting in a reflex decrease in upper airway muscle activity may explain these observations. The contribution of upper airway receptors on the reflex activa-tion of upper airway muscles is also evident when comparing the effect of nasal (mouth sealed) versus tracheal occlusion.[55] Figure 4-12 illustrates the effect of upper airway versus tracheal occlusion on diaphragmatic and posterior cricoarytenoid activity. Peak diaphragmatic activity is nearly the same in the two maneuvers. How-ever, a much greater increase in peak PCA muscle activity occurs with upper airway than tracheal occlusion, and this potentiation is ablated by sectioning the superior laryngeal nerves.

Several investigators have studied the role of upper airway receptors on efferent output to upper airway muscles by introducing static pressure changes in an isolated upper airway of spontaneously breathing, tracheostomized animals.[34,54,56,57] Sus-tained negative pressure in an isolated upper airway is associated with an increase in upper airway muscle activity (Fig. 4-13). With constant chemical drive, this reflex response is unsustained, perhaps due to receptor adaptation. The magnitude of the activation is directly proportional to the amount of negative pressure but varies

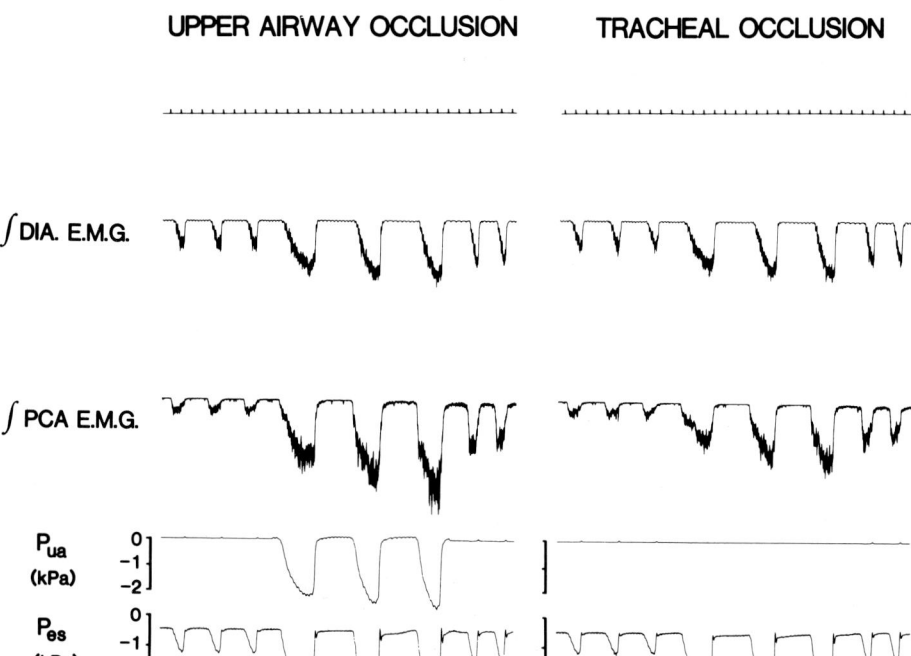

UPPER AIRWAY OCCLUSION   TRACHEAL OCCLUSION

∫ DIA. E.M.G.

∫ PCA E.M.G.

P_{ua} (kPa)

P_{es} (kPa)

Fig. 4-12. Effect of upper airway (left) and tracheal (right) occlusion on diaphragmatic and posterior cricoarytenoid (PCA) muscle activity in anesthetized dogs. Tracings are (top to bottom): time in seconds, direct and integrated diaphragmatic (DIA) electromyogram (EMG), direct and integrated PCA EMG, upper airway pressure (Pua) and esophageal pressure (Pes) in kPa. (From Sant'Ambrogio FE, Mathew OP, Clark WD, Sant'Ambrogio G: Laryngeal influences on breathing pattern and posterior cricoarytenoid muscle activity. J Appl Physiol 58:1300, 1985. With permission.)

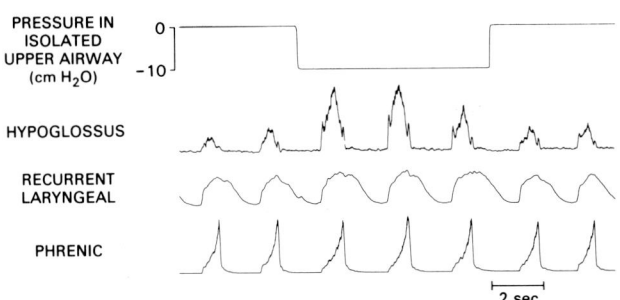

Fig. 4-13. Effect of maintained subatmospheric pressure in a sealed isolated upper airway on hypoglossal, recurrent laryngeal, and phrenic discharge in a spontaneously breathing decerebrate cat.

among the different upper airway muscles. In Figure 4-13, hypoglossal discharge increases more than the recurrent laryngeal's to changes in upper airway pressure. In the anesthetized dog, negative upper airway pressures caused an average increase of 122 percent in genioglossus muscle activity, 88 percent in alae nasi activity and 22 percent in posterior cricoarytenoid activity.[34]

The exact location of pressure, flow, and motion receptors is believed to be quite superficial in the airway wall as topical application of anesthetic inactivates their reflex activation of upper airway muscles.[34,56] Sant'Ambrogio et al have recently defined the contributing role of the different types of upper airway receptors on the above reflex.[55] They were unable to detect any significant effect of flow and motion receptors on muscle activity in the larynx during the upper airway breathing. However, they found that the changes in laryngeal muscle activity could be accounted for by the pressure receptors. Although respiratory-related receptors in the pharynx and nasal passages have not been identified, receptors similar to these laryngeal proto-types are probably located throughout the upper airway. However, afferent information from laryngeal receptors may play a preeminent role. These receptors in particular would be subjected to the dramatic changes in transmural pressure created by respiratory efforts following pharyngeal narrowing or collapse.

Upper airway receptors also affect diaphragmatic activity, but this is not demonstrable with diversion from nasal to tracheal breathing. But, when comparing nasal versus tracheal occlusion, the former is associated with a prolongation in the time of inspiration and a decrease in the rate of rise of diaphragmatic activity.[55,56a] Peak diaphragmatic activity is unchanged. Similar effects on diaphragmatic activity have been described with sustained negative pressure in the isolated upper airway.[34]

While investigating the pressure required to cause upper airway closure in anesthetized rabbits, Brouillette and Thach cut the hypoglossal nerves, the efferent output to the intrinsic and extrinsic muscles of the tongue.[57] However, closing pressure was still more subatmospheric than in sacrificed animals indicating that other muscles were also contributing to maintenance of upper airway patency. Subsequent investigations have shown that negative pressure applied to the isolated upper airway produces a reflex activation of many different muscles, including the alae nasi, genioglossi, posterior cricoarytenoids, and possibly palatal muscles.[34,56,57a] This indicates that the reflex has multiple efferent pathways.

Compartmentation of the isolated upper airway and nerve section studies reveal multiple afferent pathways as well. Application of negative pressure to the larynx alone results in a reflex activation of laryngeal muscles. This localized laryngeal reflex is ablated when the superior laryngeal nerves are cut bilaterally. Muscles in areas separated from this pressure stimulus, e.g., the alae nasi or genioglossus muscles, also exhibit an increased activity; however, even greater activation of these latter muscles occurs when the pressure stimulus is applied directly to the naso and oro-pharynx. A recent study was able to virtually eliminate the reflex activation of upper airway muscles by upper airway negative pressure only after bilateral sectioning of the superior laryngeal, glossopharyngeal, and trigeminal nerves.[58]

Upper airway receptors influence upper airway stability in sleeping adults.[59] Selective application of lidocaine and a long acting anesthetic to the oropharynx of normal men is associated with a significant increase in number of hypopneas and upper airway closures during sleep. In contrast, selective anesthesia of the nasal passages does not appear to be associated with an increased incidence of respiratory dysrhythmias during sleep. One can speculate that upper airway patency was maintained after nasal anesthesia alone because of an intact local reflex activating muscles surrounding the oropharynx. These observations provide an important clinical correlation to the animal studies, indicating that the reflex activation of upper airway muscles by upper airway receptors is not only present in man, but may play an important role in the maintenance of upper airway patency.

The effects of upper airway receptors on efferent output to the pump muscles of respiration also appears to be functional in man. Thach et al studied the effect of negative upper airway pressure in tracheostomized infants.[60] Sustained negative airway pressure (mean 27.8 cm H_2O) was applied at intermittent intervals via a face mask. This negative pressure caused pharyngeal closure, compartmentalizing the stimulus to the nasal passages and pharynx, and isolating it from the larynx. Even so, this negative airway pressure stimulus was associated with a sudden decrease in tidal volume and mean inspiratory flow rate. Extrapolating from the animal studies, one would assume that even greater effects might result if the negative airway pressure stimulus also reached the larynx.

ROLE OF HYOID MUSCLES IN MAINTENANCE OF UPPER AIRWAY PATENCY

Besides the muscles surrounding the upper airway, neck muscles also play a role in maintaining upper airway patency. Of these muscles, those attaching to the hyoid bone are felt to be of particular importance. The hyoid lacks a bony articulation. This floating bone serves as the site of attachment of certain strap muscles. Other muscles, such as the thyrohyoid, connect it to the larynx. Activation of these muscles creates a vector of force in the caudal direction (Fig. 4-14). Muscles attached to the mandible, e.g., the myohyoid and geniohyoid, also insert in the hyoid. Their activation creates a force vector in the antero-rostral direction. The net effect of these two vectors would be to displace the hyoid and ventral wall of the airway in an outward direction increasing airway patency.

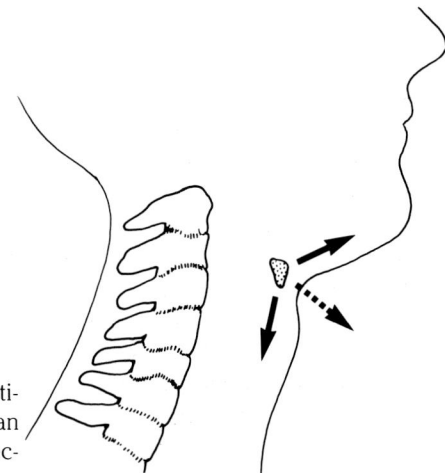

Fig. 4-14. Schematic diagram showing how activation of muscles attached to the hyoid bone can create a net vector of force in the anterior direction.

The hyoid muscles respond to chemical, vagal, and negative pressure stimuli similar to muscles surrounding the upper airway.[57,61] In anesthetized dogs, the geniohyoid, thyrohyoid, and sternohyoid have phasic respiratory activity. The sternohyoid is not consistently active and, if silent, is not recruited by chemical or mechanical stimuli. Traction of the hyoid bone ventrally or stimulation of hyoid muscles result in a large decrease in upper airway resistance. Furthermore, electrical stimulation of these muscles increases the amount of negative pressure required to induce upper airway collapse.[62] Muscles attached to the hyoid can stabilize and dilate the airway.

EFFECT OF PHARMACOLOGIC AGENTS AND STATE OF WAKEFULNESS ON UPPER AIRWAY MUSCLE ACTIVITY

Various pharmacologic agents alter upper airway muscle activity. General anesthetics, alcohol, and sedatives such as diazepam, decrease upper airway muscle activity more than diaphragmatic activity.[43,63–66] These agents decrease both phasic and tonic activity and blunt their response to increases in chemical drive. Administration of ethanol to normal subjects causes an increase in upper airway resistance.[67] Clinically, all of these agents are associated with an increased incidence of upper airway closure during sleep, not only in patients with obstructive sleep apnea, but also in normal subjects. When normal subjects are administered alcohol or flurazepam prior to sleep, they experience an increased incidence of respiratory dysrhythmias, including obstructive apneas.[68–70] In contrast, other pharmacologic agents, such as protriptyline, are associated with a differential increase in upper airway muscle activity.[63] Protriptyline ameliorates upper airway closures during sleep in patients with obstructive sleep apnea.[71,72]

The differential suppression or activation of upper airway muscles compared to the diaphragm appears to be a generalized response to a variety of stimuli. As described above, phasic volume feedback, anesthesia, alcohol, and sedatives cause a greater suppression of upper airway muscle activity, whereas increased chemical drive and protriptyline preferentially increase upper airway muscle activity. But even nonspecific stimuli, such as auditory, tactile, or sciatic nerve stimulation cause a differential increase in upper airway muscle activity.[37,73] Differential activation and suppression of upper airway motoneurons varies markedly with different states of wakefulness and sleep. Brainstem neurons that exhibit respiratory-related activity during wakefulness may be silent during sleep.[74] Both tonic and phasic upper airway muscle activity decrease with sleep onset despite a relative preservation in diaphragmatic activity.[75,76] Further decreases in upper airway muscle activity occur during REM sleep, especially during bursts of rapid eye movement. This sleep related reduction in upper airway muscle activity is associated with a concomitant increase in upper airway resistance.[77–79]

The differential effect of the state of consciousness on upper airway muscle activity suggests that the phenomenon may be mediated through the rostral pons and/or reticular activating system. Lesions in the dorsolateral pons can release brainstem inhibition of descending cortical activity during REM sleep preventing the associated decrease in upper airway muscle activity.[80] Recent data suggests that endorphins may play a role. Naloxone has a greater effect on hypoglossal and glossopharyngeal activation than on phrenic activation in anesthetized cats.[81]

DEFENSE OF UPPER AIRWAY PATENCY

From the animal and human studies described above, the concept emerges that upper airway muscles are recruited as needed to protect upper airway patency. Some upper airway muscles are located at valving sites along the respiratory tract. Activation of the alae nasi muscles prevents collapse of the nares. Posterior cricoarytenoid muscles regulate the caliber of the larynx by abducting the vocal cords. They also regulate expiratory flow and functional residual capacity.[82] Activation of these valving muscles will lead to a decrease in airway resistance and a decrease in work of breathing. The muscles located at these two valving sites are phasically active on inspiration even under conditions that otherwise favor airway patency.

Muscles surrounding the collapsible pharynx seem to behave in a slightly different manner. In an upright position at rest, many adults have tonic but very little, if any, phasic inspiratory activity of the pharyngeal muscles. Conditions may arise that result in pharyngeal narrowing. With the increase in upper airway resistance, several mechanisms can lead to an increase in upper airway muscle activity and thereby, an increase in the outward dilating force on this narrowed segment. The first line of defense appears to be mediated by the activation of upper airway receptors by increased subatmospheric pressure. Activation of these receptors causes a reflex increase in upper airway muscle activity and, simultaneously, may decrease the rate of rise in diaphragmatic discharge. Both of these effects would help shift the net balance of forces acting on the upper airway to favor its patency. If upper airway narrowing becomes significant enough to compromise tidal volume and gas exchange, the decrease in phasic volume feedback and the increase in chemical drive will result in further activation of upper airway muscles. The reflex effects defending upper airway patency are blunted during sleep, making the upper airway more susceptible to closure.

Upper airway muscles respond in a differential manner to various stimuli. In general, the genioglossus activates much more than the recurrent laryngeal or alae nasi to any particular stimulus. These differences may reflect the varying morphologic characteristics occurring in different segments of the upper airway. If the pharynx is uniformly the most compliant segment, then it would be advantageous if pharyngeal muscles were the most sensitive to activation. Although this appears to be the case, it also seems that pharyngeal muscle activity is the easiest to suppress. But upper airway muscles also perform very different functions. It seems logical that a muscle controlling a valving site in the upper airway, such as the posterior cricoarytenoid in the larynx, would require different controls than a nonvalving muscle such as the genioglossus. Finally, this differential activation of upper airway muscles appears to be more compatible with the graded rather than all or nothing mechanisms that have evolved to defend upper airway patency. With compromise of the upper airway, the initial increase in upper airway muscle activity, especially in the genioglossus muscle, helps ensure stability of the most likely site of airway collapse, the pharynx. Failure to correct the problem leads to greater activation of the genioglossus and recruitment of other upper airway and neck muscles. The initial activation of upper airway muscles against a compromised upper airway is visually imperceptible. The agonal respirations of an anesthetized animal with hypoventilation due to shock offer an example at the other end of the spectrum. The protrusion of the tongue, extension of the mandible, and elevation of the hyoid with each inspiratory effort dramatically illustrate how these defense mechanisms can combine to ensure upper airway patency.

SWALLOWING

Understanding the physiological closure of the pharnyx during swallowing provides insights into upper airway closure as a pathologic event. The action of swallowing has been subdivided into three stages: oral, pharyngeal, and esophageal.[1,83] The reflex coordination of swallowing is extraordinarily consistent. During mastication, juxtaposition of the soft palate with the elevated tongue creates a barrier posteriorly, permitting respiration and oral manipulation to occur simultaneously. The act of swallowing is initiated by activation of a group of pharyngeal muscles collectively termed the leading complex. Among others, they include the palatopharyngeus, superior constrictor, and posterior tongue muscles. Activation of the leading complex closes the nasopharynx by drawing together the lateral palatopharyngeal folds and elevating the soft palate. In the oral preparation for the swallow, the hyoid assumes a slightly elevated position as the tongue centers the bolus against the palate in the posterior part of the oral cavity. The bolus advances between the diagonal wall formed by the soft palate and the adducted palatopharyngeal folds as the body of the tongue rolls backward upon the hyoid, its posterior pedestal. As the bolus advances in the pharynx, the posterior displacement of the tongue causes a cephalad and posterior movement of the hyoid and the laryngeal structures suspended from it. Further elevation of the soft palate occurs and contact with the tongue is broken. During the oral and pharyngeal stages of swallowing, the respiratory role of the upper airway is briefly superceded. Afferents in the superior laryngeal nerve may help coordinate these events. In anesthetized animals, stimulation of the superior laryngeal nerve can initiate swallowing and can also cause a cessation of inspiratory efforts.[34,56,84]

Nonfeeding swallows occur during wakefulness and sleep.[85,86] Nonfeeding swallows are probably initiated by accumulating oropharyngeal secretions and protect the lower respiratory tract from aspiration. During sleep, swallows are initiated during all phases of the respiratory cycle. In sleeping preterm infants with idiopathic apnea, swallows are more common during the apneic episodes, especially during mixed and obstructive apneas.[85] The swallows usually precede termination of the apneic episode by 5 to 6 seconds. During the apneic episodes, swallowing is frequently associated with small inspiratory efforts occurring in the pharyngeal stage. These inspiratory efforts, or swallow breaths, occur at a time when the nasopharynx is closed. Swallow breaths have also been described in adults. Other reflex sequential events such as regurgitation and eructation also involve complex activation of upper airway muscles and a close integration with respiration. All involve active closure of the upper airway. Obstructive apnea may be initiated by activation of muscles in the leading complex.[6,87] However, electromyographic recordings of upper airway muscle activity during sleep in patients with OSA do not support this theory.[3] Similarly, the occurrance of a small respiratory effort in the face of a closed upper airway during a swallow, the swallow breath, seems analogous to the unusually small respiratory effort that characteristically occurs at the beginning of an obstructive apnea. Whether this represents a component part of the swallowing mechanism is speculative.

PATHOPHYSIOLOGIC FACTORS IN UPPER AIRWAY CLOSURE

Common experience with patients with OSA indicates that two general classes of abnormalities, those related to neural factors and those related to anatomic factors, should be included in a comprehensive view of the sequence of events that produce opening and closure of the pharyngeal airway. The tendency for the pharyngeal airway to close is obviously dependent upon the state of the central nervous system; patients displaying upper airway obstruction during sleep easily maintain a patent upper airway while awake. Another evidence of a neural component controlling airway closure is that obstructive apnea is more common and severe during REM sleep[88,89] when upper airway muscle hypotonia is most extreme.[75,76,90–93] That state-dependent reduction in efferent neural traffic is not the only event underlying airway occlusion in patients with OSA is apparent from two observations: (1) weight loss usually ameliorates OSA in obese patients;[94,95] and (2) structural abnormalities of the pharynx are common in patients with OSA.[20,96,97] In the following sections of this chapter we shall first describe the sequence of events related to periodic, repeated occlusion of the pharyngeal airway in patients with OSA, and then discuss in detail the structural and neural abnormalities in patients with OSA.

PATHOPHYSIOLOGICAL SEQUENCE OF AIRWAY CLOSURE

In most severe cases of obstructive sleep apnea, airway closure is initiated by sleep onset, i.e., by the shift in the CNS associated with falling asleep. The key feature of sleep onset that contributes to airway closure appears to be a diminution in force of oropharyngeal muscles that maintain a patent airway, such as, the genioglossus, geniohyoid, hyoglossus, and tensor palatini. This reduction of muscular forces decreases the outward pull on the ventral and lateral pharyngeal walls, thereby narrowing the airway. Because of underlying anatomic abnormalities, this narrowing greatly increases pharyngeal resistance, which produces a very low intrapharyngeal pressure during inspiration. As a result of this transpharyngeal pressure, the airway closes and subsequent respiratory efforts are blocked by the occluded pharyngeal airway. The intensity of these efforts increases progressively because of the augmenting hypoxic and hypercapnic stimuli. Such respiratory stimulation, during nonREM sleep, results in co-activation of thoracic inspiratory and upper airway dilation muscles, including alae nasi, tensor palatini, genioglossus, geniohyoid, and posterior cricoarytenoid muscles. Nonetheless, the pharyngeal airway remains collapsed because the inward pull caused by subatmospheric pressure transmitted to the pharynx during each inspiratory effort exceeds the outward pull of the pharyngeal muscles. A remarkable, but typical, feature of patients with obstructive sleep apnea is that this relative deficit of force generated by upper airway muscles persists until arousal occurs. In other words, the progressive increase in chemical and mechanical stimuli during the apneic period augments contraction of both thoracic inspiratory muscles and pharyngeal muscles, but the former increases more than the latter. As a result, the sleeping brain is unable to open the pharyngeal airway. During prolonged apneas, the respiratory control system strongly activates all respiratory muscles, but the net outcome favors airway closure even though arterial oxygen saturation falls to near-lethal levels. Only when higher neural components specifically activate upper airway muscles is the pharyngeal lumen reestablished. Exactly what causes this arousal is uncertain. The intense stimulation of chemoreceptors may play a role, but afferent traffic from lung, airway, and chest wall mechanoreceptors may also be important. While these higher neural mechanisms are active, this favorable balance between trans-mural pharyngeal pressure and contraction of pharyngeal muscles is maintained. In severe OSA, the patient takes several breaths, the chemical stimulation of breathing subsides, and sleep resumes. Typically, the cycle repeats as the reduction in pharyngeal muscle activity associated with sleep onset increases pharyngeal resistance, augments trans-pharyngeal pressure and collapses the airway.

Evidence for the foregoing sequence has been derived from a variety of sources, but until recently the pivotal roles of intrapharyngeal pressure and genioglossal force have remained somewhat speculative. An important role of each has been established by direct evidence. That pharyngeal pressure greatly influences the aperture of the highly compliant pharyngeal airway is evidenced by the effective treatment of obstructive sleep apnea by nasal airway positive pressure (NAPP).[98,99] That inspiratory contraction of pharyngeal muscles tends to open the pharyngeal airway is demonstrated by the sub-atmospheric swing in pressure of the isolated, sealed pharynx during inspiration. Taken together, these findings lay a strong foundation for the concept of the opposing action between transpharyngeal pressure generated by thoracic inspiratory muscle contraction and force generated by contraction of pharyngeal muscles during inspiration.

PHARYNGEAL MUSCLE PRESSURE

To unify the analysis of factors determining airway patency, we will employ the concept of pharyngeal muscle pressure. During inspiration, contraction of pharyngeal muscles dilates the oropharynx and hypopharynx. If the pharynx is collapsed the action of these muscles is to reestablish the lumen. The net action of these muscles to open the airway is represented by the subatmospheric pressure generated within the closed upper airway, which has been isolated from the lower airway and sealed. In such a preparation, Strohl and Fouke[13] observed that a wave of negative pressure during inspiration that resembled the electrical activity recorded from the alae nasi and genioglossus (Fig. 4-15). This pressure is produced by inspiratory contraction of pharyngeal muscles and is referred to as the net pharyngeal muscle pressure (phar P_{mus}). It is analogous to the concept of thoracic muscle pressure used to describe the net pressure generated by the thoracic respiratory muscles to move the lungs and chest wall.

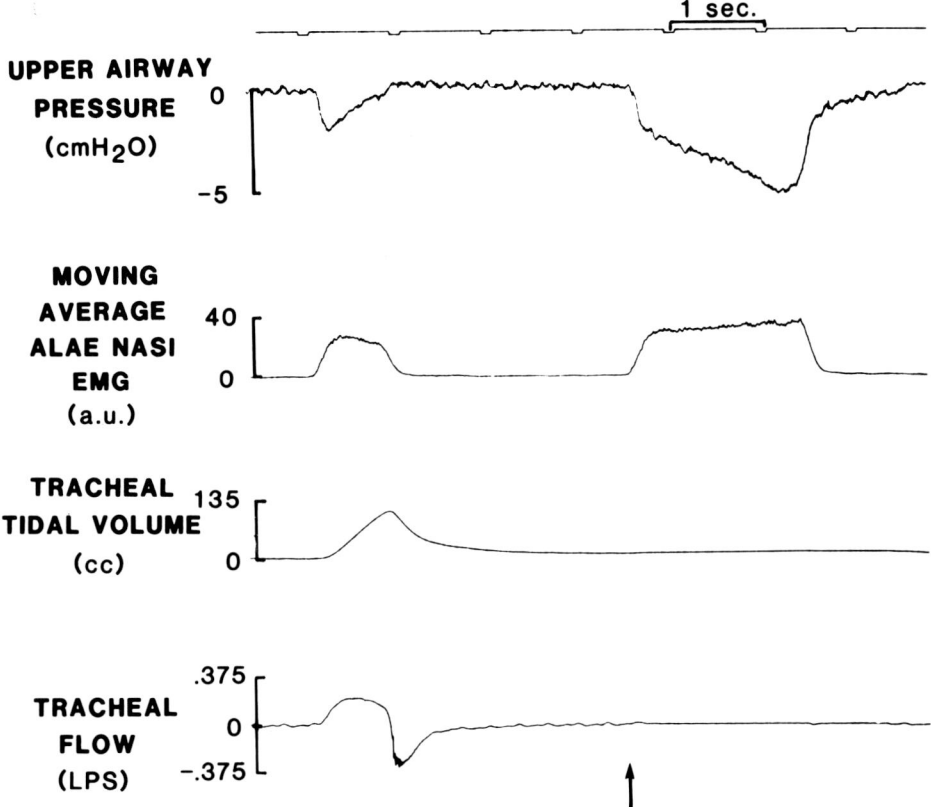

Fig. 4-15. Recording from an anesthetized dog with an isolated upper airway comparing upper airway pressure, moving average of alae nasi activation and tracheal tidal volume and flow during a control breath (unoccluded) and subsequent effort when trachea was occluded at end expiration (arrow). (From Strohl KP, Fouke JM: Dilating forces on the upper airway of anesthetized dogs. J Appl Physiol 58:454, 1985. With permission.)

The state of the airway is determined by three pressures: intrapharyngeal pressure generated by the pharyngeal muscles (phar P_{mus}), and opening/closing pressure. Opening pressure (P_{open}) is the static trans-pharyngeal pressure required to open the passive, closed pharyngeal airway; closing pressure ($P_{closing}$) is the static transpharyneal pressure at which the lumen of the open pharyngeal airway is eliminated. To open the closed pharyngeal airway, phar P_{mus} must exceed the sum of opening pressure and alveolar pressure (P_{alv}), i.e., the following must be true:

$$phar\ P_{mus} > P_{open} + P_{alv}.$$

For the open airway to close, phar P_{mus} must be less than flow-related intra-pharyngeal pressure (P_{flow}) plus the closing pressure, i.e., the following must hold:

$$phar\ P_{mus} < P_{close} + P_{flow}.$$

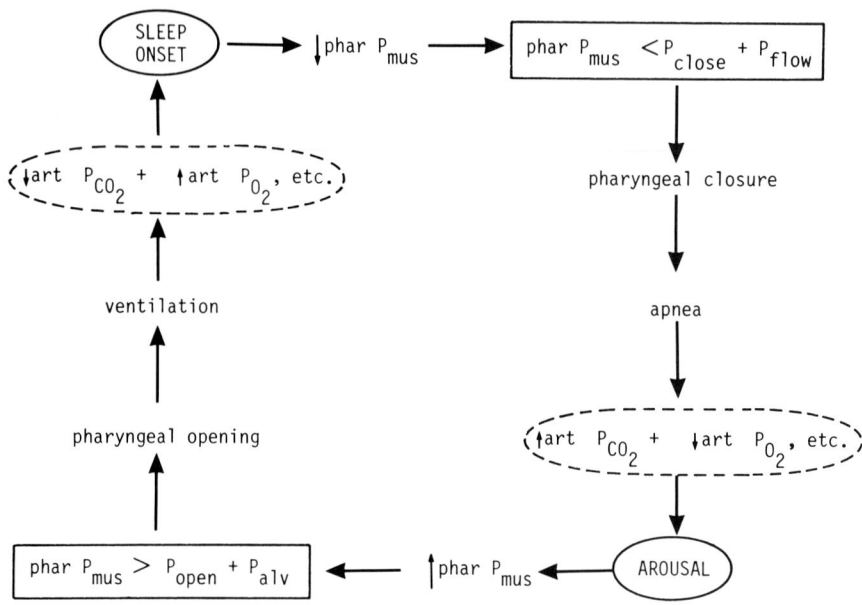

Fig. 4-16. Schematic diagram of pathophysiologic sequence of upper airway closure.

Opening and closing pressures reflect the anatomic factors that determine how easily the passive pharyngeal airway can be opened or closed. These pressures can be approximated during sleep when NAPP is applied, because the pharyngeal muscles are minimally active at this time. With sudden reductions in NAPP the airway will close, allowing direct measurement of P_{close}. This can be reversed by increasing the pressure before pharyngeal muscles become active, allowing measurement of P_{open}.

Periodic opening and closing of the airway in severe obstructive sleep apnea can be understood as a cycle involving shifts in the state of vigilance and consequent changes in phar P_{mus}, as shown in Figure 4-16. Sleep onset, with its attendant loss of genioglossal activity, decreases phar P_{mus} so that it is less than the sum of closing and flow-related pressures (top row). The pharynx occludes and the apnea causes a decrease in $P_{a_{O_2}}$ and an increase in $P_{a_{CO_2}}$ (right-hand row). The stimulation of chemoreceptors and, perhaps, mechanoreceptors related to respiratory efforts, lead to arousal. This recruitment of the higher nervous system augments phar P_{mus} (bottom row), causing it to exceed the sum of opening and alveolar pressures, thereby opening the airway. A ventilitory period ensues during which blood gases return toward normal, sleep resumes and the cycle repeats.

NEURAL ABNORMALITIES IN PATIENTS WITH OBSTRUCTIVE SLEEP APNEA

Identification of primary neural abnormalities in patients with obstructive sleep apnea has proved elusive, perhaps not because they are absent but because of the complexity of the nervous system. Secondary neural alterations, e.g., depression,

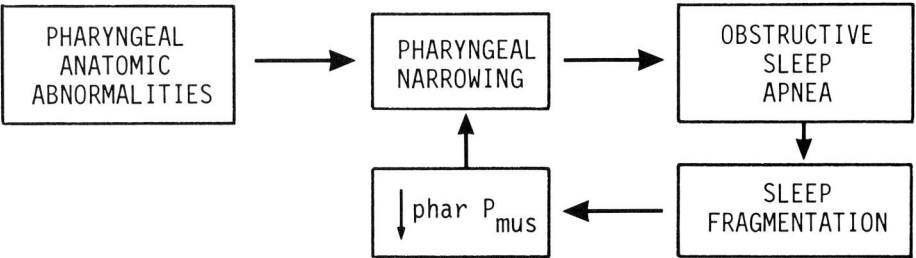

Fig. 4-17. Schematic diagram of possible interaction of anatomic and neural abnormalities in pathogenesis of OSA.

loss of memory, impotence, weakness, are commonly observed and abate after effective treatment of sleep apnea. Whether these global abnormalities result from sleep fragmentation, nocturnal hypoxia, or both, is unclear. Secondary alterations in control of breathing possibly contribute to the natural history of OSA. Sleep deprivation produces some decrease in hypercapnic ventilatory response. However, recent studies by Leiter, Knuth, and Bartlett[100] reveal loss of genioglossal response to hypercapnia with sleep deprivation in normals. This finding suggests a sequential process depicted in Figure 4-17, whereby underlying anatomic abnormalities initiate obstructive sleep apnea, which, in turn, fragments sleep. The latter suppresses phar P_{mus}, which augments obstructive sleep apnea, further enhancing the sleep disturbance. Support for this secondary cyclical feedback derives from recent observations that patients treated with NAPP for several months display less severe obstructive sleep apnea when restudied without NAPP. Another and, perhaps, contributory neural complication secondary to sleep fragmentation and/or hypoxia is an elevation in arousal threshold.[101] Sleep fragmentation may alter the sleeping nervous system such that more severe hypoxia or more pronounced mechanical alterations must occur during apnea to achieve arousal and, thereby, a state-dependent shift in the nervous system that activates upper airway muscles and increases phar P_{mus} enough to open the pharynx.

ANATOMIC ABNORMALITIES IN PATIENTS WITH OSA

The theory of cyclic, state-dependent changes in the pharyngeal airway leads to the hypothesis that these neural alterations in phar P_{mus} interact with underlying anatomic abnormalities. Such an argument develops from the failure of normals to develop pharyngeal obstruction during REM sleep, a period of virtual elimination of genioglossal activity. By contrast, patients with OSA sustain pharyngeal closure when genioglossal activity decreases only moderately at sleep onset. A related piece of evidence is that patients with OSA, while asleep and receiving NAPP, sustain airway closure when intrapharyngeal pressure is $+5-10$ cm H_2O. By contrast, closing pressure for normals under the same circumstances is atmospheric pressure or lower. A final concordant observation is that weight loss in obese patients with obstructive sleep apnea generally ameliorates the disorder, suggesting that loss of adipose tissue in critical areas of the pharynx may be important.

This type of inferential evidence pointing to underlying structural narrowing of the pharynx in patients with obstructive sleep apnea prompted the study of supraglottic impedance to airflow in patients with sleep apnea while awake.[27] A higher than normal airflow impedance was observed in patients after nasal vasoconstriction, suggesting a structural narrowing of the airway in patients. More direct support for anatomic narrowing hypothesis is provided by several direct studies of upper airway dimensions using radiographic and acoustical methods. Measurements from lateral radiographs of the head and neck reveal that a patient with OSA is likely to display bony abnormality, such as a small mandible or a caudally displaced hyoid.[102,103] Computed tomography reveals narrowing at the level of the soft palate in one study and narrowing of nasopharynx, oropharnx and hypopharnx in another.[5,104] Estimates of cross-sectional area of the pharynx by acoustic reflectance have been documented to be abnormally low in patients with obstructive sleep apnea.[46,103]

Therefore, both neural and anatomic abnormalities appear to contribute to upper airway closure in patients with OSA. Suratt et al. found that less subatmospheric pressure was required to produce upper airway closure during wakefulness in patients with OSA than in normal subjects.[105] The smaller upper airway area, an abnormally low reflex activation of upper airway muscles, or, as seems likely, a combination of the two, could explain such a finding.

SNORING

To snore is to "breathe during sleep with a rough, hoarse noise due to vibration of the uvula and soft palate" (Webster's Third New International Dictionary, 1976). This remarkably insightful definition, may be overly restrictive. Since the advent of understanding of mechanical features of OSA, snoring commonly connotes any loud respiratory sound during sleep, even the very loud snorts bordering on stridor emitted by the patient with OSA. Such sound lacks the coarse, low frequency quality, resembling feline purring, referred to by the lexicographer. In other words, the characteristics of the snoring sound in patients with sleep apnea differs from snoring sounds in otherwise normal individuals. We shall refer to the latter as benign snoring, to contrast it with a near stridorous snorts characteristic of OSA.

Recent investigations have elaborated understanding of benign snoring.[106,]* The fundamental frequency of the sound generated by snoring during nose breathing is 40–60 Hz and is somewhat higher during nose and mouth breathing. During snoring, supraglottic pressure and airflow both oscillate at this fundamental frequency. During nose/mouth snoring, airflow in the two orifices alternates with the same periodicity observed for pressure and sound. Sound is emitted in bursts, the onset of each occurring during the abrupt decompression of the pharynx. These results indicate that the soft palate oscillates in the pharyngeal airstream at the same frequency as the fundamental frequency of the sound and that this palatal oscillation constitutes the key mechanical event responsible for benign snoring.

Comparison of the spectral analyses of snoring sounds in OSA patients with benign snoring reveals that the former has less power at a fundamental frequency

---

* Perez-Padilla JR, Slawinska E, Remmers JE, DeFranceso L: Characteristics of the snoring noise in patients with and without obstructive sleep apnea. (Personal communication.)

and displays a broad envelope of power at higher frequencies (1000–3000 Hz). This difference from benign snoring is particularly apparent during the first and last of the ventilatory phase breaths, when resistance is relatively high. The relative deficiency of a low, fundamental frequency suggests that periodic oscillation of some pharyngeal structure plays a minor role in sound generation. The broad spectrum noise in the high frequency range suggests that the balance generated by a high rate of inflow through a small orifice is responsible. The hypopharynx is the most likely site for this orifice, which presumably constitutes the choke point for the entire airway.

OBSTRUCTIVE VERSUS ARRHYTHMIC APNEA: COMPARISONS AND CONTRASTS

Mechanically, two types of sleep apnea have been identified. In one the patient cannot breathe (obstructive), and in the other the patients fails to make respiratory efforts (arrhythmic). While the proximate cause and global features of obstructive and arrhythmic sleep apnea clearly differ, the same fundamental pathophysiological mechanism may underly both. This speculation rests on a variety of inferential evidences, e.g., the two types of apnea can coexist and some patients with obstructive sleep apnea display central apnea after treatment. However, in uncomplicated examples of each, the two display disparate features suggesting that the neural basis of one apnea differs substantially from that of the other. This is particularly true if one accepts hypoxic induced periodic breathing as the prototype for arrhythmic sleep apnea.

Recent experiments by Dempsey and coworkers have greatly elucidated the pathogenesis of hypoxic induced apnea in normals.[107] As summarized in Table 4-1, they observe that this apnea occurs during NREM, but not REM sleep and that it is contingent upon periodic hypocapnia. Increasing F_{ICO_2} by 1–2 percent eliminates the apnea because an apneic threshold for the CO_2 stimulus is not reached. Table 4-1 indicates that by contrast, obstructive sleep apnea displays that converse state dependency observed during REM and mild hypercapnia probably has little effect. Finally, the response to O_2 administration contrasts with that observed in arrhythmic apnea. Hypoxia is the requisite condition for initiating arrhythmic periodic breathing during sleep in normals, so that O_2 administration eliminates the condition. Obstructive sleep apnea, on the other hand, may worsen during O_2 administration, and certainly the duration of apneas are not reduced by O_2 administration.

A consideration of differences in neural and chemical controls of breathing between REM and NREM sleep may explain these disparate features of obstructive

Table 4-1
Comparison of Two Types of Apnea

	Arrhythmic	Obstructive
Respiratory efforts:	periodically abate	continuous
State dependency:	NREM only	most severe during REM can occur during NREM
Administration of 1–2% CO_2	eliminates apnea	probably no effect
Administration of 100% O_2 apnea	eliminates apnea	may prolong

and arrhythmic apnea. During NREM, the respiratory control system appears to rely heavily on automatic control process in the brain stem, having lost conscious or paraconscious supervisory function on the higher nervous system. During this stage of sleep, chemical feedback derived from central and peripheral chemoreceptors dominates and an apneic threshold for the CO_2 stimulus now appears. This means that feedback instabilities caused by alinearity of the effective hypoxic ventilatory response and/or prolonged circulation time will tend to induce periodic apnea during NREM. During REM, by contrast, higher neural influences reappear and the influence of chemical feedback assume less importance. Accordingly, the arrhythmic variety of sleep apnea being dependent upon instability in chemical feedback, can be expected to abate during REM. As described previously, obstructive sleep apnea appears during NREM in moderately severe cases, possibly because of loss of a supervisory function of the higher nervous system. However, obstructive sleep apnea will become more pronounced or, in mild cases, only appear during REM when the activity of pharyngeal muscles is preferentially reduced and thresholds for arousal increase. The foregoing speculations apply to those cases of uncomplicated arrhythmic or obstructive apnea. Patients displaying both types of apnea are not rare and in these cases a common neural basis for periodic breathing during sleep needs to be considered.

ACKNOWLEDGMENT

Funded by grants from the American Lung Association of Texas, CRC grant #236, and NIH grant #HL27520.

REFERENCES

1. Bosma J: Deglutition: pharyngeal stage. Physiol Rev 37:275–300, 1957
2. Kuhlo W, Doll E, Frank MC: Erfolgreiche behandlung eines Pickwick-Syndroms durch eine dauertrachealkanule. Dtsch Med Wschr 94:1286–1290, 1969
3. Guilleminault C, Hill MW, Simmons B, Dement WC: Obstructive sleep apnea: electromyographic and fiberoptic studies. Exp Neurol 62:48–67, 1978
4. Lugaresi E, Cocagna G, Cirignotta P: Polygraphic and cineradiographic aspects of obstructive apneas occurring during sleep: physiopathological implications, in von Euler C, Lagercrantz H (eds): Central Nervous Control Mechanisms in Breathing. Oxford, Pergamon Press, 1979, pp 495–501
5. Suratt PM, Dee P, Atkinson RL, et al: Fluoroscopic and computed tomographic features of the pharyngeal airway in obstructive sleep apnea. Am Rev Respir Dis 127:487–492, 1983
6. Weitzman FD, Pollak CP, Borowiecki B, et al: The hypersomnia-sleep apnea syndrome: site and mechanism of upper airway obstruction, in Guilleminault C, Dement WC (eds): Sleep Apnea Syndromes. New York, Alan R Liss Inc, 1978, pp 235–248
7. Remmers JE, deGroot WJ, Sauerland EK, et al: Pathogenesis of upper airway occlusion during sleep. J Appl Physiol 44:931–938, 1978
8. Remmers JE, Anch AM, deGroot WJ: Respiratory disturbances during sleep. Clinics Chest Medicine 1:57–71, 1980
9. Kurtz D, Krieger J, Stierly JC: EMG activity of cricothyroid and chin muscles during wakefulness and sleeping in the sleep apnea syndrome. Electroenceph Clin Neurophysiol 45:777–784, 1978
10. Suratt PM, McTier R, Wilhoit SC: Alae nasi electromyographic activity and timing in obstructive sleep apnea. J Appl Physiol 58:1252–1256, 1985

11. Wilson SL, Thach BT, Brouillette RT, Abu-Osba YK: Upper airway patency in the human infant: influence of airway pressure and posture. J Appl Physiol 48:500–5–4, 1980

12. Glenn W, Gee JB, Cole DR, et al: Combined central alveolar hypoventilation and upper airway obstruction. Am J Med 64:50–60, 1978

13. Strohl KP, Fouke JM: Dilating forces on the upper airway of anesthetized dogs. J Appl Physiol 58:452–458, 1985

14. McCaffrey TV, Kern EB: Response of nasal airway resistance to hypercapnia and hypoxia in man. Ann Otol 88:247–252, 1979

15. Strohl KP, O'Cain CF, Slutsky AS: Alae nasi activation and nasal resistance in healthy subjects. J Appl Physiol 52:1432–1437, 1982

16. Gottfried SB, Strohl KP, Van de Graaff WB, et al: Effects of phrenic stimulation on upper airway resistance in anesthetized dogs. J Appl Physiol 55:419–426, 1983

17. Reed WR, Roberts JL, Thach BT: Factors influencing regional patency and configuration of the human infant upper airway. J Appl Physiol 58:635–644, 1985

18. Block AJ, Faulkner JA, Hughes RL, et al: Factors influencing upper airway closure. Chest 86:114–122, 1984

19. Issa FG, Sullivan CE: Upper airway closing pressures in obstructive sleep apnea. J Appl Physiol 57:520–527, 1984

20. Roberts JL, Reed WR, Mathew OP, et al: Assessment of pharyngeal airway stability in normal and micrognathic infants. J Appl Physiol 58:190–299, 1985

21. Fouke JM, Galbraith FM, Strohl KP: Effect of subject position on upper airway geometry. Fed Proc 44:A2498, 1985

22. Shelton RL Jr, Bosma JF: Maintenance of the pharyngeal airway. J Appl Physiol 17:209–214, 1962

23. Sauerland EK, Mitchell SP: Electromyographic activity of intrinsic and extrinsic muscles of the human tongue. Texas Rep Bio Med 33:1945–1955, 1975

24. Morikawa S, Safar P, DeCarlo J: Influence of the head-jaw position upon upper airway patency. Anesthesia 22:265–270, 1981

25. Safar P, Escarraga LA, Chang F: Upper airway obstruction in the unconscious patient. J Appl Physiol 14:760–764, 1959

26. Stark AR, Thach BT: Mechanisms of airway obstruction leading to apnea in newborn infants. J Pediatrics 89:982–985, 1976

27. Anch AM, Remmers JE, Bunce H III: Supraglottic airway resistance in normal subjects and patients with occlusive sleep apnea. J Appl Physiol 53:1158–1163, 1982

28. Lavie PR, Gertner R, Zomer J, Podoskin L: Breathing disorders in sleep associated with microarousals in patients with allergic rhinitis. Acta Otolaryngol 92:529–533, 1981

29. Taasan VC, Wynne JW, Cassisi N, Block AJ: The effect of nasal packing on sleep disordered breathing and nocturnal oxygen desaturation. Laryngoscope 19:1163–1172, 1981

30. Zwillich CW, Pickett C, Hanson RN, Weil JV: Disturbed sleep and prolonged apnea during nasal obstruction in normal men. Am Rev Respir Dis 124:158–160, 1981

31. Cohen MI: Phrenic and recurrent laryngeal discharge patterns and the Hering-Breuer reflex. Am J Physiol 228:1489–1496, 1975

32. Onal E, Lopata M, O'Connor T: Diaphragmatic and genioglossal electromyogram responses to CO_2 rebreathing in humans. J Appl Physiol 50:1052–1055, 1981

33. Strohl KP, Hensley MJ, Hallett M, et al: Activation of upper airway muscles before onset of inspiration in normal humans. J Appl Physiol 49:638–642, 1980

34. Van Lunteren E, Van de Graaff WB, Parker DM, et al: Nasal and laryngeal reflex responses to negative upper airway pressure. J Appl Physiol 56:746–752, 1984

35. Sica AL, Cohen MI, Donnelly DF, Zhang H: Hypoglossal motoneuron responses to pulmonary and superior laryngeal afferent inputs. Respir Physiol 56:339–357, 1984

36. Van Lunteren E, Strohl KP, Parker DM, et al: Phasic volume-related feedback on upper airway muscle activity. J Appl Physiol 56:730–736, 1984

37. Brouillette RT, Thach BT: Control of genioglossus muscle inspiratory activity. J Appl Physiol 49:801–808, 1980

38. Fukuda Y, Honda Y: Roles of vagal afferents on discharge patterns and CO_2-responsiveness of efferent superior laryngeal, hypoglossal, and phrenic respiratory activities in anesthetized rats. Jap J Physiol 32:689–698, 1982

39. Kuna ST: Inhibition of inspiratory upper airway motoneuron activity by phasic volume feedback. Am Rev Respir Dis 131:A300, 1985

40. Younes MK, Remmers JE, Baker J: Characteristics of inspiratory inhibition by phasic volume feedback in cats. J Appl Physiol 45:80–86, 1978

41. DiMarco AF, von Euler C, Romaniuk JR, Yamamoto Y: Positive feedback faciliation of external intercostal and phrenic inspiratory activity by pulmonary stretch receptors. Acta Physiol Scand 113:375–386, 1981

42. Pack AI, DeLaney RG, Fishman AP: Augmentation of phrenic neural activity by increased

rates of lung inflation. J Appl Physiol 50:149–161, 1981

43. Bonora M, Shields GI, Knuth SL, et al: Selective depression by ethanol of upper airway respiratory motor activity in cats. Am Rev Respir Dis 130:156–161, 1984

44. Bruce NB, Mitra J, Cherniack NS: Central and peripheral chemoreceptor inputs to phrenic and hypoglossal motoneurons. J Appl Physiol 53:1504–1511, 1982

45. Haxhiu MA, Lunteren E van, Mitra J, et al: Responses to chemical stimulation of upper airway muscles and diaphragm in awake cats. J Appl Physiol 56:397–403, 1984

46. Hoffstein V, Zamel N, Phillipson EA: Lung volume dependence of pharyngeal cross-sectional area in patients with obstructive sleep apnea. Am Rev Respir Dis 130:175–178, 1984

47. Onal E, Lopata M, O'Connor T: Diaphragmatic and genioglossal electromyogram responses to isocapnic hypoxia in humans. Am Rev Respir Dis 124:215–217, 1981

48. Parisi RA, Neubauer JA, Frank M, et al: Correlation between genioglossal and diaphragmatic responses to hypercapnia in sleeping goats. Am Rev Respir Dis 131:A295, 1985

49. Weiner D, Mitra J, Salamone J, Cherniack NS: Effect of chemical stimuli on nerves supplying upper airway muscles. J Appl Physiol 52:530–536, 1982

50. Fukuda Y, Honda Y: Effects of hypocapnia on respiratory timing and inspiratory activities of the superior laryngeal, hypoglossal, and phrenic nerves in the vagotomized rat. Jap J Physiol 33:733–742, 1983

51. Mathew OP, Sant'Ambrogio G, Fisher JT, Sant'Ambrogio FB: Laryngeal pressure receptors. Respir Physiol 57:113–122, 1984

52. Sant'Ambrogio G, Mathew OP, Fisher JT, Sant'Ambrogio FB: Laryngeal receptors responding to transmural pressure, airflow and local muscle activity. Respir Physiol 54:317–330, 1983

53. Sant'Ambrogio G, Mathew OP, Sant'Ambrogio FB, Fisher JT: Laryngeal cold receptors. Respir Physiol 59:35–44, 1985

54. Mathew OP, Abu-Osba YK, Thach BT: Influence of upper airway pressure changes on genioglossus muscle respiratory activity. J Appl Physiol 52:438–444, 1982

55. Sant'Ambrogio F, Mathew OP, Clark WD, Sant'Ambrogio G: Laryngeal influences on breathing pattern and posterior cricoarytenoid muscle activity. J Appl Physiol 58:1298–1304, 1985

56. Mathew OP, Abu-Osba YK, Thach BT: Genioglossus muscle responses to upper air-

way pressure changes: afferent pathways. J Appl Physiol 52:445–450, 1982

56a. Mathew OP, Farber JP: Effect of upper airway negative pressure on respiratory timing. Respir Physiol 54:259–268, 1983

57. Brouillette RT, Thach BT: A neuromuscular mechanism maintaining extrathoracic airway patency. J Appl Physiol 46:772–779, 1979

57a. Mathew OP: Upper airway negative-pressure effects on respiratory activity of upper airway muscles. J Appl Physiol 56:500–505, 1984

58. Hwang J, St. John WM, Bartlett D Jr: Afferent pathways for hypoglossal and phrenic responses to changes in upper airway pressure. Respir Physiol 55:341–354, 1984

59. McNicholas WT, Coffey M, McDonnell T, et al: Abnormal respiration during sleep in normal subjects following selective topical oropharyngeal and nasal anaesthesia. Am Rev Respir Dis 131:A302, 1985

60. Thach BT, Menon PA, Schefft G: Negative upper airway pressure decreases inspiratory airflow and tidal volume in tracheostomized sleeping human infants. Am Rev Respir Dis 131:A295, 1985

61. Van de Graaff WB, Gottfried SB, Mitra J, et al: Respiratory function of hyoid muscles and hyoid arch. J Appl Physiol 57:197–204, 1984

62. Roberts JL, Reed WR, Thach BT: Pharyngeal airway-stabilizing function of sternohyoid and sternothyroid muscles in the rabbit. J Appl Physiol 57:1790–1795, 1984

63. Bonora M, St. John WM, Bledsoe TA: Differential elevation by protriptyline and depression by diazepam of upper airway respiratory motor activity. Am Rev Respir Dis 131:41–45, 1985

64. Hwang J, St. John WM, Bartlett D Jr: Respiratory-related hypoglossal nerve activity: Influence of anesthetics. J Appl Physiol 55:785–792, 1983

65. Krol RC, Knuth SI, Bartlett D Jr: Selective reduction of genioglossal muscle activity by alcohol in normal human subjects. Am Rev Respir Dis 129:247–250, 1984

66. Nishino T, Shirahata M, Yonezawa T, Honda Y: Comparison of changes in the hypoglossal and phrenic nerve activity in response to increasing depth of anesthesia in cats. Anesthesiology 60:19–24, 1984

67. Robinson RW, White DP, Zwillich CW, et al: Effects of alcohol on upper airway resistance. Am Rev Respir Dis 131:A104, 1985

68. Dolly FR, Block AJ: Effect of flurazepam on sleep-disordered breathing and nocturnal

oxygen desaturation in asymptomatic subjects. Am J Med 73:239–242, 1982

69. Mendelson WB, Garnett D, Gillin JC: Flurazepam-induced sleep apnea syndrome in a patient with insomnia and mild sleep-related respiratory changes. J Nerv Ment Dis 169:261–264, 1981

70. Taasan VC, Block AJ, Boysen PG, et al: Alcohol increases sleep apnea and oxygen desaturation in asymptomatic men. Am J Med 71:240–245, 1981

71. Brownell LG, West P, Sweatman P, et al: Protriptyline in obstructive sleep apnea: a double blind trial. New Engl J Med 307:1037–1042, 1982

72. Clark RW, Schmidt MS, Schoal SF, et al: Sleep apnea: treatment with protriptyline. Neurology 29:1287–1292, 1979

73. Haxhiu MA, Lunteren E van, Mitra J, et al: Comparison of the responses of the diaphragm and upper airway muscles to central stimulation of the sciatic nerve. Respir Physiol 58:65–76, 1984

74. Orem J, Montplaisir J, Dement WC: Changes in the activity of respiratory neurons during sleep. Brain Research 82:109–315, 1974

75. Orem J, Lydic R: Upper airway function during sleep and wakefulness: experimental studies on normal and anesthetized cats. Sleep 1:49–68, 1978

76. Sauerland EK, Harper RM: The human tongue during sleep: electromyographic activity of the genioglossus muscle. Exp Neurol 51:160–170, 1976

77. Lopes JM, Tabachnik E, Muller NL, et al: Total airway resistance and respiratory muscle activity during sleep. J Appl Physiol 54:773–777, 1983

78. Orem J, Netick A, Dement WC: Increased upper airway resistance to breathing during sleep in the cat. Electro Clin Neurophys 43:14–22, 1977

79. Skatrud JB, Dempsey JA: Airway resistance and respiratory muscle function in snorers during NREM sleep. J Appl Physiol 59:328–335, 1985

80. Hendricks JC, Morrison AR, Mann GL: Different behaviors during paradoxical sleep without atonia depend on pontine lesion site. Brain Res 239:81–105, 1982

81. Overholt JL, Mitra J, Lunteren E van, et al: Naloxone affects upper airway respiratory muscle response to CO_2. Am Rev Respir Dis 131:A294, 1985

82. Bartlett D Jr, Remmers JE, Gautier H: Laryngeal regulation of respiratory airflow. Respir Physiol 18:194–204, 1973

83. Shelton RL Jr, Bosma JF, Sheets BV: Tongue,

hyoid and larynx displacement in swallow and phonation. J Appl Physiol 15:283–288, 1960

84. Doty R: Neural organization of deglutition, in Cole CF (ed): Handbook of Physiology, Section 6: Alimentary Canal, volume IV. Washington DC, Amer Physiol Soc, 1968, pp 1861–1902

85. Menon AP, Schefft GL, Thach BT: Frequency and significance of swallowing during prolonged apnea in infants. Am Rev Respir Dis 130:969–973, 1984

86. Wilson SL, Thach BT, Brouillette RT, Abu-Osba YK: Coordination of breathing and swallowing in human infants. J Appl Physiol 50:851–858, 1981

87. Sherrey JH, Megirian D: Analysis of the respiratory role of pharyngeal constrictor motoneurons of cat. Exp Neurol 49:839–851, 1975

88. Findley LJ, Wilhoit SC, Suratt PM: Apnea duration and hypoxemia during REM sleep in patients with obstructive sleep apnea. Chest 87:432–436, 1985

89. Lugaresi E, Copcagna G, Mantovani M, et al: Hypersomnia with periodic breathing: periodic apneas and alveolar hypoventilation during sleep. Bull Europ Physiopath Resp 8:1103–1113, 1972

90. Harper RM, Sauerland EK: The role of the tongue in sleep apnea, in Guilleminault C, Dement WC (eds): Sleep Apnea Syndromes. New York, Alan Liss, 1978, pp 219–234

91. Megirian D, Cespuglio R, Jouvet M: Rhythmical activity of the rat's tongue in sleep and wakefulness. Electroenceph Clin Neurophysiol 44:8–13, 1978

92. Sherrey JH, Megirian D: State dependence of upper airway respiratory motoneurons: Functions of the cricothyroid and nasolabial muscles of the unanesthetized rat. Electroenceph Clin Neurophysiol 43:218–228, 1977

93. Sherrey JH, Megirian D: Respiratory EMG activity of the posterior cricoarytrnoid, cricothyroid and diaphragm muscles during sleep. Respir Physiol 39:355–365, 1980

94. Browman CP, Sampson MG, Yolles SF, et al: Obstructive sleep apnea and body weight. Chest 85:435–436, 1984

95. Harman EM, Wynne JW, Block AJ: The effect of weight loss on sleep-disordered breathing and oxygen desaturation in morbidly obese men. Chest 82:291–294, 1982

96. Conway WA, Bower GC, Barnes ME: Hypersomnolence and intermittent upper airway obstruction: Occurrence caused by micrognathia. JAMA 237:2740–2742, 1977

97. Mangat E, Orr WC, Smith RO: Sleep apnea,

hypersomnolence and upper airway obstruction secondary to adenotonsillar enlargement. Arch Otolaryngol 103:383–386, 1977

98. Remmers JE, Sterling JA, Thorarinsson B, Kuna ST: Nasal airway positive pressure in patients with obstructive sleep apnea. Am Rev Respir Dis 130:1152–1155, 1984

99. Sullivan CE, Issa RQ, Berthon-Jones M, Eves L: Reveral of obstructive sleep apnoea by continuous positive airway pressure applied through the nares. Lancet 1:862–865, 1981

100. Leiter JC, Knuth SL, Bartlett D Jr: The effect of sleep deprivation on activity of the genioglossus muscle in man. Am Rev Respir Dis 132:1242–1245, 1985

101. Guilleminault C, Rosekind M: The arousal threshold: sleep deprivation, sleep fragmantation, and obstructive sleep apnea syndrome. Bull Europ Physiopath Resp 17:341–349, 1981

102. Guilleminault C, Riley R, Powell N: Obstructive sleep apnea and abnormal cephalomet-ric measurements: implications for treatment. Chest 86:793–794, 1984

103. Rivlin J, Hoffstein V, Kalbfleisch J, et al: Upper airway morphology in patients with idiopathic obstructive sleep apnea. Am Rev Respir Dis 129:355–360, 1984

104. Haponik EF, Smith PL, Bohlman ME, et al: Computerized tomography in obstructive sleep apnea. Am Rev Respir Dis 127:221–226, 1983

105. Suratt PM, Wilhoit SC, Cooper K: Induction of airway collapse with subatmospheric pressure in awake patients with sleep apnea. J Appl Physiol 57:140–146, 1984

106. Perez-Padilla JR, Remmers JE: Dynamics of pressure, airflow and noise production during simulated snoring. Am Rev Respir Dis 131:A106, 1985

107. Skatrud JB, Dempsey JA: Interaction of sleep state and chemical stimuli in sustaining rhythmic ventilation. J Appl Physiol 55:813–822, 1983

Richard J. Martin

5

Medical Treatment for the Sleep Apnea Syndrome

In treating respiratory disorders during sleep, objective goals must be set whether medical or surgical intervention is followed. It is very easy to repeat a polysomnographic evaluation and say the apnea time was improved by 80 percent. However, does the patient still have significant oxygen desaturation or arrhythmias with the remaining apneas? If systemic hypertension, pulmonary hypertension, erythrocytosis, impotency, etc. were initial findings, are these problems improving or resolved? Finally, the most bothersome symptom the patient has is usually daytime somnolence. Is this objectively improved? Although in most instances improvement in the apneas will improve the above mentioned symptoms and signs, this should not be taken for granted.

This chapter will discuss medical treatment options for upper airway obstruction (cessation of airflow with continued respiratory effort), central apnea (cessation of airflow without respiratory effort), mixed apnea (cessation of airflow without respiratory effort initially and then effort being made in the same apneic episode), and primary alveolar hypoventilation (decreased airflow and decreased respiratory effort). Primary alveolar hypoventilation is not a true apnea, but can produce the same signs and symptoms as seen with the other types of apneas. Primary alveolar hypoventilation should be considered in the differential diagnosis of patients presenting with possible respiratory abnormalities during sleep.

UPPER AIRWAY OBSTRUCTION

A review of the pathophysiology of the upper airway obstruction helps in understanding the various treatment interventions that have been developed.[1] Additionally, a detailed description of the pathophysiology of apnea can be found in Chapter 4 of this text.

ABNORMALITIES OF RESPIRATION DURING SLEEP
ISBN 0-8089-1812-5

Copyright © 1986 by Grune & Stratton, Inc.
All rights of reproduction in any form reserved.

Correctable Processes

The first principle in considering appropriate treatment for patients with upper airway obstruction during sleep is to be absolutely positive that a correctable cause does not exist. This point tends to be overlooked in the treatment process. Not uncommonly, simple treatment modalities or nontracheostomy surgical procedures can correct the problem. The following are correctable causes of upper airway obstruction:

1. Tonsils/Adenoids
    Children and adults
2. Endocrine
    Hypothyroidism
    Acromegaly
    Cushings
3. Micrognathia/Retrognathia
4. Alcohol
    Before sleep
5. Respiratory Depressants
    Sedatives
    Narcotics
6. Beta-blockers
7. Obesity

Hypertrophied tonsils and adenoids, even in the adult, can produce this syndrome and surgical excision is curative.[2] Although this is not a medical intervention, it must be stressed here. This "simple" procedure compared to other extensive surgical interventions is all too frequently overlooked. The tonsils do not necessarily need to occlude the airway on visual examination to produce upper airway obstruction during sleep. Upper airway obstruction can be produced if the oropharynx is slightly small with only a moderate increase in tonsillar size.

Several endocrine problems are associated with sleep apnea. Thyroid function studies should be checked routinely in patients with upper airway obstruction as hypothyroidism is another correctable cause to be considered.[3,4] There are several possible mechanisms that could relate hypothyroidism and obstructive apnea. First is the mechanical effect of an enlarged tongue producing a smaller oropharyngeal area. Second is the decreased chemosensitivity and neural output in these individuals, which, although it has not been studied during sleep, could potentiate apneic patterns. Third is a potential myopathy of the upper airway muscles as the Creatinine Phosphokinase (CPK) has been noted to be increased. Correction of the hypothyroid state may lead to reversal of the apneas. Since it takes time to fully reverse this syndrome in hypothyroid patients, other temporary interventions listed below may need to be considered if the process is severe or life threatening.

Acromegaly probably causes upper airway obstruction because of the thick tongue that develops.[5] It appears that with treatment for this disease, the sleep apnea is improved in some patients.[6] However, that study did not have polysomnographic tracings and the authors stated that the patients had "narcolepsy." An acromegalic patient seen in our laboratory with severe sleep apnea did not have improvement in the sleep apnea or daytime symptoms six months after pituitary ablation. Cushings syndrome can produce sleep apnea. One patient was seen in our laboratory with iatrogenic Cushings due to excessively high prednisone administration. Prior to the initiation of prednisone, the patient was asymptomatic regarding signs and symptoms of sleep apnea. After becoming cushingoid, he developed sleep apnea. Once this patient was tapered off the steroids, the sleep apnea syndrome subsided both objectively and subjectively.

Two therapeutic interventions that can prevent worsening of sleep apnea are the elimination of alcohol and other respiratory depressive agents, particularly before bedtime. Alcohol has been shown to increase the duration and frequency of the obstructive episodes associated with a marked increase in the degree of hypoxemia.[7] In fact, two subjects who had chronic snoring without total occlusive episodes developed frank obstructive sleep apnea following alcohol ingestion. In a placebo controlled and randomized study of asymptomatic males, alcohol ingestion increased the incidence of arterial oxygen desaturation and apneic events.[8] Of interest, the worsening of the oxygen desaturation persisted for an additional night, even when alcohol was not consumed. It appears that alcohol induces oropharyngeal muscle hypotonia producing the apneas and increases the duration of the episodes by further depressing the arousal mechanisms. In a study of the effects of ethyl alcohol on cats, it was shown that a significant reduction of hypoglossal and recurrent laryngeal nerve activities occurred at doses that had little or no effect on phrenic nerve discharge.[9] Figure 5-1 shows the dose-related reduction in recurrent laryngeal nerve activity secondary to alcohol as the phrenic activity remains constant. Thus, selective inhibition of the upper airway musculature due to alcohol occurs with continued diaphragmatic activity. This type of situation will potentiate apneas. Alcohol also inhibited the responsiveness of the upper airway muscle activity to hypercapnia and normocapnic hypoxemia. Thus, alcohol potentiates sleep apnea and depresses the normal responses of opening the upper airway in the presence of altered blood gas tensions. Similarities of action exist between sedatives and alcohol in the potentiation of apnea. Respiratory depressants, such as sleeping pills, also produce increased periodic breathing as demonstrated in a normal population.[10] As with alcohol, diazepam induces a reduction of hypoglossal and recurrent laryngeal nerve activity at doses that do not alter phrenic nerve discharge.[11] This is important knowledge to have as many apneic patients may complain of "insomnia" or restless sleep and the physician will prescribe sedatives that then will potentiate the primary problem. Since the incidence of apnea and oxygen desaturation increases with age and/or weight, appropriate history and examination should be undertaken before these agents are prescribed.

Although little is known about the effects of pre- and post-operative medication, one can surmise from the above discussion that these sedatives and analgesics could potentiate apneas and/or oxygen desaturation in certain patients. If a patient has a history or physical status compatible with sleep related respiratory disorders, then these agents need to be used with care. Along the same lines, extubation in these patients should not occur until he or she is fully awake.

Beta adrenergic receptor blockers (propranolol, etc.) may have a deleterious effect on sleep apnea.[12] The exact mechanism is not understood, but death related to propranolol overdose is secondary to respiratory arrest. Alternately, in a double blind

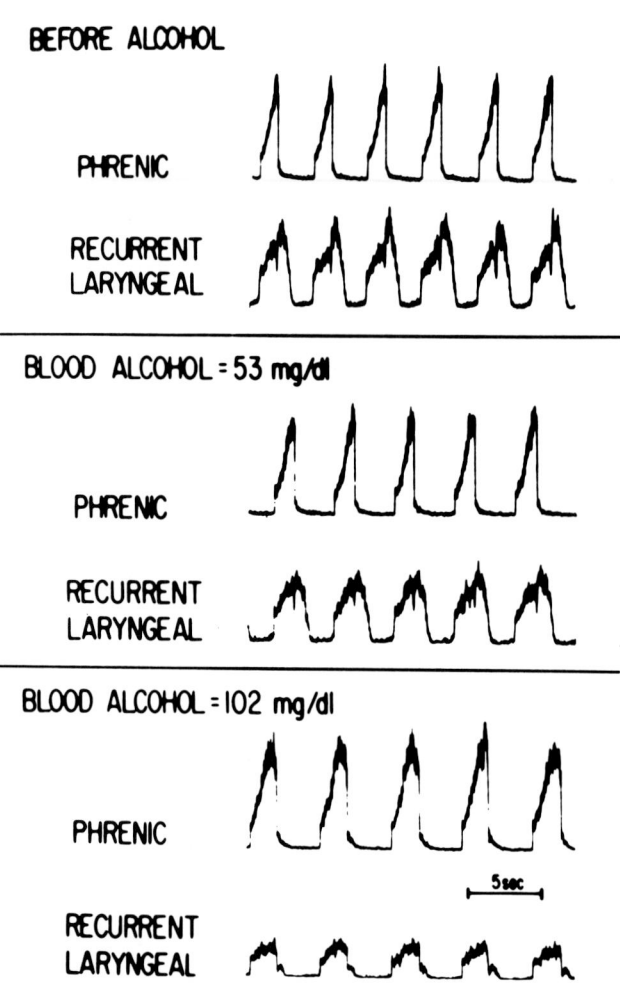

Fig. 5-1. Integrated electrical activity of the phrenic and recurrent laryngeal nerves in a decerebrate, vagotomized cat demonstrating the effect of different intravenous doses of alcohol. Alcohol has no apparent effect upon phrenic nerve activity while progressively suppressing activity in the nerves supplying the upper airway, a situation that would favor the development of apnea. See ref. 9. (From Bonora M, Shields GI, Knuth SL, et al: Selective depression by ethanol of upper airway respiratory motor activity in cats. Am Rev Respir Dis 130:156–161, 1984. With permission.)

study,[13] propranolol did not worsen sleep apnea. If after the institution of beta-blockers, sleep apnea signs and symptoms are produced, the physician must be cognizant of the possible interaction.

Unfortunately, weight loss in the obese sleep apnea patient is difficult to voluntarily accomplish and is not always an effective means of overcoming the sleep-related upper airway obstruction. Furthermore, about 20–30 percent of sleep apnea patients are not grossly overweight and weight loss would not be a therapeutic alternative. In one study,[14] patients with essentially continuous apnea were placed on an 800-calorie per day reducing diet achieving weight loss of over 30 kg each, but no symptomatic or objective improvement was noted. An additional, small group of patients with only non-rapid-eye-movement sleep apneas showed no improvement after weight loss. The one group of patients that does appear to respond to weight reduction are those who have intermittent apneas throughout the night. The mean apnea index was 32 per hour before weight loss and 14 after the diet regimen. There was not a total reversal of either symptoms or signs of sleep apnea, but considerable improvement occurred in this group.

Harman et al[15] showed that massive weight reduction (53–155 Kg) in four subjects significantly reduced the number of apneas per hour (78 to 0.37) and the oxygen desaturation (65.5 percent to 84 percent) following bypass surgery. The two subjects with daytime somnolence and hypercapnia prior to weight loss showed the most dramatic improvement in desaturation. In a single obstructive sleep apnea patient whose weight fluctuated within a range of 26 Kg over a three year period, sleep studies were monitored on five different occasions.[16] The number of apnea per hour varied dramatically from 60 at 111 Kg to 3 at 85 Kg. The relation between the apneas per hour and weight was a logarithmic function (Fig. 5-2). In this study, which is not universally shown, a modest decrease in weight was associated with a disproportionately larger decrease in apnea rate. The level of oxygen saturation also had a logarithmic relation with weight. Important to note was that the sinus bradycardia associated with the apneas and the post-apneic tachycardia were only present at the highest weight. These two reports suggest that weight loss is beneficial in at least a subset of sleep apnea patients.

When dietary therapy for apnea is considered, one must be sure that the potential for sudden death due to ventricular arrhythmias is not evident on the polysomnographic evaluation. Also, if the patient's work depends on a rapid resolution of the symptoms, weight loss is not the primary mode of therapy. Under these circumstances, one should consider other interventions, e.g., tracheostomy or nasal continuous positive airway pressure (CPAP). Then a weight loss program can be embarked upon and if successful (including improved polysomnographic evaluation) the initial intervention can be terminated.

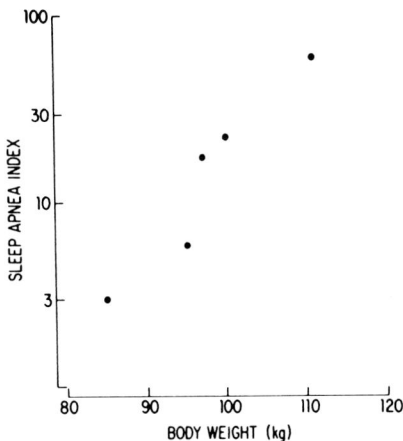

Fig. 5-2. Apnea index (printed in log scale) on the ordinate and body weight on the abscissa of a single sleep apnea patient who underwent massive weight loss. Sleep recordings were made on five occasions during the weight loss period. There appeared to be an initial "threshold" weight at which a large portion of the apneas disappeared. (From Browman CP, Sampson MG, Yolles SF, et al: Obstructive sleep apnea and body weight. Chest 85:435, 1984. With permission.)

Improved Neurorespiratory Input

There are several agents that have been shown to be beneficial in upper airway obstruction to varying degrees: oxygen, protriptyline, progesterone ±, strychnine ±, and nicotine ±. Two of the more successful are supplemental oxygen and protriptyline while medroxyprogesterone acetate may have limited benefit in a very select group of these patients. A fourth agent, strychnine, has been shown to produce beneficial effects in upper airway obstruction. Although this drug will be discussed, its place in clinical practice is yet to be determined. A fifth agent, nicotine, has recently been shown to be of benefit in obstructive apnea, but only during the early hours of sleep. Other agents (see below) have had limited testing or success.

Oxygen

Although it appears that the oscillations in saturation are of primary importance in the formation and cessation of the upper airway obstruction, the picture is not that simple. Martin et al[17] showed that both acute and chronic hyperoxia when compared to room air breathing resulted in a significant decrease in the total number of apneic episodes as well as the percent apnea time (duration of apneas divided by sleep time). The length of the apneas on oxygen was slightly longer, but the number was significantly decreased. In the eight patients studied, the response was generally positive. In addition, there was a subset who dramatically improved and another subset who remained the same or worsened. When improvement was seen, it was reflected in improvement of the symptoms of somnolence, fatigue, and general well being.

Several hypotheses were considered to explain the respiratory improvement in apneas while breathing oxygen.[17] Each hypothesis involves the relationship between the depressant effect of hyperoxia on peripheral chemoreceptor function and other stimulatory or beneficial effects of oxygen. Hypoxia per se can have a direct central depressant effect on ventilation in addition to the initial stimulatory effect that is seen, which is mediated by the peripheral arterial chemoreceptors. The prolonged effect of hyperoxic breathing in normals is stimulatory after a transient decrease in ventilation. In sleep apnea, hyperoxia may decrease the number of apneas by centrally relieving hypoxic ventilatory depression and/or by hyperoxic stimulation. Along similar lines, hyperoxia may relieve a hypoxic dependent disruption in central nervous system function by an alteration in the concentration of some oxygen tension-sensitive metabolite. Two other possible explanations for the hyperoxic effect are interruption of a negative hypoxic-hypecapnic interaction, which can occur at very low levels of oxygen tension, and a smoothing out of oscillations in the central respiratory system by diminishing the gain of the carbon dioxide sensor.

It appears that once the cycle of apnea and hypoxia is initiated, hypoxia plays a divergent role. As the apnea progresses, the patient becomes more hypoxemic, which could well be the stimulus for arousal, increased genioglossal activity, and cessation of the apnea. On the other hand, the marked hypoxia can lead to a detrimental central nervous system effect of ventilatory suppression and potentiate apneic breathing in general. With hyperoxia, the apneas tend to be longer but are less frequent (in a subset population), which would suggest that there is a central mechanism operating with upper airway obstruction.

Two other recent studies support the finding that oxygenation improves the ventilatory pattern during sleep. In a man with primary alveolar hypoventilation and central sleep apneas, but without responsiveness to exogenous respiratory stimulants, low-flow nocturnal oxygen improved his sleep pattern.[18] There was a marked decrease in the number and duration of apneas and an increase in the level of ventilation that was sustained for the five-month followup period. In another study of five post-tracheostomy sleep apnea patients, a dramatic decrease in overall apnea index was seen (tracheostomy tube plugged for repeat studies).[19] Before surgery, the lowest oxygen saturation ranged between 29–68 percent, while five weeks post tracheostomy the lowest saturation was 86–89 percent. Of interest, the ventilatory response to carbon dioxide improved in all cases following surgery. These findings, again, suggest that hypoxic brainstem depression develops with the sleep apnea syndromes and improvement occurs when proper oxygenation is maintained.

Although prediction of which patient will respond to supplemental oxygen cannot be made at the present time, it appears that a one-half to one hour testing period on oxygen in the laboratory will determine the long-term response.[17] Thus, patients who improved by more than 60 percent during the brief testing period in the laboratory with respect to the apnea time also responded similarly on a long-term basis. In addition, daytime symptoms were markedly improved. Home oxygen can be given via nasal prongs at a flow rate of three to four liters per minute. Patients should not be sent home for a trial of oxygen without proper evaluation in the laboratory because it may worsen the apneas in certain individuals.

Another study confirmed the potential benefits of supplemental oxygen therapy for sleep apnea.[20] These investigators found that in nonrapid-eye-movement (NREM) sleep, breathing 3 L/minute of oxygen significantly decreased both rate of sleep-disordered breathing and the peak fall in oxygen saturation. Additionally, the percentage of central and mixed apneas was also reduced. During rapid-eye-movement (REM) sleep the disordered breathing was improved, but the oxygen desaturation did not improve. Although the sleep architecture improved and 7 of 12 patients felt more alert, there was no overall improvement in multiple sleep latency testing.

A major drawback to oxygen therapy is the cost. This will range between $150–$400 per month. This cost factor needs to be balanced against the beneficial effects. Objective data needs to be obtained from both the polysomnogram as well as the daytime symptoms and signs of this syndrome. Thus, supplemental oxygen should not just be prescribed without a definite end point for success or failure. Additionally, long term research studies are needed to see if improvement in cardiopulmonary hemodynamics are obtained.

Protriptyline

Protriptyline is a nonsedating tricyclic antidepressant that appears to relieve upper airway obstruction during sleep in occasional patients. Tricyclics have been used in narcolepsy-cataplexy syndromes with good results and were thus tried in sleep apnea. In 1 study, protriptyline had a lasting beneficial effect in 8 of 14 sleep apnea patients over 7 to 15 months of observation.[21] It appears that the responders had the lowest percentage of total sleep time spent in apnea. In personal communications with other laboratories, success rate with protriptyline is lower. The exact reason for the beneficial effect seen with protriptyline is unknown. In cats, both hypoglassal and recurrent laryngeal nerve activities were consistently increased after protriptyline administration, whereas phrenic nerve discharge was not altered.[11] This drug additionally improves ventilatory response to carbon dioxide, but patients with normal ventilatory responses may also have decreased apneas on protriptyline. Improvement in oxygen saturation during the apnea has been documented.[22] This agent does decrease the amount of NREM sleep, which may be one way the apnea index is reduced, but will also improve REM apneas. A major drawback to tricyclic antidepressants is the cardiovascular toxicity that has the potential to develop. This includes arrhythmias and blood pressure abnormalities. Additionally, urinary retention limits the dose that can be used. Therefore, low doses should be used initially (5 mg) and increased as needed to levels of 20–30 mg. The medication is given as a once-a-day dose about one hour before bedtime.

One patient in our laboratory had a minimal response to both oxygen and protriptyline each used alone. When we used oxygen and protriptyline in combination, his sleep apnea syndrome was improved. This is obviously an anecdotal case and further study needs to be done.

Progesterone

Another therapeutic agent that has been tried in patients with upper airway obstruction is medroxyprogesterone acetate. Lyons and Huang[23] and Sutton et al[24] have shown the efficacy of progesterone in a group of patients with probable respiratory abnormalities during sleep. Since polysomnographic studies were not done, the exact type of abnormality is not known. Another study of patients with upper airway obstruction showed a response to progesterone in four of nine subjects.[25] It appears that the responders were separated from the nonresponders by a lower resting awake PaO_2 level and a tendency toward an elevated $PaCO_2$ level. From this, it would appear that the chemical control of breathing in the responder group would be less responsive to lowered oxygen or elevated carbon dioxide tensions and perhaps progesterone had a beneficial stimulatory effect. Orr et al[26] showed no overall response to progesterone in seven patients with sleep-related upper airway obstruction. Although the apnea time was lower in 5 patients, 4 of these individuals still had between 259 and 456 apneic episodes per night. Even though their daytime hypersomnolence improved slightly, it still interfered with normal routine functioning. Similar results of progesterone unresponsiveness were demonstrated in 13 eucapneic male sleep apneic patients.[27]

Progesterone has several different effects in normal human subjects. First, it is a respiratory stimulant that increases minute ventilation. There are progesterone (hormonal) receptors concentrated in the hypothalamus and hippocampus. These sites appear to work in a feedback system for hormonal control and may also either directly or indirectly enhance ventilation. Progesterone also increases the glomerular filtration rate and has an anti-aldosterone diuretic effect. This would tend to improve elements of cardiac decompensation in sleep apnea patients.

Clinical experience at our institution has shown medroxyprogesterone therapy to be a successful treatment regimen in patients with primary alveolar hypoventilation or central apneas (see below). It appears that a subgroup of upper airway obstruction patients may also respond to this therapy. Further investigation is needed for better definition of the responders because of contradicting evidence in the literature about its efficacy in upper airway obstruction patients.

The dose of progesterone is 20–40 mg P.O. t.i.d. The more common side effects in the male population are hair loss and decreased libido. The decreased libido can be overcome by monthly testosterone injections. Diabetes mellitus can become clinically evident if a patient had a predisposition for this prior to initiation of the progesterone.

Strychnine

The tensor palatini (as well as other oropharyngeal muscles) has been noted to decrease or cease action in the sleeping patient during an obstructive apnea.[28] This loss is much more pronounced in apneic individuals than the mild or moderate decline in activity during quiet sleep in normals. During sleep, this abnormal decrease in activity may be produced with a preferentially diminished excitatory projection to the tensor palatini motoneurons (disfactilitation) or by enhancing neurally mediated inhibition. During sleep motoneurons become hyperpolarized, which is a manifestation of postsynaptic inhibition, and can be blocked by strychnine.

Remmers et al[28] demonstrated in one patient that 0.2 mg/kg of strychnine given through a nasogastric catheter helped alleviate obstructive sleep apnea. One hour after strychnine administration, the duration of apnea was reduced and the duration of the ventilatory phase had increased. Accompanying this change were longer bursts of tensor palatini activity. Two hours after strychnine, rhythmic inspiratory tensor palatini bursts were observed and apnea did not occur. Three hours post-drug, the tensor palatini electromyogram returned nearly to the awake value. Thus, remembering the pathophysiologic discussion on obstructive apnea, strychnine augmented the activity of the oropharyngeal muscles without a comparable increase in diaphragmatic activity. This combination promotes upper airway patency and helps to eliminate obstructive apnea. However, since strychnine has a low therapeutic/toxic ratio it is not suitable for clinical use.

Nicotine

Nicotine tends to stimulate ventilation, but increases the activity of muscles that dilate the upper airway to a greater extent. Using the nicotine gum, Gothe et al[29] analyzed the first two hours of sleep (peak blood levels are decreased by one third in 60 minutes) in eight obstructive sleep apnea patients. The number of obstructive and mixed apneas were significantly decreased during the 2 hour period. If a longer acting preparation can be produced, then this form of therapy could possibly be an important step in stimulating the muscle of the upper airway to maintain patency during sleep.

Other Agents

Many other respiratory stimulants have been tried with limited success or numbers in sleep apnea patients. These include almitrine, L-tryptophane, naloxone, bromocriptine, and theophylline. Whereas, in adults theophylline has not been of proven benefit, in the treatment of recurrent apnea of prematurity it is the treatment of choice.[30] Additionally, theophylline appears to be of benefit in other sleep related apneas in children. Almitrine is an investigational drug with stimulatory action on the peripheral chemoreceptors.[31] It has been shown to decrease the mean duration of hypopneas, obstructive, and mixed apneas in NREM sleep.[32] Of interest is a lack of effect in reducing the frequency or duration of central apneas.

Mechanical Methods to Alleviate the Upper Airway Obstruction

Below is a list of the many different types of devices that have been developed to help overcome the sleep related upper airway occlusion:

- Nasal Continuous Positive Airway Pressure (CPAP)
- Expiratory Positive Airway Pressure (EPAP)
- Continuous Nasal Airflow
- Nasopharyngeal Intubation ±
- Tongue-Retaining Device?
- Position Change

Nasal Continuous Positive Airway Pressure (CPAP)

Nasal CPAP has recently been shown to reduce or abolish both upper airway obstruction and mixed apnea in several studies.[33–39] This is an interesting concept that, although it appears to have a high degree of success, the exact mechanism of action is not entirely clear. Some investigators claim this form of therapy is essentially 100 percent effective, which is an overstatement. The success rate of nasal CPAP is probably 70–80 percent, which is the best nontracheostomy form of therapy yet described.

The theoretical background for nasal CPAP comes from the evidence that upper airway obstruction is a passive phenomenon. To highlight the physiology (Fig. 5-3), during an upper airway obstruction, the subatmospheric pressure in the airway during an inspiratory attempt pulls the oropharyngeal structures into greater apposition. Also, there is evidence that the dilator action of pharyngeal muscle during the upper airway obstruction is malfunctioning.[40] With increasing upper airway resistance, more negative intrathoracic pressure would need to be applied in an attempt to generate flow. As stated above, this only potentiates the occlusion. An additional force that favors collapse is gravity affecting the weight of the heavier structures, e.g., tongue and jaw. The theory of nasal CPAP is that giving a positive pressure to the oropharynx would act as a "pneumatic splint" and prevent the upper airway obstruction by pushing the soft palate and tongue forward and away from the posterior oropharyngeal wall. Figure 5-3 shows a pictorial representation of the effects of negative intra-airway pressure and gravity producing an upper airway occlusion. With the application of nasal CPAP, positive airway pressure is maintained causing the airway to remain open.[33]

In all reported studies the results are dramatic.[33–39] The use of nasal CPAP significantly reduces the number of upper airway obstruction and mixed apnea (both the central and obstructive components) as well as the oxygen desaturation during sleep. Figures 5-4 and 5-5 demonstrate the effect of apneas and oxygenation of nasal CPAP. This improvement in respiration occurs both during NREM sleep as well as during REM sleep. Nasal CPAP does not alter the central apnea frequency if that type of pattern is present. Sullivan et al also demonstrated the improvement in the overall sleep architecture[39] as shown in Figure 5-6. Some reports state patients have used this device with beneficial results for 6–13 months.

Certain problems do occur with nasal CPAP. About 20 percent cannot tolerate the device. This can be due to the feeling of suffocation, a dry nose, and inability to sleep with the device. In a rare patient, more than the 5–15 cmH$_2$O of CPAP is needed

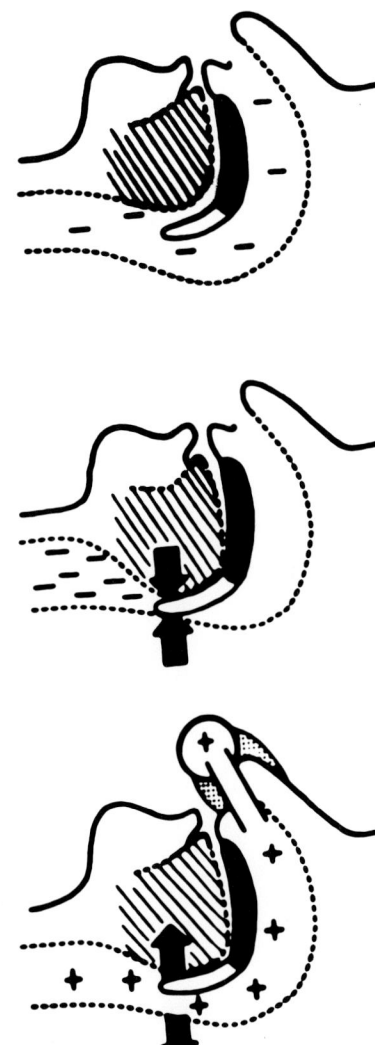

Fig. 5-3. Schematic representation of the effect of CPAP on the upper airway in obstructive sleep apnea. The top panel demonstrates that negative airway pressure is generated during inspiration and that muscle tone is needed to prevent airway collapse. The middle panel represents airway occlusion resulting from negative intra-airway pressure exceeding muscle forces tending to maintain airway patency. The lower panel shows the theoretical effect of reversing the negative airway pressure with continuous positive pressure. (From Sullivan CE, Berthon-Jones M, Issa FG, et al: Reversal of obstructive sleep apnea by continuous positive airway pressure applied through the nares. Lancet 1:862–865, 1981. With permission.)

to open the airway. In one patient from our laboratory, 35 cmH$_2$O CPAP was required during a controlled study. These high levels should not be used clinically as barotrauma could potentially be a serious problem. Another potential problem is perforation of the tympanic membrane.

The various types of nasal CPAP delivery systems all use the same principle of a mask system, a blower unit and an expiratory valve (Fig. 5-7) to produce the positive pressure.[33–39] The design of the mask appears to differ the most. Anything from a soft occlusive nasal mask to an individually molded system (Fig. 5-8) is used. Catheters projecting from the mask into the nose may or may not be used.

Expiratory Positive Airway Pressure (EPAP)

Mahadevia et al[41] showed that with 10 cmH$_2$O of EPAP, sleep apnea patients significantly reduced the apnea index, duration of apnea, and oxygen desaturation

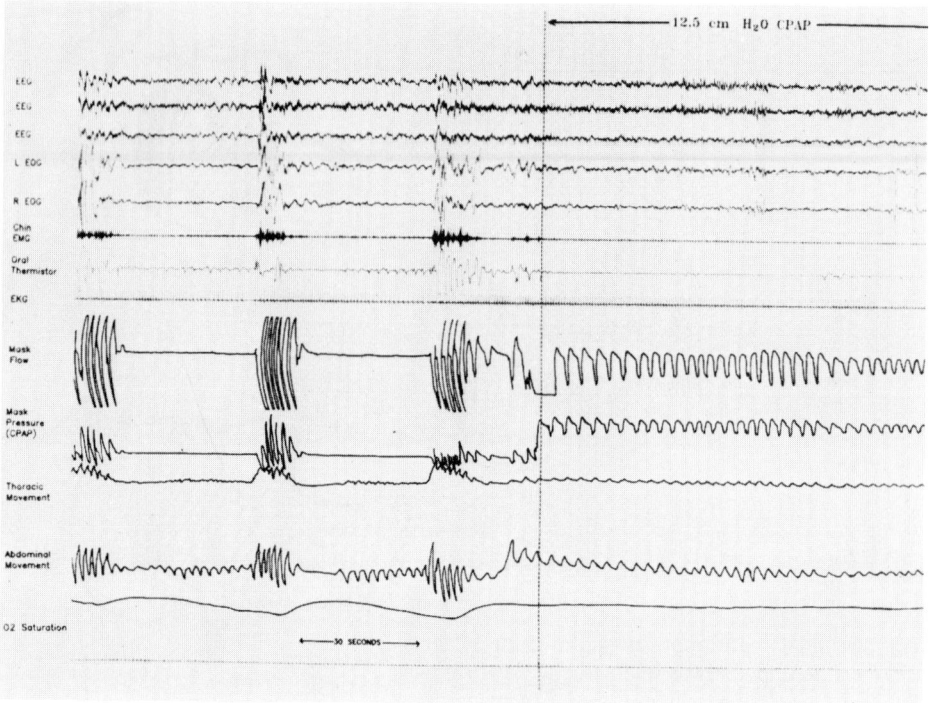

Fig. 5-4. Polysomnographic sleep tracing of a patient with obstructive apnea during the application of nasal CPAP. The left half of the tracing shows typical obstructive apneas with cessation of mask flow but continued abdominal wall movement and desaturation. The application of positive pressure represented by the dotted line, causes immediate disappearance of the apneas. (From Rapoport DM, Geroy, Goldring RM: Nasal CPAP in obstructive sleep apnea: mechanisms of action. Bull europ Physiopath Respir 19:616–620, 1983. With permission.)

while improving the quality of sleep. Whereas the initial hypothesis of nasal CPAP was to give a "pneumatic splint" to the airway on inspiration, with the information from this study the effect of EPAP and CPAP are probably multifactorial. The effects are more than likely an increase in the neural drive to the upper airway muscles, an increase in functional residual volume with a decrease in the intrathoracic pressure thus lessening the forces of upper airway collapse, and some type of upper airway splinting mechanism.

If the EPAP method proves to be tolerated by the patient and of long term benefit, then it may be more useful than CPAP. The EPAP application does not necessitate specially designed devices and an air compressor is not needed.[41] Thus, it could be more cost effective and transportable than the CPAP system.

Continuous Nasal Airflow (CNA)

Another variation of CPAP is CNA delivered into the nostrils via nasal prong catheters used for oxygen delivery. Foam cylinders or wax are placed over the nasal prongs so that a tight air seal is formed. Compressed air is delivered through the

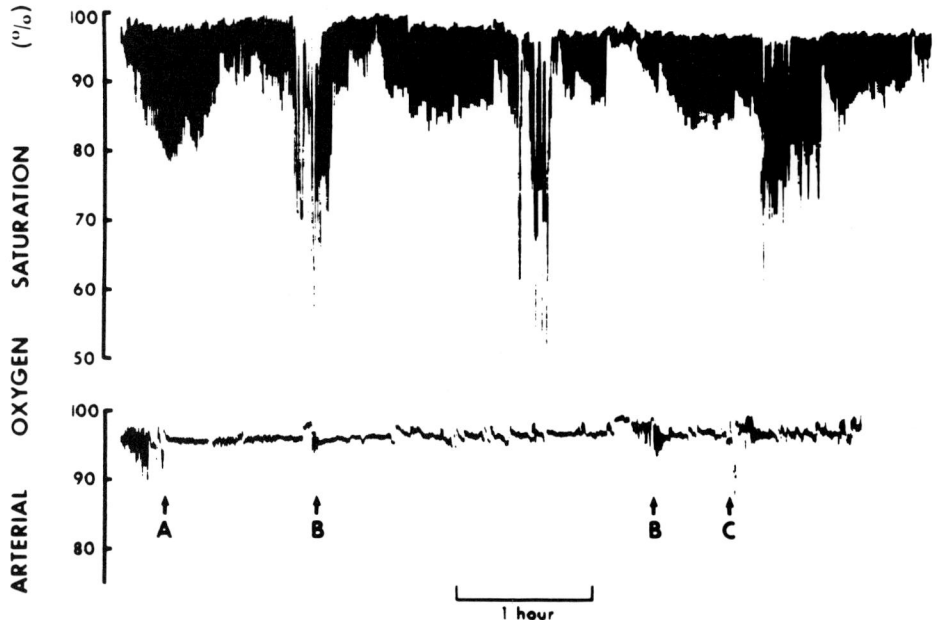

Fig. 5-5. A slow speed (overnight) recording of oxyhemoglobin saturation in a single patient with severe obstructive sleep apnea. The top panel shows marked falls in saturation below 50 percent associated with repetitive apneas. The bottom panel shows the same patient on another night while nasal CPAP is applied. A = nasal CPAP turned on; B = brief central apneas; C = obstructive apnea in REM sleep during adjustment of the CPAP pressure. (From Sullivan CE, Issa FG, Bertron-Jones M, et al: Home treatment of obstructive sleep apnoea with CPAP applied through a nose-mask. Bull europ Physiopath Resp 49–54, 1984. With permission.)

catheter into the patients nose. The flow rate is between 7–15 L/minute and expiration is through the mouth.

Wilhoit et al[42] showed that in six patients with obstructive sleep apnea the amount of oxygen desaturation and daytime somnolence was improved in the mild to moderate apnea patients. Additionally, this device was better tolerated in one patient than was nasal CPAP.

The above three devices (CPAP, EPAP, and CNA) need further evaluation to determine if any one is superior or if all three have their place in the treatment of upper airway obstruction and mixed apnea.

Nasopharyngeal Intubation and Tongue-Retaining Devices

Two types of mechanical devices that have been reported to have some beneficial results in upper airway obstruction will only receive brief mention here as their role in the treatment of sleep apnea has not been established. Nasopharyngeal intubation has been shown in limited trials to be of benefit. In a recent report[43] of two patients, there was improvement in the clinical picture over a six month period. The problem with repeated nasal intubation in our laboratory as well as others is that over time the patients complain of increasing nasal pain. Usually topical xylocaine is

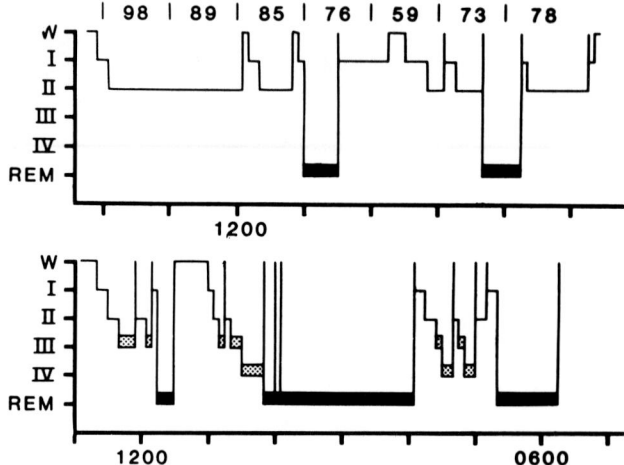

Fig. 5-6. Sleep architecture histograms of a patient with obstructive apnea on two different nights. The top panel demonstrates a disturbed pattern with predominant stage two and no slow wave sleep. The numbers at the top show movement arousals. The lower panel shows the same patient breathing with nasal CPAP. Note the appearance of slow wave sleep and the apparent REM rebound. (From Sullivan CE, et al: Home treatment of obstructive sleep apnoea with CPAP applied through a nose-mask. Bull europ Physiopath Resp 49–54, 1984. With permission.)

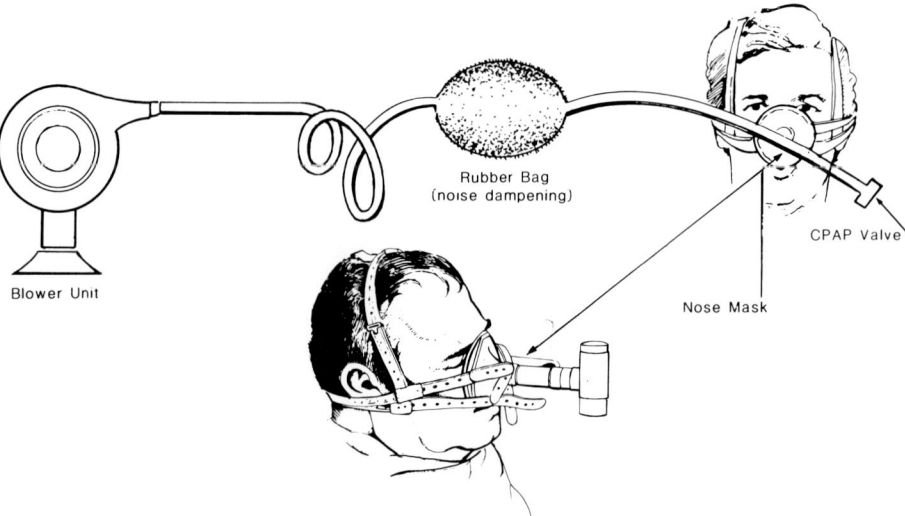

Fig. 5-7. Drawing of a typical CPAP apparatus. A blower unit is used to generate airflow past the patient's face mask. A CPAP valve provides some resistance to airflow, generating positive pressure. The amount of pressure is regulated by adjusting the "pop off" pressure of the valve. The rubber bag is optional but may help to reduce vibration of the air column and decrease noise.

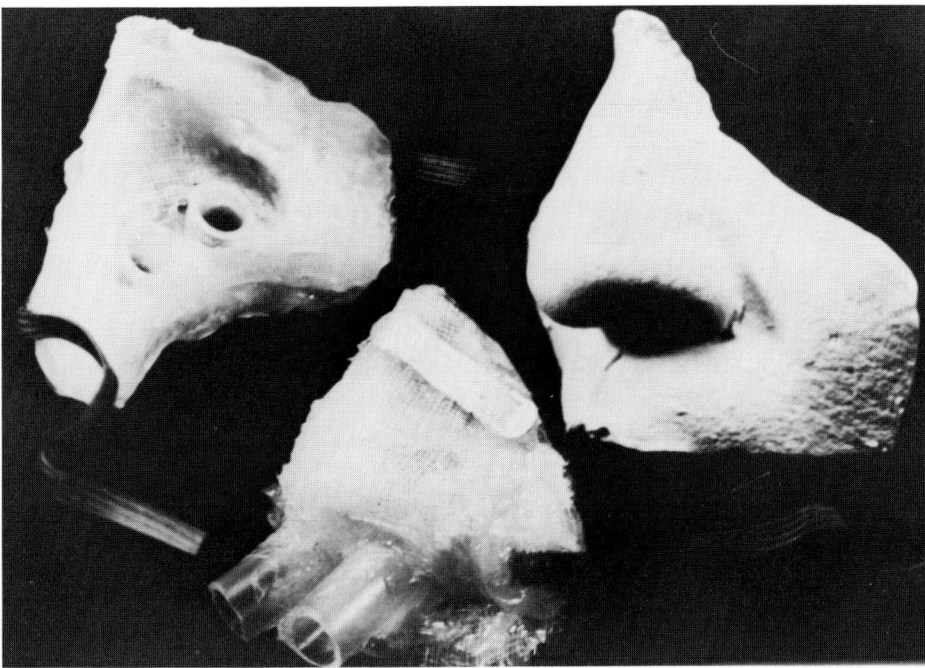

Fig. 5-8. Molded face mask used to seal the nose and allow generation of CPAP pressure. The tight seal is achieved by custom molding the mask over the patient's face using materials similar to those used in dental work. Photograph courtesy of Samuel T. Kuna, M.D.

used but eventually cocaine is needed for insertion. This was not the case in the above report. Additionally, patients may have the occlusion occurring distal to the nasopharyngeal tube and thus no benefit occurs. A tongue-retaining device has been designed to increase the unobstructed dimension of the breathing passage during sleep.[44] This device holds the tongue in a forward position by slight negative pressure. Using this system, there was significantly improved sleep with fewer and shorter apneic events in 14 obstructive sleep apnea patients. Discomfort is associated with this device and only 50 percent of patients continue to wear it over time. Additionally, the device may not be worn the entire night, eliminating whatever benefit that was derived when worn. Repeated and long term studies are needed to better evaluate this procedure.

Position Change

It is important that the patient's position is recorded in relation to apneas as on occasion a patient will only have apneas in a certain position. If this is the case, then the supine position is the predominant apnea position. However, we have had a few patients where either the left or right decubitus position was where the apneas occurred. If the apnea is position related, then tennis balls sewn into the pajama back will force the patient onto a side. If the side is the problem position, then any type of solid device to force the patient to the supine or opposite position will be of benefit. We have used wooden or sponge wedges about four feet in length. Overall, this type of position apnea is rare.

MIXED APNEAS

Mixed apneas are defined as episodes of cessation of airflow for at least ten seconds in which there occurs both a lack of respiratory effort and respiratory muscle attempts at ventilation. Thus, there are components of both central apneas and upper airway obstruction during a given apneic episode. Usually the central component precedes the obstructive component. When there are respiratory disorders during sleep, the occurrence of mixed apneas is quite common and is seen frequently throughout the night in conjunction with upper airway obstruction. The clinical presentation is similar to upper airway obstruction.

One would expect mixed apneas to be a common event in the sleep apnea syndrome. If the drive to the neuron in the tractus solitarius is reduced, a cessation of diaphragmatic activity is produced, resulting in central apneas. If there is a decreased stimulus to an area just a few microns away, the upper motorneurons for the upper airway will be affected and the result is decreased tone to the muscles that maintain extrathoracic airway patency. There is a possibility that since the anatomical regions of control are quite close, the physiologic control may be similar and, as a result, mixed apneas could easily develop. Even in an upper airway obstruction episode, there is decreased neural output to the respiratory muscles preceeding the apneas.[45]

The therapy for mixed apneas is similar to those discussed above for upper airway obstruction. Occasionally a respiratory stimulant (see Central Apneas) needs to be added to the regimen.

CENTRAL APNEAS

Patients with central apneas presenting as the predominant type of sleep-related respiratory problem are fewer than 10 percent in comparison to the number of patients having predominantly upper airway obstruction during sleep. A central apnea is defined as a cessation of airflow for at least ten seconds during which no respiratory effort is made. The disorders that can be associated with central apneas are:

- No defined etiology
- Brainstem
    Infarct
    Neoplasm
- Cervical Cordotomy
- Encephalitis
- Bulbar poliomyelitis
- Spinal surgery

Most commonly, clinical diseases cannot be found. Although patients with central apneas may not always have hypersomnolence,[14] all of the symptoms and signs associated with upper airway obstruction can occur. Rarely, the central apneas are so severe that they occur during waking hours in addition to sleep. In this setting, cyanosis and severe hypoxia develops because the patient does not perceive the need to breathe and consequently seizures may occur.

Since this type of apnea is not as common as the upper airway obstruction, investigation into the pathophysiology is not as extensive. In addition, central apneas, primary alveolar hypoventilation, and upper airway obstruction are frequently combined, or the terminology is interchanged in many reports, making precise separation and analysis difficult.

It appears that the chemical control of breathing (ventilatory responses to hypercapnic hyperoxia and eucapnic hypoxia) is reduced in this group of patients.[46–48] Whether the defect in ventilatory control is the primary cause of central apneas is not known. There are many other patient groups who have abnormalities in ventilatory control but do not have central apneas during sleep. There is a possibility that this group is predisposed to the development of central apneas. Thus during sleep, when the ventilatory responses are normally suppressed the hypoxia that develops possibly leads to further central blunting of the respiratory drive. This hypothesis is indirectly supported by several observations. Martin et al[17] and McNicholas et al[18] showed in adults that central apneas were totally eliminated or markedly improved by the use of supplemental oxygen, and Hunt[49] reported that an infant with tetralogy of Fallot was cured of central apneas and repeated "near miss sudden infant death" episodes when oxygenation returned to normal following surgery for the congenital heart defects.

Normal subjects develop periodic breathing and central apneas when taken to higher altitudes from sea level.[50–51] This type of breathing was abolished with the use of supplemental oxygen during sleep at altitude[50] and recurred about eight minutes after cessation of oxygen. Acetazolamide, a carbonic anhydrase inhibitor, also produced improvement in the ventilatory pattern and oxygenation in high altitude sleep.[51] Acetazolamide does not heighten the slope of the ventilatory response to hypoxia but, rather, produces a parallel shift in the response curve so that ventilation is augmented at all levels of hypoxia.[52] Perhaps in this situation the subject is more responsive to a decrease in oxygen and increases respiration, which prevents the "critical level" of hypoxia from developing and inducing periodic breathing.

Treatment for symptomatic patients with central apneas (Table 5-1) should start with the easiest trials. The carbonic anhydrase inhibitor, acetazolamide 250 mg po qid or dichlorphenamide 50 mg P.O. b.i.d. can be used. The side effects to be aware of are hypokalemia and the potential for significant acidosis. In one study, six

Table 5-1
Treatment of Central Apneas and Primary Alveolar Hypoventilation

Both	Central Apnea	Primary Alveolar Hypoventilation
Carbonic Anhydrase Inhibitors	Gamma hydroxybutyrate	Weight Loss
Dichlorphenamide		
Acetazolamide		
Progesterone		
Oxygen		
Negative Pressure Ventilators		
Rocking Bed		
Phrenic Nerve Pacing		

patients with predominantly central apneas improved on acetazolamide.[53] Progesterone (discussed under upper airway obstruction, above) reverses central apneas and is usually given in a dose between 20–40 mg P.O. or sublingual t.i.d. Side effects that may occur (infrequent) are impotency and alopecia in the male and glucose intolerance. There are anecdotal reports of tolerance developing to these oral agents with return of the central apnea or hypoventilation. The incidence or cause of this is unknown, but the physician needs to be aware of its potential for developing. Since home oxygen therapy is very expensive, it should be used initially in conjunction with drug therapy when hypoxemia is considered to have potentially harmful effects. It appears that one form of therapy may be beneficial in a given patient while another is not.

If these therapeutic interventions fail to improve the patient, then a negative pressure ventilation[48] or a rocking bed can be used at night. Both these forms of therapy are uncomfortable and take time to become accustomed to. At times a given patient will not tolerate these interventions. The last form of therapy that should be tried is phrenic nerve pacing.[46–47,54] Electrodes are placed around one phrenic nerve with a receiver unit that is inserted subcutaneously. At night, an antenna is placed on the skin over the receiver. A transmitter is then turned on to stimulate the phrenic nerve and, in turn, the diaphragm. Different rates and amplitudes of stimulations can be given to develop the proper rate and volume of breathing. There are major drawbacks to this system, which include the morbidity from any routine surgical procedure, malfunctioning of the unit, and fibrosis of the phrenic nerve. The latter complication is reduced if the unit is used for less than 12 hours per day, or bilaterial implants are used with alternating sides.

A special note needs to be added regarding the common association between the narcolepsy-cataplexy syndrome and central apneas. Narcoleptics frequently present respiratory pauses during sleep, particularly rapid-eye movement sleep. The possibility exists that these patients could also develop the hemodynamic alterations that occur in other sleep apnea patients. One case report[55] showed that gammahydroxybutyrate relieved the major symptoms of narcolepsy and significantly decreased the number of apneic periods.

PRIMARY ALVEOLAR HYPOVENTILATION

Primary alveolar hypoventilation is defined as decreased alveolar ventilation leading to increased carbon dioxide retention that is not associated with apneas. This disorder is usually present during both the awake and sleep states but is greatly exacerbated during sleep. Primary alveolar hypoventilation may present only during sleep. All of the signs and symptoms associated with the sleep apnea syndromes may be associated with primary alveolar hypoventilation.[56–61]

The ventilatory responses to the chemical control of breathing are abnormal in primary alveolar hypoventilation.[56–62] This includes both the diminished response to hyperoxic hypercapnia and eucapnic hypoxia. The hypercapnia may occur only with sleep or while awake with further sleep related worsening. Patients with primary alveolar hypoventilation usually have normal pulmonary function tests. The development of arterial hypoxemia can be explained by the elevation in carbon dioxide levels. These patients can voluntarily hyperventilate and decrease the $PaCO_2$ toward normal resulting in a proportional increase in PaO_2. Usually one minute of supervised hyperventilation while drawing a blood gas during the hyperventilation episode will be enough to document the reversal of the carbon dioxide and oxygen tensions.

Treatment may be successful with one therapeutic modality or a combination may be needed. Respiratory stimulants are quite useful in primary alveolar hypoventilation. These include progesterone or a carbonic anhydrase inhibitor (see Central Apneas, above). Supplemental oxygen may be needed to prevent the severe nocturnal hypoxemia that develops.[57,58] Weight loss may be very beneficial if excessive obesity is present. If a rocking bed is tolerated, the $PaCO_2$ and PaO_2 can be reversed during sleep. Not all patients can tolerate such a device. If these fail, another intervention that may be tried is a negative-pressure ventilator. Lastly, phrenic nerve pacing is successful[46,47] but the possibility of significant complications exists (see Central Apneas, above).

REFERENCES

1. Martin RJ: Sleep-related respiratory disorders associated with daytime somnolence: Sleep apnea and hypoventilatory syndromes, in Cardiorespiratory Disorders During Sleep. Mount Kisco, NY, Futura Publishing Co., 1984, 65–117

2. Orr WC, Martin RJ: Obstructive sleep apnea associated with tonsillar hypertrophy in adults. Arch Intern Med 141:990–992, 1981

3. Yamamoto T, Hirose N, Miyoshi K: Polygraphic study of periodic breathing and hypersomnolence in a patient with severe hypothyroidism. Eur Neurol 15:188–193, 1977

4. Orr WC, Males JL, Imes, NK: Myxedema and obstructive sleep apnea. Am J Med 70:1061–1066, 1981

5. Mezon BJ, West P, MaClern JP: Sleep apnea in acromegaly. Am J Med 69:615–618, 1980

6. Barnes AJ, Pallis C, Joplin GF: Acromegaly and narcolepsy. Lancet 2:332–333, 1979

7. Issa FG, Sullivan CE: Alcohol, snoring and sleep apnoea. J Neurol Neurosurg Psychiat 45:353–59, 1982

8. Taasan VC, Blovic AJ, Biysen PG, Wynne JW: Alcohol increases sleep apnea and oxygen desaturation in asymptomatic men. Am J Med 71:240–245, 1981

9. Bonora M, Shields GI, Knuth SL, et al: Selective depression by ethanol of upper airway respiratory motor activity in cats. Am Rev Respir Dis 130:156–161, 1984

10. Hedemark L, Kronenberg R: Ventilatory responses to hypoxia and CO_2 during natural and flurazepim-induced sleep in normal adults. Chest 80:366, 1981

11. Bonora M, St. John WM, Bledsoe TA: Differential elevation by protriptyline and depression by diazepam of upper airway respiratory motor activity. Am Rev Respir Dis 131:41–45, 1985

12. Boudoulas H, Schmidt H, Geleris P, et al: Case reports on deterioration of sleep apnea during therapy with propranolol—preliminary studies. Res Comm Chem Pathol Pharmocol 39:3–10, 1983

13. Fletcher E, Lovoi, Miller J, Schaaf J: Propranolol and sleep apnea. Am Rev Respir Dis 131:A103, 1985

14. Guilleminault C, Van de Hoed J, Mitler MM: Clinical overviews of the sleep apnea syndromes, in Guilleminault C, Dement WC (eds): Sleep apnea syndromes. New York, Alan R. Liss, Inc. 1978, pp. 1–12

15. Harmen EM, Wynne JW, Block AJ: The effect of weight loss on sleep-disordered breathing and oxygen desaturation in morbidly obese men. Chest 82:291–294, 1982

16. Browman CP, Sampson MG, Yolles SF, et al: Obstructive sleep apnea and body weight. Chest 85:435–436, 1984

17. Martin RJ, Sanders MH, Gray BA et al: Acute and long-term ventilatory effects of hyperoxia in the adult sleep apnea syndrome. Am Rev Respir Dis 125:175–180, 1982

18. McNicholas WT, Carter JL, Rutherford R, et al: Beneficial effect of oxygen in primary alveolar hypoventilation with central sleep apnea. Am Rev Respir Dis 125:773–775, 1982

19. Guilleminault C, Cummiskey J: Progressive improvement of apnea index and ventilatory response to CO_2 after tracheostomy in obstructive sleep apnea syndrome. Am Respir Dis 126:14–20, 1982

20. Smith PL, Haponik EF, Bleecker ER: The ef-

fects of oxygen in patients with sleep apnea. Am Rev Respir Dis 130:958–963, 1984

21. Clark RW, Schmidt HS, Schaal SF, et al: Sleep apnea: Treatment with protriptyline. Neurol 29:1287–1292, 1979

22. Brownell LG, West P, Sweatman P, et al: Protriptyline in obstructive sleep apnea: A double blind trial. N Engl J Med 307:1037–1042, 1982

23. Lyons HA, Huang CT: Therapeutic use of progesterone in alveolar hypoventilation associated with obesity. Am J Med 44:881–888, 1968

24. Sutton FD, Zwillich CW, Creagh CE, et al: Progesterone for outpatient treatment of Pickwickian syndrome. Ann Intern Med 83:476–479, 1975

25. Strohl KP, Hensley MJ, Saunders NA, et al: Progesterone administration and progressive sleep apneas. J Am Med Assoc 245:1230–1232, 1981

26. Orr WC, Imes NK, Martin RJ: Progesterone therapy in obese patients with sleep apnea. Arch Intern Med 139:109–111, 1979

27. Rajagopal KR, Abbrecht PH, Jabbari B, Tellis CJ: The use of medroxyprogesterone acetate in obstructive sleep apnea. Chest 86:332, 1984

28. Remmers JE, Arch AM, deGroat WJ, et al: Oropharyngeal muscle tone in obstructive sleep apnea before and after strychnine. Sleep 447–453, 1980

29. Gothe B, Strohl KP, Levin S, Cherniack NS: Nicotine: A different approach to treatment of obstructive sleep apnea. Chest 87:11–17, 1985

30. Aranda JV, Turmen T: Methylxanthines in apnea of prematurity. Clin Perinatal 6:87–108, 1979

31. Laubie M, Schmitt H: Long lasting hyperventilation induced by almitrine: Evidence for a specific effect on carotid and thoracic chemoreceptors. Eur J Pharm 61:125–136, 1980

32. Krieger J, Mangin P, Kurtz D: Effects of almitrine in the treatment of sleep apnea syndrome. Bull Eur Physiopath Resp 19:630, 1983

33. Sullivan CE, Berthon-Jones M, Issa FG, Eves L: Reversal of obstructive sleep apnea by continuous positive airway pressure applied through the nares. Lancet 1:862–865, 1981

34. Sanders MH, Moore SE, Eveslage J: CPAP via nasal mask: A treatment for occlusion sleep apnea. Chest 83:144–145, 1983

35. Rapoport DM, Surkin B, Gasay SM, Goldring RM: Reversal of the "Pickwickian Syndrome" by long term use of nocturnal nasal airway pressure. N Engl J Med 307:931–933, 1982

36. Sullivan CE, Berthon-Jones M, Issa FG: Remission of severe obesity-hypoventilation syndrome after short-term treatment during sleep with continuous positive airway pressure. Am Rev Respir Dis 128:177–181, 1983

37. Sanders MH: Nasal CPAP effect on patterns of sleep. Chest 86:839–844, 1984

38. Rapoport DM, Geroy, Goldring RM: Nasal CPAP in obstructive sleep apnea: Mechanism of action. Bull Eur Physiopath 19:616–620, 1983

39. Sullivan CE, Issa FG, Bertron-Jones M, et al: Treatment of obstructive sleep apnea with continuous positive airway pressure applied through a nose-mask. Bull Eur Physiopath Resp 20:49–54, 1984

40. Guilleminault C, Hill MW, Simmons FB, Dement WC: Obstructive sleep apnea: Electromyographic and fiberoptic studies. Exp Neurol 62:48–67, 1978

41. Mahadevia AK, Oral E, Lopata M: Effects of expiratory positive airway pressure on sleep-induced respiratory abnormalities in patients with hypersomnia sleep apnea syndrome. Am Rev Respir Dis 128:708–711, 1983

42. Wilhoit SC, Brown ED, Suratt PM: Treatment of obstructive sleep apnea with continuous nasal airflow delivered through nasal prongs. Chest 85:170–73, 1984

43. Afzelius LE, Almqvist D, Houyaard K, et al: Sleep apnea syndrome—an alternative treatment to tracheostomy. Laryngoscope 41:285–291, 1981

44. Cartwright RD, Samelson CF: The effects of a non-surgical treatment for obstructive sleep apnea. The tongue retaining device. J Am Med Assoc 248:705–709, 1982

45. Martin RJ, Pennock BE, Orr WC, et al: Respiratory mechanics and timing during sleep in occlusive sleep apnea. J Appl Physiol: Respirat Environ Exercise Physiol 48:432–437, 1980

46. Farmer WC, Glenn WWL, Gee JBL: Alveolar hypoventilation syndrome. Am J Med 64:39–49, 1978

47. Glenn WWI, Gee JBL, Cole DR, et al: Combined central alveolar hypoventilation and upper airway obstruction. Am J Med 64:50–60, 1978

48. Man GCW, Jones RL, MacDonald GF, et al: Primary alveolar hypoventilation managed by negative-pressure ventilators. Chest 76:219–220, 1979

49. Hunt CE: Reversible central apnea in an infant with cyanotic heart disease. Chest 77:565–567, 1980

50. Reite M, Jackson D, Cahoun RL, et al: Sleep physiology at high altitude. Electroencephalogr Clin Neurophysiol 38:463–471, 1975

51. Sutton JR, Gray GW, Houston CS: Effects of duration at altitude and acetazolamide on ventilation and oxygenation during sleep. Sleep 3:454–455, 1980

52. Sutton JR, Lasser N: Pathophysiology of acute mountain sickness and high altitude pulmonary oedema: A hypothesis. Bull Eur Physiolpathol Resp 15:1045–1052, 1979

53. White DP, Zwillich C, Pckett CK, et al: Central sleep apnea: Improvement with acetazolamide therapy. Arch Int Med 142:1816–1819, 1982

54. Glenn WWL: Diaphragm pacing: Present status. Pace 1:357–370, 1978

55. Mamelak M, Webster P: Treatment of narcolepsy and sleep apnea wih gamma-hydroxybutyrate: A clinical and polysomnographic case study. Sleep 4:105–111, 1981

56. Naughton J, Block R, Welch M: Central alveolar hypoventilation. Am Rev Respir Dis 103:557–565, 1971

57. Bubis MJ, Anthonisen NR: Primary alveolar hypoventilation treated by nocturnal adminis-tration of oxygen. Am Rev Respir Dis 118:947–953, 1978

58. Barlow PB, Bartlett D, Hauri P, et al: Idiopathic hypoventilation syndrome: Importance of preventing nocturnal hypoxemia and hypercapnia. Am Rev Respir Dis 121:141–145, 1980

59. Rhoads GG, Brody JS: Idiopathic alveolar hypoventilation: Clinical spectrum. Ann Int Med 71:271–277, 1969

60. Lugliani R, Whipp BJ, Wasserman K: Doxapram hydrochloride. A respiratory stimulant for patients with primary alveolar hypoventilation. Chest 76:414–419, 1979

61. Hyland RH, Jones NL, Powles ACP, et al: Primary alveolar hypoventilation treated with nocturnal electrophrenic respiration. Am Rev Respir Dis 117:165–172, 1978

62. Wolkove N, Altose MD, Kelsen SG, et al: Respiratory control abnormalities in alveolar hypoventilation. Am Rev Respir Dis 122:163–167, 1980

Martin A. Cohn

6
Surgical Treatment in Sleep Apnea Syndrome

This chapter will deal with several important areas related to the surgical treatment of obstructive sleep apnea including physiological function and clinical evaluation of the upper airway; specific ear, nose, and throat surgical procedures to consider regardless of the presence or absence of specific anatomic pathologies; surgical approach to the treatment of obesity; and pre- and post-operative patient management. Surgery for obstructive sleep apnea is only one of several treatment choices available (Table 6-1), the selection of which will depend on many factors particular to each patient. Surgery may be the first treatment choice (i.e., tracheostomy in life-threatening disease), the last (i.e., uvulopalatopharyngoplasty [UPPP] after failure of nonsurgical treatment in milder sleep apnea), or combined with medical or additional surgical approaches (i.e., nasal septoplasty, UPPP, tracheostomy, and weight reduction diet). Surgical approaches for treating obstructive sleep apnea are relatively recent, the first use of tracheostomy being described in 1969.[1] These surgical approaches are often combined with medical therapy, and their novelty explain the paucity of well-designed, controlled, clinical studies to determine the efficacy of these procedures. Eventually, information from large cooperative multi-center studies will help the clinician define the patient subgroups most likely to respond to a particular surgical procedure and reduce the number of treatment failures. With continued research and development of more specific medical treatment choices (such as nasal continuous positive airway pressure), surgical approaches will play a lesser role in the management of such patients.

ABNORMALITIES OF RESPIRATION DURING SLEEP
ISBN 0-8089-1812-5 Copyright © 1986 by Grune & Stratton, Inc.
All rights of reproduction in any form reserved.

Table 6-1
Treatment of Obstructive Sleep Apnea

I. Nonsurgical
   1. Oxygen
   2. Protriptyline
   3. Medroxyprogesterone
   4. Weight Reduction
   5. Avoidance of Supine Sleeping Position
   6. Tongue Retaining Device
   7. Nasopharyngeal Airway
   8. Nasal Continuous Positive Airway Pressure (CPAP)
II. Surgical
   1. Nasal Surgery
   2. Tonsillectomy and Adenoidectomy
   3. Uvulopalatopharyngoplasty
   4. Tracheostomy
   5. Mandibular, Maxillary, and Hyoid Bone Reconstruction

ANATOMY AND PHYSIOLOGY OF THE UPPER AIRWAY: SURGICAL CONSIDERATIONS

The upper airway is divided into the naso-, oro-, and hypo-pharynx. The first two are separated by the soft palate and the latter two by the tip of the epiglottis. To understand the physiology of obstructive sleep apnea, the upper airway may be considered a Y-shaped tube whose patency is dependent on the tone of muscles within its collapsible walls (Fig. 6-1). The naso- and oro-pharynx make up the two arms of the "Y" and the hypo-pharynx the base of the "Y". They meet at a common focal point consisting of the distal uvular tip of the soft palate, posterior pharyngeal wall, and base of the tongue. In addition to maintaining rigidity of its wall, other muscles act as valves controlling flow through the two arms of the "Y". The anterior nares have the smallest total cross-sectional area in the respiratory tract, patency being controlled by the alae nasi muscles.[2] The large number of muscles of the soft palate allow fine control of movement control shifting from nasal to oral breathing.[3] Such control has been shown to differ in males and females, the latter being unable to elevate their palate to the same degree as males.[4] In addition, the thickness and length of the soft palate help determine its position relative to the base of the tongue and degree of obstruction at the crucial focal point of the "Y" configuration. In this respect, the soft palate may be considered to function as a fine needle valve such that the slightest displacement towards or away from the "Y" greatly affects airflow resistance and, thus, collapsibility.

Although an oversimplification, obstructive sleep apnea is primarily an inspiratory pathologic event. Inspiratory airflow results from the generation of subatmospheric pressure within the thoracic cavity produced by the contraction of the diaphragm and accessory muscles of respiration. The resultant airflow through the upper airway and tracheobronchial tree conforms with aerodynamic principles relating airflow resistance to pressure and flow; i.e., airflow is directly related to the pressure gradient across a tube and inversely related to its resistance. As described

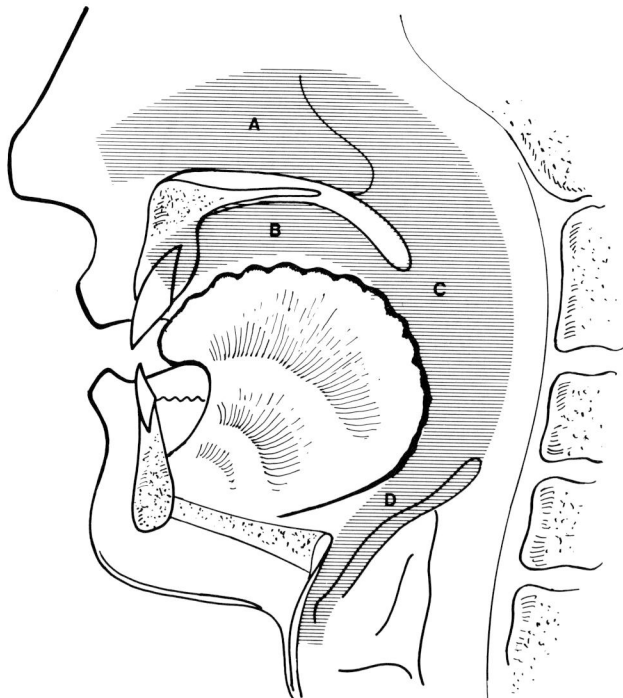

Fig. 6-1. Drawing of the upper airway showing relationship of the various anatomic divisions. A = nasal passage; B = oral cavity; C = area where naso and oro pharynx join; D = opening to larynx. See text for explanation.

above, portions of the upper airway may be considered a collapsible tube with the rigidity of its walls dependent upon the tone of the palate, pharynx, and tongue muscles. To maintain patency it must overcome the intrapharyngeal subatmospheric pressure that tends to collapse the tube at its narrowest part.

In addition, since the magnitude of inspiratory downstream subatmospheric pressure is determined by the most upstream point of obstruction, correction of the latter may reduce or eliminate the downstream airway "collapse." For example, during nasal breathing the increase in airflow resistance produced with nasal obstruction will result in a more negative subatmospheric downstream pressure for a given airflow and, thus, a greater tendency for upper airway collapse and obstruction. Relief may require the opening of the mouth or active dilatation of the oropharynx through participation of the muscles of the soft palate. Such nasal obstruction may be physiologic, i.e., associated with recumbency[5–8] or with the nasal cycle.[9] Indeed, is it likely that pathologic fixed unilateral nasal obstruction in combination with closure of the nonpathologic nasal passage during sleep may result in complete bilateral nasal obstruction and the appearance of obstructive sleep apnea events.

That nasal obstruction can contribute to the development of obstructive sleep apnea is well established.[10–13] Medically and surgically treatable causes of nasal obstruction include allergic and vasomotor rhinitis,[14] adenoid hypertrophy,[15–17] nasal septal deviation,[18] nasopharyngeal stenosis, craniofacial anomalies, choanal atresia, polyps, and tumors.[19] In newborn infants, nasal obstruction in relation to viral naso-pharyngitis has been implicated in sudden infant death syndrome ("crib death"; see Chapter 11).[20] The newborn is believed to be an "obligate nose breather" (although recent evidence refutes this claim[21]) and is unable to switch easily from nasal to oral breathing in the face of nasal obstruction. Therefore, nasal obstruction theoretically could be potentially lethal, presumably via the development of obstructive sleep apnea,[22] leading to hypoxia and fatal cardiac arrhythmias.

The oropharynx (from the mouth to the end of the soft palate) is most suscepti-ble to inspiratory collapse at the focal point where the base of the tongue and uvular portion of the soft palate meet. Since airflow resistance through a circular tube is related to the fourth power of its radius, small changes in the latter markedly affect the degree of subatmospheric pressure generated as well as the inward pulling pressure produced by the venturi effect. Thus, treatment to increase luminal diame-ter a few millimeters (medically or surgically) may result in marked physiologic and clinical improvement.

On occasion, the hypopharynx (from the tip of the soft palate to the larynx) may be the only contributing point of inspiratory obstruction due to increased airflow resistance from an enlarged or posteriorly displaced tongue (retrognathia), hypertro-phied lingular tonsils, or other abnormal tissue (lingual cyst, lymphoma).

Clinical evaluation of the upper airway in sleep apnea patients is extremely important since specific surgical correction of recognized obstructing lesions is usually the preferred treatment. History of nasal obstruction (due to epistaxis, aller-gic rhinitis, fractures, mouth breathing) may aid in choosing medical or surgical treatment since improving nasal patency is often necessary to allow maximal pa-tency downstream. Indeed, surgical outfracture of the nasal turbinates is often re-quired to achieve adequate improvement from UPPP (see below). A hypopharyngeal level of obstruction is suggested by a history of frequent sore throats and tonsillitis in children and young adults with sleep apnea. Tonsillectomy alone may be corrective in such patients, especially children.[23]

Physical examination of the naso- and oro-pharynx for obstructing tissue may reveal obvious pathology. Often, however, the obstruction is only apparent during sleep or while the patient is under anesthesia prior to surgery.

Several diagnostic techniques have been used for evaluating and defining the level of pharyngeal obstruction. For example, fiberoptic endoscopy of the nasophar-ynx (during sleep and voluntary respiratory maneuvers while awake), lateral neck fluoroscopy, and computed tomography of the pharynx may help determine the likelihood of success of UPPP. Similarly, cephalometric assessment of maxillary, mandibular, and hyoid bone relationships may help support the indication for man-dibular and/or hyoid bone reconstructive surgery (see below).

SURGICAL PROCEDURES

When specific obstructing pathologic tissue is recognized, its removal is often curative.[24-27] Usually, however, the sleep-induced upper airway obstruction is appar-ent only during sleep, a time when the tone of the pharyngeal musculature de-creases.

SEPTOPLASTY

It is well demonstrated that nasal obstruction induces or worsens apnea in asymptomatic individuals.[10,28] There may be several reasons why this happens. Airflow and pressure changes over the nasal mucosa have been shown to increase pharyngeal and genioglossus muscle electromyogram (EMG) activity.[29] Absence of airflow may do the opposite. Thus, reduced airflow through the nasal passages could increase the pressure/EMG relationship by reducing EMG activity.[30] Alternatively, simple mechanical obstruction could lead to an increased pharyngeal resistance, a *more* negative intraairway pressure, and an increased pressure/EMG ratio. Several reports have shown that correction of nasal obstruction by septoplasty and submucosal resection has resulted in amelioration or cure of the apnea.[26,31] However, cases are also reported where elimination of the obstruction did not correct the apnea.[32]

TRACHEOSTOMY

Prior to a few years ago, tracheostomy was the only long term treatment available for patients with severe disease or who failed medical approaches. Tracheostomy is essentially curative for obstructive sleep apnea regardless of location of the upstream obstruction.[33–35] Any associated components of sleep-induced respiratory failure (hypoventilation or central apneas) may or may not improve following surgery.[36,37] For example, patients with a combination of obstructive sleep apnea and chronic obstructive lung disease may also require supplemental oxygen in order to eliminate any REM-sleep associated hypoxia unrelated to upper airway obstruction.[38]

Tracheostomy is not without post-operative complications and psychosocial difficulties.[39] A tracheostomy requires patient and family cooperation in cleaning and caring for the stoma, which can be complicated by infection, bleeding (usually inconsequential), and granulation tissue with subsequent obstruction. Such obstruction may interfere with respiration around the tube, speech, or eventual decannulation and require laser surgery for correction. Tracheostomy tubes often promote secretion production, which becomes malodorous.

With a readily available nasal continuous positive airway pressure (CPAP) system (SleepEasy®, Respironics, Inc., 530 Seco Road, Monroeville, PA), patients (with severe disease in whom nasal CPAP is shown to be effective during sleep) may be removed from the danger list, thus, allowing more time for medical or other surgical procedures that are more acceptable than tracheostomy, to take effect. However, a tracheostomy may still be needed in select patients with severe obstructive sleep apnea. For example, it should be considered in patients with (1) moderate to severe symptoms including somnolence, cerebral dysfunction with impaired social functioning or work ability; (2) secondary pulmonary hypertension or cor pulmonale; (3) life threatening arrhythmias (heart block, ventricular irritability) resulting from the upper airway obstruction; (4) strong patient motivation to have immediate cure along with capability of cleaning and caring for stoma and tube; and (5) severe desaturation or very high apnea index on polysomnography. The definition of "severe" is arbitrary but would include patients considered at risk for sudden death during sleep. For example in a massively obese (over 100 pounds above ideal body weight) with frequent apneas (over 50 per hour), were desaturation (below 60 percent) and signs of cor pulmonale, tracheostomy may be a more appropriate choice than nasal CPAP. The compliance with long term CPAP may fall to 50 percent of apnea patients tried (personal observation M. Cohn). In the severe patient it may be safer to institute curative treatment (tracheostomy) early. More recently tracheostomy is used to temporize and protect the airway during anesthesia while other surgical procedures for sleep apnea are carried out (UPP, mandibular advancement, etc.).

Surgical techniques vary from surgeon to surgeon and depend partly on the type of tracheostomy tube to be selected. Some prefer to use a skin flap to enable patency of the opening without the use of any tube. All tracheostomy tubes have advantages and disadvantages. In general, a tube with a removable inner cannula is preferable since it allows for easy removal and cleaning. The standard silver tube is readily available and reusable, but it is expensive to replace lost parts and the tube is not provided with a plug or cap. A Dow-Corning Silastic® (Dow-Corning Corporation, Midland, MI) tracheostomy tube is flexible, more comfortable than rigid tubes, and is approximately two centimeters longer than comparable size tubes, an advantage in morbidly obese patients. The Shiley® (Shiley, Inc., Irvine, CA) tracheostomy tubes provide lock-on caps and come with or without fenestrations and/or cuffs. Cuffs are necessary for post-operative positive pressure ventilation via respirators and helpful in preventing aspiration of oral secretions and feedings. A fenestrated tube has a small hole in the distal end of the tube such that when the tube is capped, flow of air through the trachea occurs through the fenestration as well as around the tube. However, in obese patients, the fenestration may be positioned within the soft tissue of the neck and become fixed by granulation tissue, making removal difficult. By using the smallest diameter tube (#6 with a 10mm outer diameter), there is usually sufficient distance between the walls of the trachea and tube to allow for unrestricted airflow, thus avoiding the necessity of a fenestrated tube. Alternatively, the "button" type of tube (which does not project fully within the lumen of the trachea) may be used (Montgomery Tracheal Cannula, Boston Medical Products, Inc., Boston, MA). However, patients may find removal and reinsertion more difficult than when using conventional tubes.

Several immediate post-operative complications of tracheostomy tubes are particularly likely in the obese sleep apnea patient. Accidental dislodgement of the tracheostomy tube may occur shortly after surgery and may be related to an inadequate length of tube such that soft tissue swelling may result in the tube tip being pulled out from the lumen of the trachea. If this occurs during the first three days after surgery, it is best for the surgeon to replace the tube since reinsertion is difficult prior to establishment of a fistulous tract.

UVULOPALATOPHARYNGOPLASTY

More recently, uvulopalatopharyngoplasty (UPPP), originally described for the treatment of snoring,[40] has been applied to obstructive sleep apnea. The technique varies somewhat among the different surgeons,[41–43] but all have the goal of shortening the soft palate and increasing the lateral dimensions of the pharynx at the tonsillar level (Fig. 6-2). If necessary, redundant posterior pharyngeal tissue may be removed to enlarge the posterior pharyngeal space. A UPPP takes approximately one hour to complete and has little morbidity and rare mortality.[44] Post-operative pain

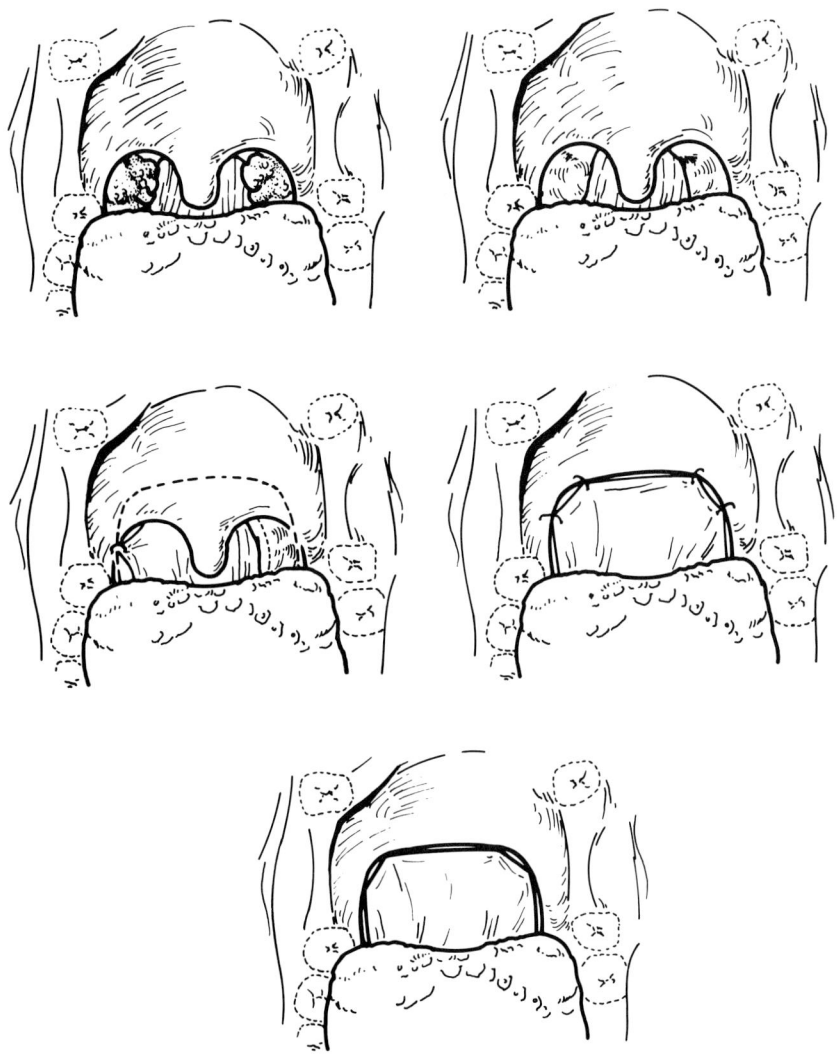

Fig. 6-2. Representation of the surgical steps involved in uvulopalatopharyngoplasty. Upper Left: view of oropharynx from the oral cavity. Upper Right: tonsilar tissue has been removed. Middle Left: tonsilar fossa closed, posterior pharyngeal wall "stretched," and soft palate marked for resection. Middle Right: membranous portion of the soft palate is resected. Bottom: finished procedure. Drawing courtesy of Dr. Stanley E. Thawley. (From Thawley SE, Shepard JW, Jr: Understanding the sleep apnea syndrome: Causes and treatment. VA Practitioner January: 60–83, 1985. With permission.)

subsides gradually over several weeks during which swallowing may be difficult or associated with nasal regurgitation. Permanent palatal incompetence has been described only rarely and is usually minimized if the patient swallows carefully. The patient's voice is usually not affected although there may be some concern about its effect on certain sounds.[45] In addition to relief of loud snoring in most patients, the effect of UPPP on symptoms can be as dramatic as tracheostomy with improvement in the severity of obstructive sleep apnea events and daytime sleepiness in many. The post-operative response to surgery can be measured by subjective assessment of amelioration of symptoms and objective changes in severity of upper airway obstruction during polysomnography.

Table 6-2 summarizes published reports of the short-term results of UPPP showing an overall reduction in the apnea/hypopnea index (AHI, number of events per hour sleep) from 57.8 pre-operatively to 30.5 post-operatively. The percent of UPPP surgeries reducing the AHI to less than 50 percent of the pre-operative baseline averaged 56.8 percent. This compares favorably to a report* of 254 UPPP patients from contributing Sleep Disorders Centers (Jackson, MI; Miami Beach, FL; St. Louis, MO; Stanford, CA; Oklahoma City, OK; Detroit, MI), 117 (46 percent) of whom achieved similar benefit. And it is this group of responders that appears to have the greatest improvement in sleepiness as measured by the multiple sleep latency test.[47] It should also be noted from the table that if patients are followed clinically without follow-up polysomnography there appears to be a much greater success rate of UPPP, i.e., about 85 percent. Indeed, probably only a minority (less than 50 percent) of patients are actually "cured" (i.e., less than 5–10 apneas per hour) by UPPP.

Long term follow-up studies suggest that relapse in symptoms and sleep apnea events may occur and may be associated with subsequent weight gain. Zorick[59] reported a continued improvement in symptoms and sleep apnea events in 12-month follow-up of 20 "responders" with stable body weight. However, Schoen[60] showed progressive relapse in sleep apnea events in 8 patients restudied 6 months and 12 months post-operatively and associated this with weight gain.

Since UPPP response has been shown to be so variable, various attempts have been made to pre-operatively predict those patients who are most likely to respond. Simple inspection of the pharyngeal aperture's size is insufficient to predict response[43] and massively obese patients appear to have poor surgical results.[51]

Ear, Nose, Throat (ENT) Exam including Fiberoptic Nasopharyngoscopy.[61–63]   A small fiberoptic scope may be passed through the nose and positioned above the velopharyngeal sphincter. This area is observed during quiet respiration and during Muller maneuvers with the physician partially then completely occluding the nasal airway by squeezing the external nares. The scope is then advanced to the area above the base of the tongue where the same maneuvers are used (Fig. 6-3). The tendency of these areas to collapse during negative airway pressure is an indication of where the obstruction is likely to occur during sleep. Correlation with UPPP success is lacking.

Computerized Tomography.   During computerized tomography (CT) the patient is scanned in the supine position, awake, from the nasopharyngeal area using 1 cm cuts through the lower hypopharyngeal area. Airway cross sectional area is calculated using a computer wand. First used in apneics in 1982, it has proven several things.[64,65] Apneic groups can be separated from control groups based upon awake determination of airway size but apnea cannot be diagnosed by this method (Fig. 6-3). Tissue of fat density *does not* play a physical role in the pharyngeal airway narrowing of apneics.

Attempts are being made to correlate surgical therapy with CT changes (Fig. 6-4). There is a change in airway diameter following UPPP but the CT has not yet

---

*Presented by Dr. Tom Roth at the 50th Scientific Assembly of the American College of Chest Physicians, Dallas, Texas, October 12, 1984.

Table 6-2
Uvulopalatopharyngoplasty—A Review of Results

Reference	Number of Subjects	Multiple Sleep Latency Test (min)		Subjective Improvement		Apnea/Hypopnea Index		Over 50% Reduction in Apnea/Hypopnea Index	
		Pre-Op	Post-Op	N	(%)	Pre-Op	Post-Op	Number	(% of Total)
Fujita[41]	12	—	—	11	(92%)	54.0	27.7	8	75%
Hernandez[42]	10	—	—	10	(100%)	—	—	—	—
Simmons[43]	18	—	—	15	(83%)	45.4	28.7	9	45%
Silvestri[46]	14*	3.7‡	5.3	14	(100%)	45.9	36.1	7	50%
Zorick[47]	31	3.9	6.6	—	—	61.9	29.9	16	52%
(16 responders)		(3.4)	(9.6)	—	(94%)	(64.4)	(11.7)	—	—
(15 nonresponders)		(4.4)	(3.7)	—	(58%)	(59.2)	(49.4)	—	—
Walsh[48]	11	—	—	5	(45%)	73.8	58.7	—	—
Cohn[49]	92	—	—	72	(81%)	65.8§	34.4	—	—
Smith[50]	7	3	4	7	(100%)	64.0	25.0	—	—
Guilleminault[51]	35†	—	—	31	(89%)	—	—	27	69%‖
Fujita[52]	66	—	—	—	—	—	—	33	50%
(33 responders)						58.3	9.5		
(33 nonresponders)						60.2	55.4		
Schoen[53]	13	—	—	—	—	58	22	10	77%
Thorpy[54]	15	—	—	15	(100%)	92	27	—	—
Santamaria[55]	24	—	—	—	—	34	13	15	63%
Askenasy[56]	10	—	—	—	—	—	—	4	40%
Norman[57]	43	—	—	—	—	52.5	40.5	19	44%
Scrima[58]	15	—	—	—	—	43.7	18.4	9	60%
Total	416	—	—	180	(85%)	57.8	30.5	157	56.8%

* = Heavy snorers with only hypopneas excluded.
† = Severe patients requiring tracheostomy excluded.
‡ = 5 patients.
§ = 19 patients.
‖ = Estimated from data.

125

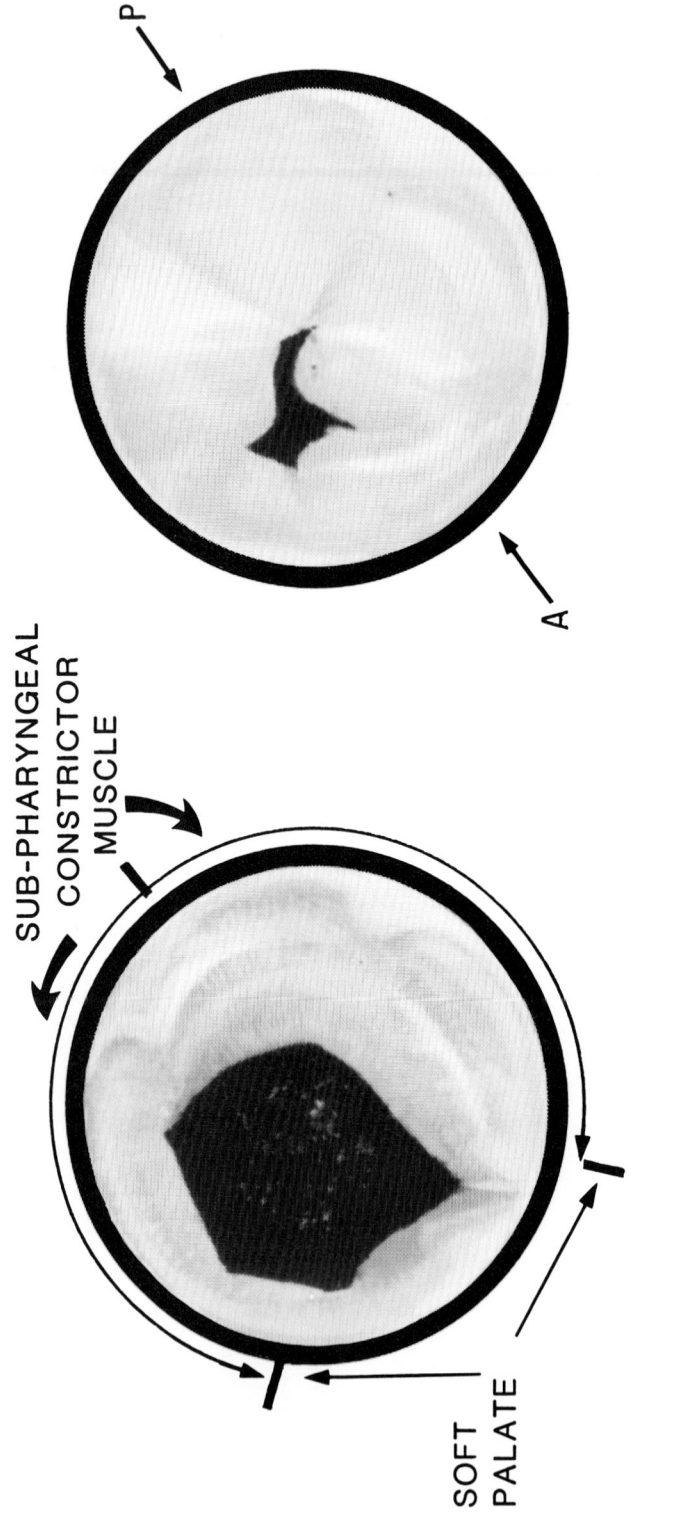

SUB-PHARYNGEAL
CONSTRICTOR
MUSCLE

SOFT
PALATE

EARLY EXPIRATION

BEGIN INSPIRATION

Fig. 6-3. Velopharyngeal constrictor viewed from above through fiberoptic scope. The soft palate is located at the lower left side of both figures. During inspiration against a closed mouth and nose, the soft palate and posterior pharyngeal tissue collapse, simulating an obstructive apnea at the level of the naso-oral-pharyngeal junction.

126

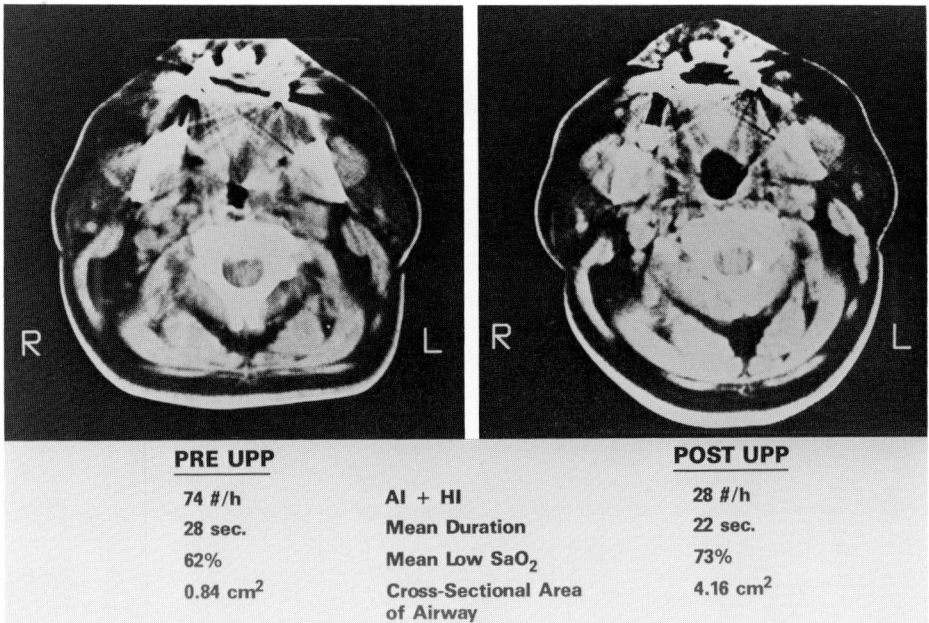

PRE UPP		POST UPP
74 #/h	AI + HI	28 #/h
28 sec.	Mean Duration	22 sec.
62%	Mean Low SaO$_2$	73%
0.84 cm^2	Cross-Sectional Area of Airway	4.16 cm^2

Fig. 6-4. Computerized tomography at the level of the naso-oro-pharynx, before and after uvulopalatopharyngoplasty, in the same patient. The apnea plus hypopnea index was reduced from 74 to 28 per hour, corresponding to an increase in airway cross sectional diameter from 0.84 cm^2 to 4.16 cm^2. Photograph courtesy of John W. Sheppard, Jr., M.D.

been used to determine those in whom UPPP will be successful. One author has been able to detect changes in the resting awake cross sectional area of the various levels of the upper airway by CT before and after UPP. The CT's success in predicting the outcome of UPP in an individual subject was less than perfect.[66]

Somnofluoroscopy. A recent approach that appears promising is fluoroscopy of the neck. Somnofluoroscopy was previously used in studying soft palate mechanics.[67] Smirne[68] described the thick, elongated uvula in a patient with Pickwickian Syndrome using lateral neck x-rays. Several authors[69–72] described fluorocopic observations of the lateral neck as a diagnostic tool in children with sleep apnea. Weitzman[73] observed that airway closure during sleep apnea in adults occurred between the top of the tongue and the junction between the naso-pharynx and the oro-pharynx. Suratt[74] compared lateral neck fluoroscopy during obstructive apneas to computed tomographic scans of the pharynx. Cross table lateral fluoroscopy is obtained with the patient supine and hopefully, asleep. The retro-palatal area and retro-glossus area can be clearly observed. The first area to obstruct during an apnea would be the area most likely to benefit from surgery. For example, a patient whose obstruction begins by closure of the area between the tongue and posterior pharyngeal wall is unlikely to benefit from UPPP alone. A patient whose apnea begins with apposition of the soft palate against the posterior pharyngeal wall followed by "sucking" of the soft palate and tongue inward might benefit from UPPP. Correlation with success of UPPP is lacking. Walsh[75] applied a similar technique[76] in order to predict UPPP success and showed that those patients with initial collapse above the hypopharyngeal level demonstrated a good response to UPPP. Using more quantitative approaches to assess functional relationships of anatomic structures[77] may further improve predictability of response to UPPP.

Cephalometrics. This technique was previously used for analysis of facial growth and development and dental and skeletal abnormalities (Fig. 6-5). The modified measurements felt to be important in apneics[78] appear in Figure 6-4. Angle SNA (maxilla) and SNB (mandible)—should be 82 ± 2 degrees and 80 ± 2 degrees, respectively. Lesser angles indicate maxillary or mandibular deficiencies that may be contributing to apnea. PAS (posterior airway space)—in normals is 11 ± 1 mm. Apneics with a 3–4 mm PAS may not benefit from UPPP alone since the obstruction is behind the tongue. PNS-Pg (soft palate)—in normals is 37 ± 3 mm (PNS-Pg). A longer soft palate may indicate that UPPP would be helpful (Fig. 6-6). MPH (hyoid position)—in normals is 15.4 ± 3 mm below a perpendicular along the inferior border of the mandible. A low hyoid usually accompanies a small PAS and implies poor results from UPPP alone.[79]

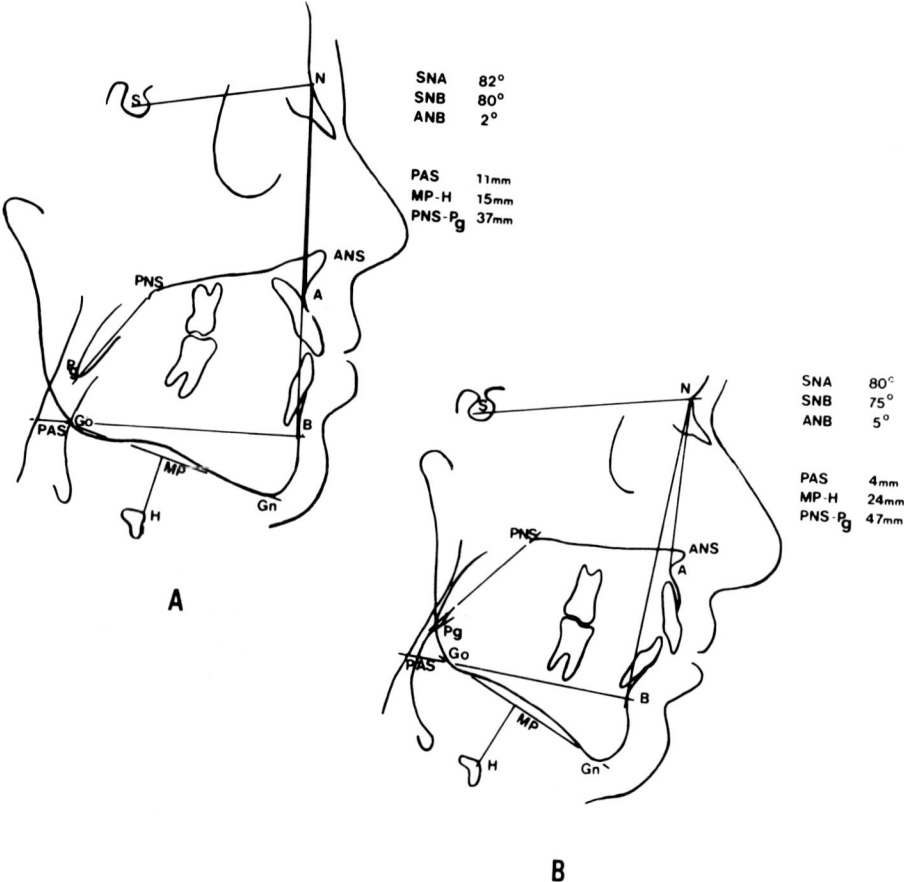

Fig. 6-5. Diagramatic representation of cephalometric measurements in normal subject (A) and one with slight retroagnathia (B). Note the narrow posterior airspace (PAS) and long soft palate (PNS-Pg) in example B. See text for explanation and normal values. (From Riley R, et al: Sleep 6(4):303–11, 1983. With permission.)

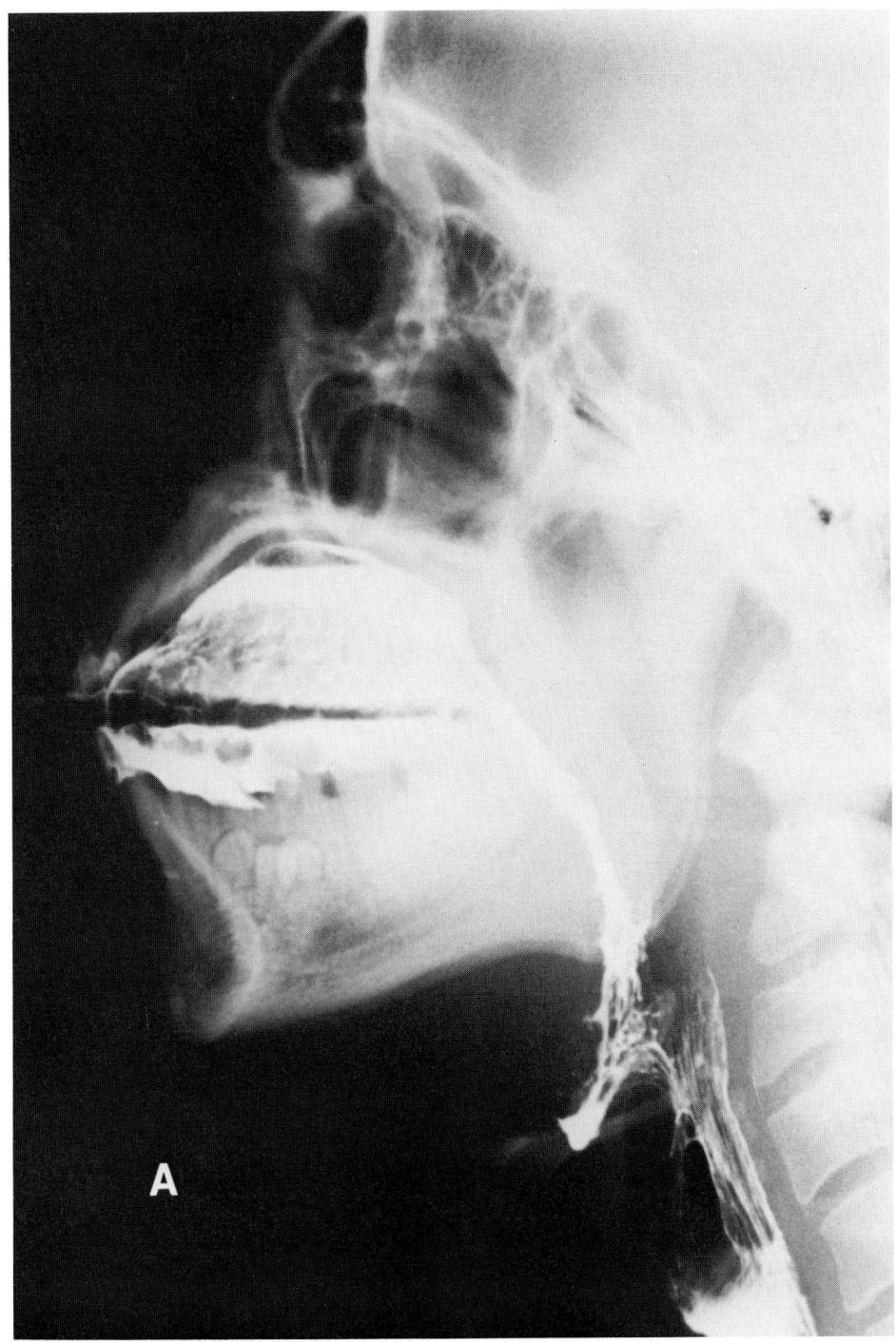

Fig. 6-6. (*Continues on next page.*)

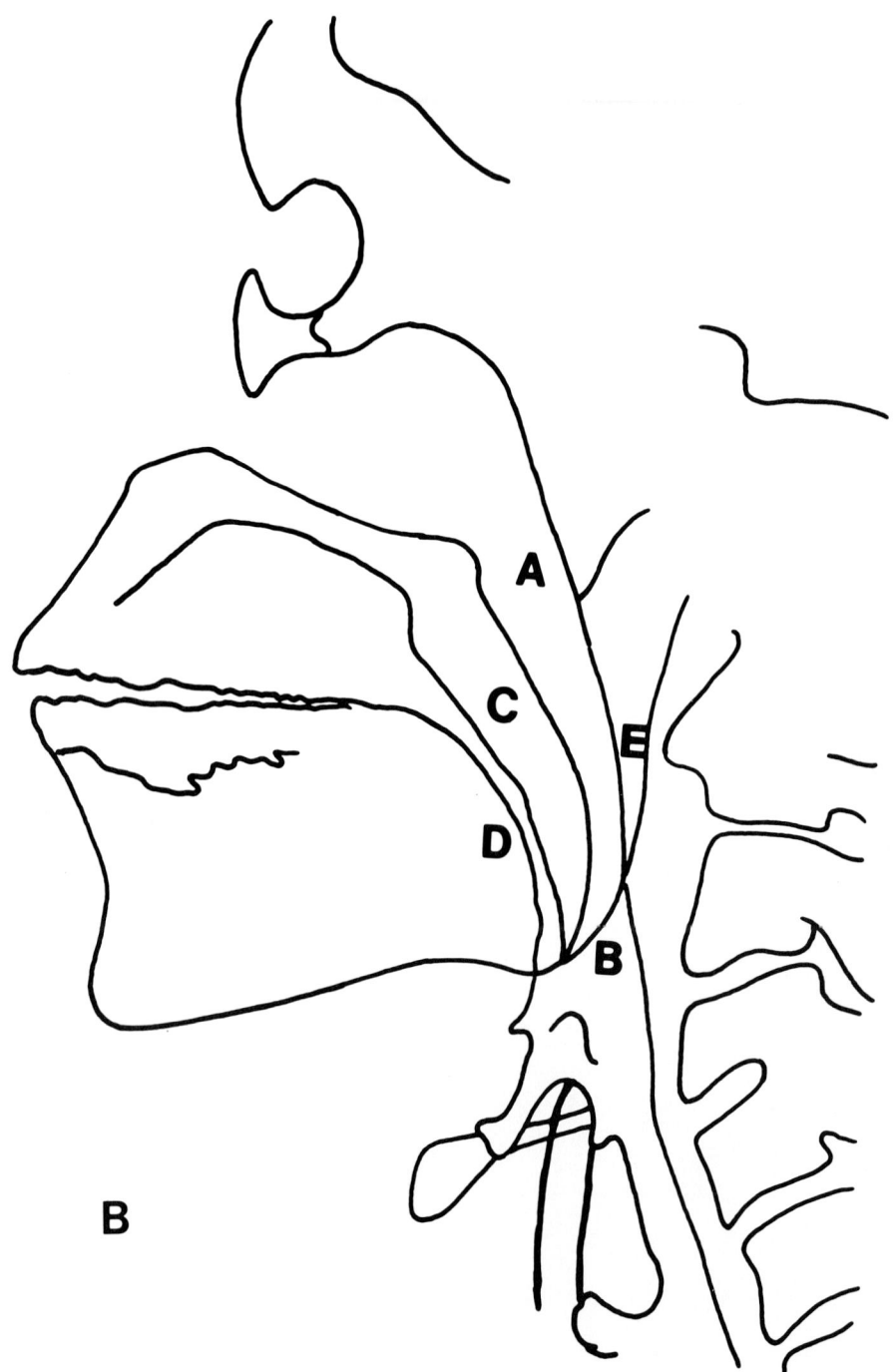

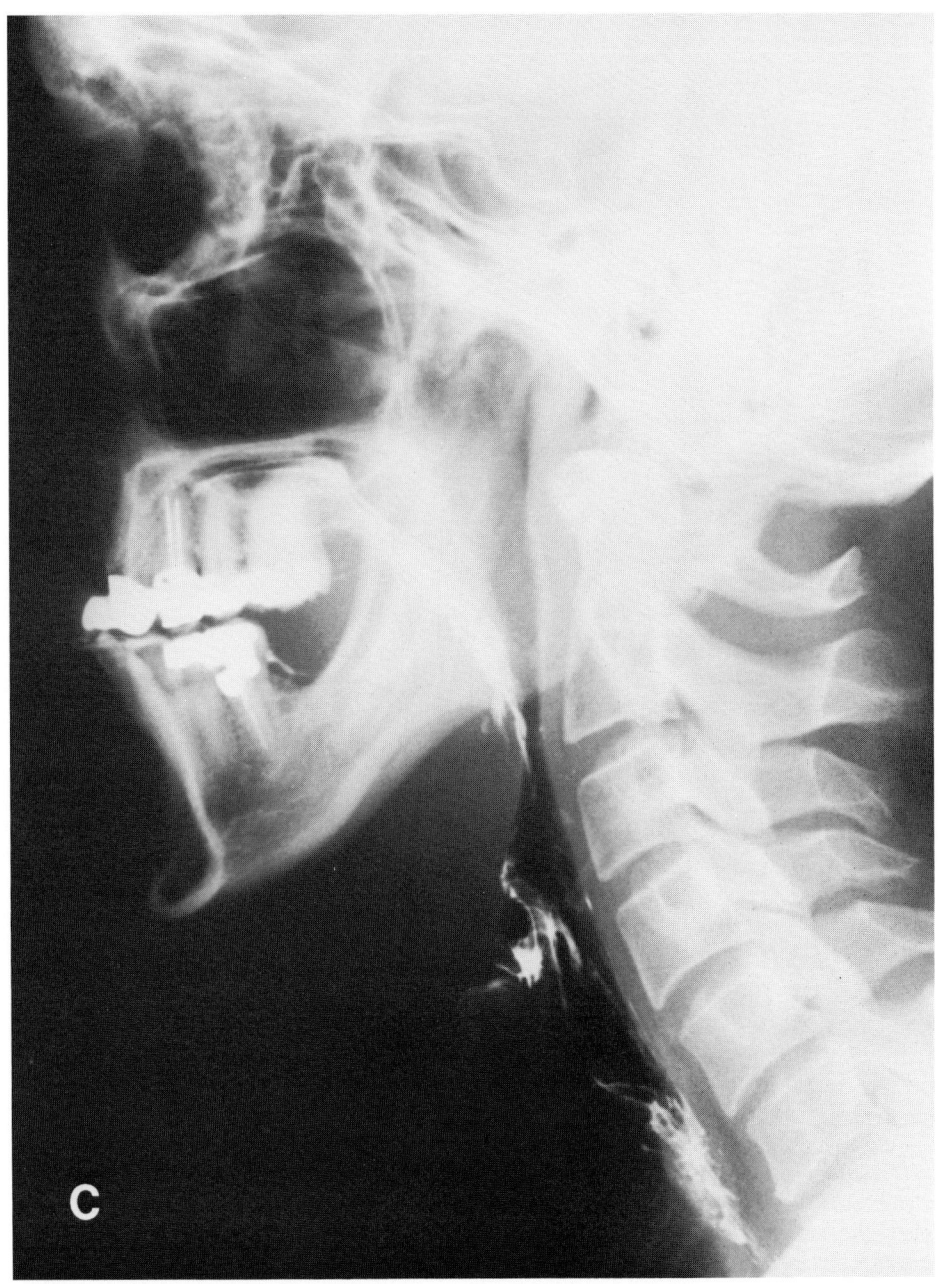

Fig. 6-6. (*Continues on next page.*)

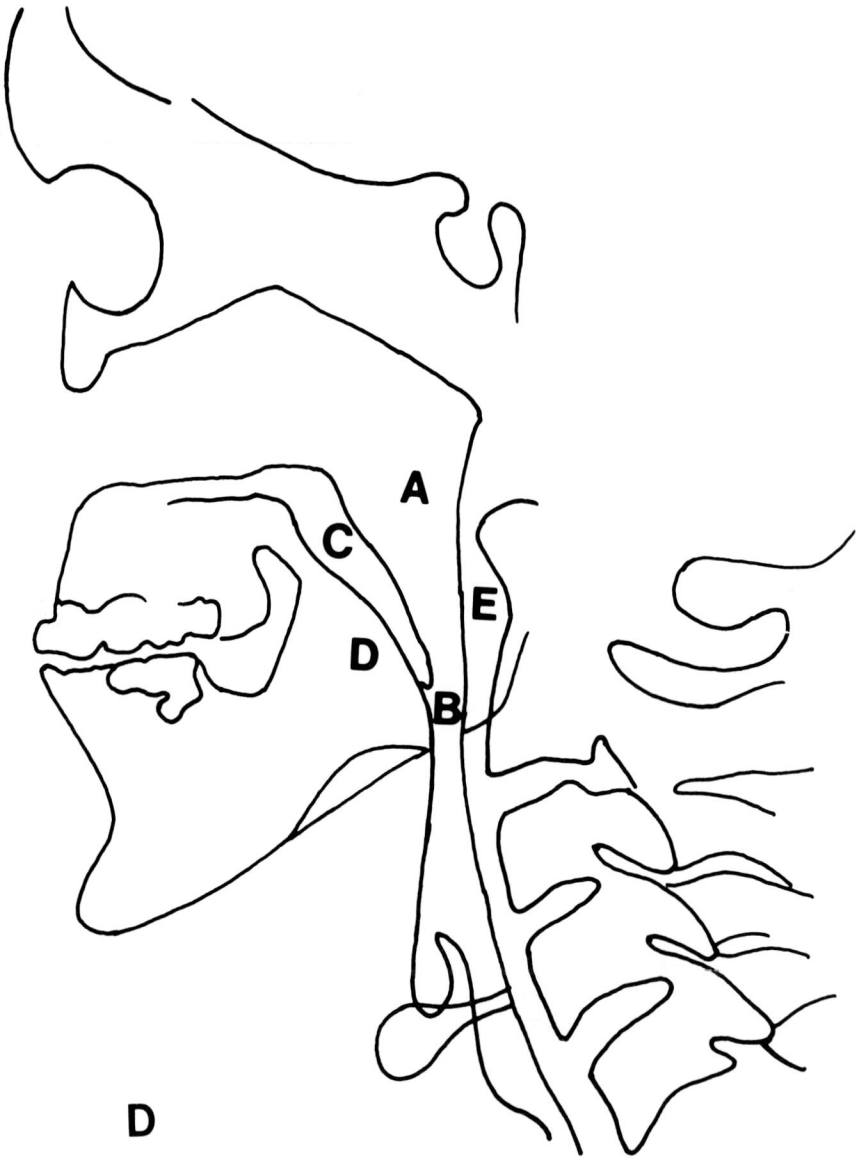

D

Fig. 6-6. (*Continued.*) (A) Lateral head cephalometric roentgenogram in a patient with severe obstructive sleep apnea. A = nasopharynx, B = posterior airspace (width, 20 mm), C = soft palate and uvula (length, 74 mm), D = tongue, E = posterior pharyngeal wall. Notice normal size of the posterior airspace behind the tongue and the large uvula. This patient was felt to be an excellent candidate, and underwent uvulopalatopharyngoplasty with good results. (B) Lateral head cephalometric roentgenogram in a patient with severe obstructive sleep apnea. A through E represent same structures as in figure 6A. The soft palate was only slightly above normal in size (length, 42 mm) but the posterior airway was small throughout the length of the pharynx including the hypopharynx (width, 3 mm). This patient was not considered a uvulopalatopharyngoplasty candidate and instead, was treated with continuous positive airway pressure (CPAP). Photographs and cases courtesy of Eugene C. Fletcher M.D.

Acoustic Reflection.   This is a recently developed research technique[80] that is completely noninvasive. Sound from a loud speaker is reflected by pharyngeal and glottic structures. The returning waves are detected and analyzed by computer to give the cross sectional area of the pharynx at all levels. Studies have documented increased pharyngeal cross sectional airway after a 68 kg weight loss in an apneic patient who went from 117 apneas/hr to 8 apneas/hr.[81]

MANDIBULAR RECONSTRUCTION

Posterior displacement of the tongue in association with micrognathia and retrognathia can cause obstructive sleep apnea.[82–87] Kuo[88] and Bear[89] successfully corrected the obstructive sleep apnea in such patients via surgical advancement of the mandible. Spire[90] suggested lateral cephalometric radiographic assessment of all obstructive sleep apnea patients to detect significant retrognathia that might not be clinically apparent. Riley[91] demonstrated mandibular deficiencies not recognized clinically in 6 of 10 obstructive sleep apnea patients. Powell[78] described a technical modification to further enlarge the hypopharyngeal space in three patients with obstructive sleep apnea and retrognathia. Patton[92] described an expansion hyoid-plasty in dogs, a new technique to open the hypopharyngeal space and decrease its collapsibility (Figs. 6-7 and 6-8). Kaya[93] performed sectioning of the hyoid bone in three patients with obstructive sleep apnea with dramatic results. Riley[94] modified this technique by suspending the hyoid bone with fascia (hyoidmyotomy suspension) combined with mandibular osteotomy in a patient with severe obstructive sleep apnea and obtained excellent response (Fig. 6-9).

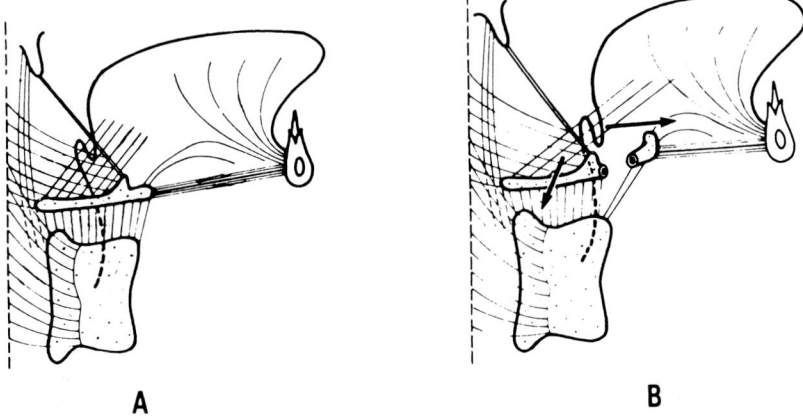

A   **B**

Fig. 6-7.   (A) Lateral view of the musculoskeletal anatomy of the pharynx showing the relationship of the tongue, genioglossus muscle, hyoid, and larynx. (B) Similar view following expansion hyoidoplasty. The base of the tongue is displaced foreward with the anterior portion of the hyoid following anteriorly. Anterior movement of the dotted line represents widening of the cross sectional area of the hypopharynx. (From Patton TJ, Thawley SE, Waters RC, et al: Expansion hyoidplasty: A potential surgical procedure designed for selected patients with obstructive sleep apnea syndrome. Experimental canine results. Laryngoscope 93:1387–1396, 1983. With permission.)

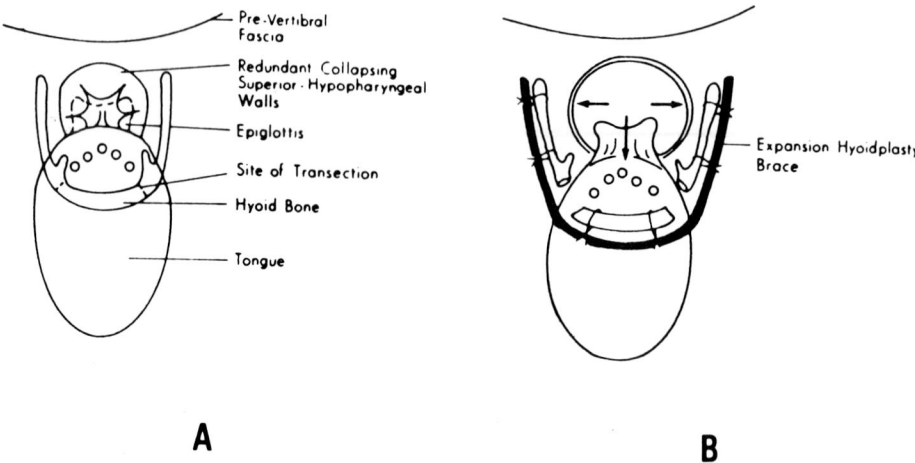

A   **B**

Fig. 6-8. Pre (A) and post (B) operative view of hyoid bone following expansion hyoidoplasty to enlarge the hypopharyngeal airspace. The heavy line in B represents a metal stint used to expand the sectioned hyoid. Reproduced by permission (From Patton TJ, Thawley SE, Waters RC, et al: Expansion hyoidplasty: A potential surgical procedure designed for selected patients with obstructive sleep apnea syndrome. Experimental canine results. Laryngoscope 93:1387–1396, 1983. With permission.)

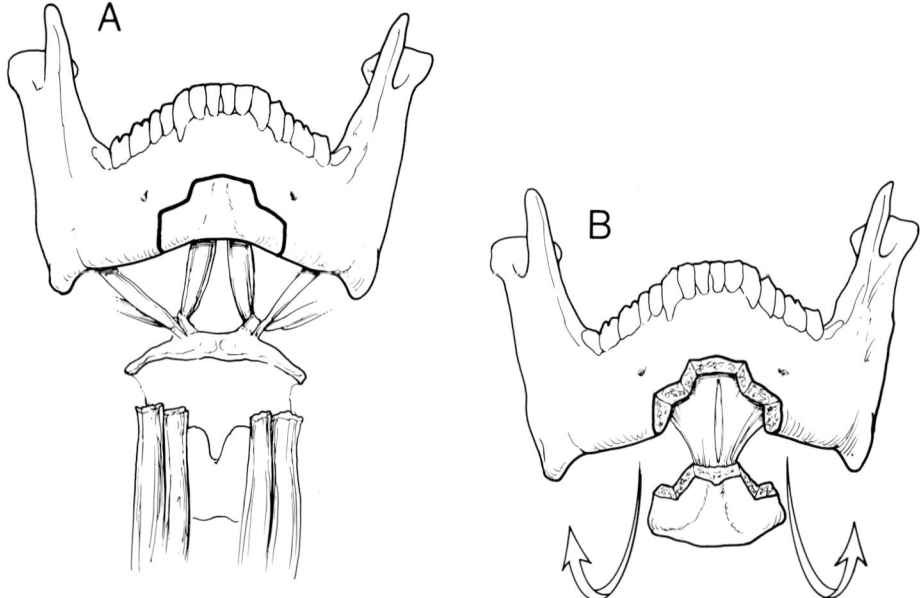

Fig. 6-9. Midline mandibular osteotomy represents one example of a technique for advancement of the tongue to enlarge the posterior airspace. (A) The anterior inferior portion of the mandible is sectioned and pulled foreward, carrying with it, the anterior insertion of the genioglossus muscle. (B) This triangular piece of bone is hooked over the remaining mandible and secured in place by wire. This may enlarge the posterior airspace by 3 to 5 mm.

Further developments and studies of such techniques are needed to assess the extent they will play in the treatment of sleep apnea.

SURGICAL TREATMENT OF OBESITY

The morbidly obese obstructive sleep apnea patient is less likely to respond to UPPP surgery than the less obese, leaving life-long tracheostomy or nasal CPAP the main treatment alternatives. If such treatment is refused or the patient is noncompliant, then the obesity represents a more life-threatening problem to the patient. Weight reduction can dramatically improve the severity of the obstructive sleep apnea.[95] If medical dietary approaches fail, then surgical treatment of obesity may be indicated. Sugerman[96] performed gastroplasty in patients with obesity-hypoventilation syndrome with marked improvement in hypercapnia following weight reduction. Victor[97] performed gastric bypass surgery in two morbidly obese patients with obstructive sleep apnea and following weight reduction resolved the obstructive events. However, bariatric surgery should not be taken lightly since pulmonary embolism post-operatively is seen often enough to suggest prophylactic inferior vena caval ligation at the time of surgery.[98]

PRE- AND POST-OPERATIVE MANAGEMENT

Acceptance of recommended surgery is highly dependent on pre-operative patient and family education with regard to alternative treatments and the purposes and risks of surgery. Unfortunately, patients with severe disease or in whom medical treatment is unsuccessful may refuse surgery out of fear or ignorance. Some eventually return for treatment after progression of the disease and symptoms, others presumably have died.

Once recommendation for surgery is made and accepted by the patient, consideration of concurrent medical conditions and their treatment is made. For example, patients with chronic obstructive pulmonary disease may need intensive respiratory care initiated several days before surgery in order to maximize pulmonary function and reduce risk of post-anesthesia respiratory failure and excessive bronchial secretions. The latter especially makes post-tracheostomy care and acceptance more difficult. Congestive heart failure or cardiac arrhythmias may need to be controlled prior to any surgical procedures.

Other medical illnesses such as diabetes mellitus or hypertension may need to be evaluated and controlled pre-operatively.

Since central nervous system (CNS) depressants may worsen or produce upper airway obstruction, hospitalization and preoperative prescribing of anxiolytics and hypnotics should be avoided. *Sedation is best given by the anesthesiologist in the operating room prior to or at the time of intubation.* Once the airway is under control and the patient ventilated, risk of intraoperative problems such as arrhythmias or hypoxemia is minimized.

Post-operative management is critical since the CNS depression effect of anesthesia may not wear off for many hours. Patients with respiratory disease are at greater risk of respiratory failure during this time. Patients having UPPP without concurrent tracheostomy may develop acute upper airway obstruction immediately post-operatively or within several days of surgery. Thus, close observation during the initial 24 to 48 hours is essential, preferably in an intensive care unit under cardiac monitoring. Because of this risk, especially in the morbidly obese, concurrent tracheostomy is often recommended at the time of UPPP. With tracheostomy, patients are assured of immediate cure of the obstructive sleep apnea events resulting in rapid clinical improvement in their sleepiness as well as assurance of an airway in case of post-UPPP pharyngeal swelling. Nasal CPAP in such patients may be a substitute for tracheostomy as long as nasal surgery with nasal packing is not also contemplated. However, nasal CPAP will not be beneficial for patients in whom post-operative respiratory failure is expected, i.e., severe hypercapnic COPD patients. Such patients are best managed with cuffed tracheal tubes to allow for ventilator support.

Usually, uncomplicated UPPP patients without tracheostomies can be discharged within a few days, determined primarily by their ability to swallow liquids. Patients with tracheostomies usually require a four or five day hospital stay to allow for development of a fistula, which is necessary for easy removal and reinsertion of the tube. Patients are instructed on antiseptic techniques of cleaning the tube and taught how to handle the different tube parts. Most are able to learn to change the entire tracheal tube themselves. This is usually required once per week to prevent accumulation of mucus around the tube, growth of bacteria, wound infection, and odor.

Another potential post-operative problem is pulmonary embolus, especially in the morbidly obese. Early ambulation and post-operative "mini-heparin" may reduce the risk for this severe complication.

Success of any treatment modality is dependent on close patient follow-up care. Since long term response to UPPP surgery and ability to eventually remove the tracheostomy tube probably depends on post-operative weight reduction or avoidance of weight gain, abstinence from alcohol, and cessation from smoking, close follow-up of patients is important. Norman[99] described a methodology to ensure patient compliance in following multiple treatment through ongoing, supportive, and educational follow-up care. Treatment of the post-operative period is no less important in achieving a final treatment success than the diagnosis or actual surgery itself.

REFERENCES

1. Kuhlo W, Doll E, Frame M: Exfolgreich behandlung eines Pickwick syndrome durch eine dauertracheal kanule. Dtsch Med Wochenschr 94:1286–1290, 1969
2. Proctor DF: The upper airways. I. Nasal physiology and defense of the lungs. Am Rev Respir Dis 115:97–129, 1977
3. Fritzell B: The velopharyngeal muscles in speech. Acta Oto-Laryng Suppl 250:1–49, 1969
4. McKerns D, Bzoch KR: Variations in velopharyngeal valving: the factor of sex. Cleft Palate J 7:652–662, 1970
5. Hudgel DW, Robertson DW: Nasal resistance during wakefulness and sleep in normal man. Acta Otolaryngol (Stockh) 98:130–135, 1984
6. Hasegawa M: Nasal cycle and postural variations in nasal resistance. Ann Otol 91:112–114, 1982
7. Rao S, Potdar A: Nasal airflow with body in various positions. J Appl Physiol 28:162–165, 1970
8. Cohn MA, Starz K, Nay KN, et al: Non-invasive monitoring of the human nasal cycle and oronasal ventilation during sleep. Sleep Res 13:199, 1984
9. Eccles R: Cyclic changes in human nasal resistance to air flow. J Physiol 272:75P–76P, 1977
10. Zwillich CW, Pickett C, Hanson FN, Weil JV: Disturbed sleep and prolonged apnea during nasal obstruction in normal men. Am Rev Respir Dis 124:158–160, 1981

11. Taasan V, Wynne JW, Cassisi N, Block AJ: The effect of nasal packing on sleep-disordered breathing and nocturnal oxygen desaturation. Laryngoscope 91:1163–1172, 1981

12. Lavie P, Fischel N, Zomer J, Eliaschar I: The effects of partial and complete mechanical occlusion of the nasal passages on sleep structure and breathing in sleep. Acta Otolaryngol 95:161–166, 1983

13. Lavie P: Nasal breathing during sleep, in Guilleminault C, Lugaresi E (eds): Sleep/Wake Disorders: Natural History, Epidemiology, and Long-Term Evolution. New York, Raven Press, 1983, pp 151–162

14. McNicholas WT, Tarlo S, Cole P, et al: Obstructive apneas during sleep in patients with seasonal allergic rhinitis. Am Rev Respir Dis 126:625–628, 1982

15. Orr WC, Martin RJ: Obstructive sleep apnea associated with tonsillar hypertrophy in adults. Arch Intern Med 141:990–992, 1981

16. Licht JR, Smith WR, Glauser FL: Tonsillar hypertrophy in an adult with obesity-hypoventilation syndrome. Chest 70:672–674, 1976

17. Kravath RE, Pollak CP, Borowiecki B: Hypoventilation during sleep in children who have lymphoid airway obstruction treated by nasopharyngeal tube and t and a. Pediatrics 59:865–871, 1977

18. Heimer D, Scharf SM, Lieberman A, Lavie P: Sleep apnea syndrome treated by repair of deviated nasal septum. Chest 84:184–185, 1983

19. Stool SE: What is causing the child's noisy nasal breathing? J Respir Dis 4:55–60, 1983

20. Shannon DC, Kelly DH: Sids and near-sids. N Engl J Med 306:959–965, 1982 (Part 1). 306:1022–1028, 1982 (Part 2)

21. Rodenstein D, Perlmutter N, Stanescu D: Infants are not obligatory nose breathers. Am Rev Respir Dis 131:343–348, 1985

22. Guilleminault C, Ariagno R, Korobkin R, et al: Mixed and obstructive sleep apnea and near miss for sudden infant death syndrome: 2. comparison of near miss and normal control infants by age. Pediatrics 64:882–891, 1979

23. Guilleminault C, Eldridge FL, Simmons FB, Dement WC: Sleep apnea in eight children. Pediatrics 58:23–30, 1976

24. Mauer KW, Staats BA, Olsen KD: Upper airway obstruction and disordered breathing in children. Mayo Clin Proc 58:349–353, 1983

25. Eliaschar I, Lavie P, Halperin E, et al: Sleep apneic episodes as indications for adenotonsillectomy. Arch Otolaryngol 106:492–496, 1980

26. Rubin A-HE, Eliaschar I, Joachim Z, et al: Effects of nasal surgery and tonsillectomy on sleep apnea. Bull europ Physiopath resp 16:612–615, 1980

27. Sukerman S, Healy GB: Sleep apnea syndrome associated with upper airway obstruction. Laryngoscope 89:878–885, 1979

28. Olsen KD, Kern EB, Westbrook PR: Sleep and breathing disturbance secondary to nasal obstruction. Otolaryngol Head Neck Surg 89:804–810, 1981

29. Mathew OP, Abu-Osba YK, Thach BT: Influence of upper airway pressure changes on genioglossus muscle respiratory activity. J Appl Physiol 52:438–444, 1982

30. Remmers JL, DeGroot WJ, Sauerland EK, Anch AM: Pathogenesis of upper airway occlusion during sleep. J Appl Physiol 44:931–938, 1978

31. Heimer D, Scarf M, Lieberman A, Lavie P: Sleep apnea syndrome treated by repair of deviated nasal septum. Chest 84:184–190, 1983

32. Simmons FB, Guilleminault C, Dement WC, et al: Surgical management of airway obstructions during sleep. Laryngoscope 87:326–338, 1977

33. Weitzman ED, Kahn E, Pollak CP: Quantitative analysis of sleep and sleep apnea before and after tracheostomy in patients with the hypersomnia-sleep apnea syndrome. Sleep 3:407–423, 1980

34. Guilleminault C, Simmons FB, Motta J, et al: Obstructive sleep apnea syndrome and tracheostomy. Arch Intern Med 141:985–989, 1981

35. Simmons FB: Tracheostomy in obstructive sleep apnea patients. Laryngoscope 89:1702–1703, 1979

36. Aubert-Tulkens G, Willems B, Veriter C, et al: Increase in ventilatory response to CO_2 following tracheostomy in obstructive sleep apnea. Bull europ Physiopath resp 16:587–593, 1980

37. Guilleminault C, Cummiskey J: Progressive improvement of apnea index and ventilatory response to CO_2 after tracheostomy in obstructive sleep apnea syndrome. Am Rev Respir Dis 126:14–20, 1982

38. Brown DL, Fletcher EC: Nocturnal oxyhemoglobin desaturation following tracheostomy for obstructive sleep apnea. Am J Med 79:35–42, 1985

39. Conway WA, Victor LD, Magilligan Jr DJ, et al: Adverse effects of tracheostomy for sleep apnea. JAMA 246:347–350, 1981

40. Ikematsu T: Study of snoring, 4th report. Therapy (in Japanese). J Jap Oto-Rhino-Laryngol 64:434–435, 1964

41. Fujita S, Conway W, Zorick F, Roth T: Surgical correction of anatomic abnormalities in obstructive sleep apnea syndrome: uvulopala-

topharyngoplasty. Otolaryngol Head Neck Surg 89:923–934, 1981

42. Hernandez SF: Palatopharyngoplasty for the obstructive sleep apnea syndrome: technique and preliminary report of results in ten patients. Am J Otolaryngol 3:229–234, 1982

43. Simmons FB, Guilleminault C, Silvestri R: Snoring, and some obstructive sleep apnea, can be cured by oropharyngeal surgery. Arch Otolaryngol 109:503–507, 1983

44. Kramer M, Anand VK, Schoen L, Draper E: Death associated with uvulopalatopharyngoplasty: a case report. Sleep Res 14:180, 1985

45. Samelson CF: Sequelae and complications of palatopharyngoplasty: impact on vocal trill. Sleep 7:83–84, 1984

46. Silvestri R, Guilleminault C, Simmons FB: Palatopharyngoplasty in the treatment of obstructive sleep apneic patients, in Guilleminault C, Lugaresi E (eds): Sleep/Wake Disorders: Natural History, Epidemiology, and Long-Term Evolution. New York, Raven Press, 1983, pp 163–169

47. Zorick F, Roehrs T, Conway W, et al: Effects of uvulopalatopharyngoplasty on the daytime sleepiness associated with sleep apnea syndrome. Bull europ Physiopath resp 19:600–603, 1983

48. Walsh JK, Katsantonis GP, Schweitzer PK, Donovan TJ: Assessing the effect of uvulopalatopharyngoplasty: two week vs. five week follow-up. Sleep Res 12:293, 1983

49. Cohn MA, Hernandez S, Foster AC, et al: Uvulo-palatopharyngoplasty (upp) in obstructive sleep apnea: clinical evaluation in 92 consecutive patients. Chest 83:336, 1983

50. Smith PL, Gehris C, Haponik EF, et al: Uvulo-palatopharyngoplasty in sleep apnea. Am Rev Respir Dis 127 (Part 2):85, 1983

51. Guilleminault C, Hayes B, Smith L, Simmons FB: Palatopharyngoplasty and obstructive sleep apnea syndrome. Bull europ Physiopath resp 19:595–599, 1983

52. Fujita S, Conway W, Zorick F, et al: Evaluation of the effectiveness of uvulopalatopharyngoplasty. Sleep Res 12:248, 1983

53. Schoen L, Kramer M, Anand VK, Weisenberger S: Efficacy of uppp in patients with obstructive sleep apnea. Sleep Res 13:164, 1984

54. Thorpy MJ, Sher A, Spielman AJ: Uvulo-palato-pharyngoplasty (uppp) for obstructive sleep apnea: II. early results. Sleep Res 3:171, 1984

55. Santamaria JD, Blokmanis A, Dickson RI, Fleetham JA: Treatment of obstructive sleep apnea by uvulopalatopharyngoplasty. Am Rev Respir Dis 131 (Suppl):A105, 1984

56. Askenasy JJ, Rosen A, Marshak G: Uvulopalatopharyngoplasty in apneic and nonapneic snoring. Sleep Res 14:144, 1985

57. Norman S, Hesla PE, Nay KN, et al: Quantitative changes of sleep parameters and symptoms in obstructive sleep apnea: effect of uvulopalatopharyngoplasty (upp). Sleep Res 14:194, 1985

58. Scrima L, Wetmore S, Lucas E, Hiller C: Indices to evaluate success of surgical correction of obstructive sleep apnea. Sleep Res 14:214, 1985

59. Zorick F, Fujita S, Conway W, et al: Uvulopalatopharyngoplasty: one year followup. Sleep Res 13:176, 1984

60. Schoen LS, Weisenberger S, Anand VK, et al: Long term effectiveness of uvulopalatopharyngoplasty. Sleep Res 14:212, 1985

61. Borowiecki B, Sassin JF: Surgical treatment of sleep apnea. Arch Otolaryngol 109:508–512, 1983

62. Borowiecki B, Pollak CP, Wietzman ED, et al: Fiberoptic study of pharyngeal airway during sleep in patients with hypersomnia obstructive sleep-apnea syndrome. Laryngoscope 88:1310–1313, 1978

63. Rojewski TE, Schuller DE, Clark RW, et al: Synchronous video recording of the pharyngeal airway and polysomnograph in patients with obstructive sleep apnea. Laryngoscope 92:246–250, 1982

64. Haponik EF, Smith PL, Bohlman ME, et al: Computerized tomography in obstructive sleep apnea. Am Rev Respir Dis 127:221–226, 1983

65. Bohlman ME, Haponik EF, Smith PL, et al: CT demonstration of pharyngeal narrowing in adult obstructive sleep apnea. A J Roent 140:543–548, 1983

66. Shepard Jr JW, Yoo R, Grither D, et al: Evaluation of the upper airway by computerized tomography in patients undergoing uvulopalatopharyngoplasty for obstructive sleep apnea. Chest 86:333, 1984.

67. Skolnick ML: Videofluoroscopic examination of the velopharyngeal portal during phonation in lateral and base projections—a new technique for studying the mechanics of closure. Cleft Palate J 7:803–816, 1970

68. Smirne S, Comi G: The obstructive mechanism in pickwickian syndrome: a serial x-ray study. Sleep Res 4:237, 1975

69. Smith TH, Baska RE, Francisco CB, et al: Sleep apnea syndrome: diagnosis of upper airway obstruction by fluoroscopy. J Pediatr 93:891–892, 1978

70. Felman AH, Loughlin GM, Leftridge Jr CA,

Cassisi NJ: Upper airway obstruction during sleep in children. AJR 133:213–216, 1979

71. Richardson MA, Seid AB, Cotton RT, et al: Evaluation of tonsils and adenoids in sleep apnea syndrome. Laryngoscope 90:1106–1110, 1980

72. Loughlin GM: Obstructive sleep apnea in older children. J Respir Dis 3:10–19, 1982

73. Weitzman E, Pollack CP, Borowiecki B, et al: The hypersomnia-sleep apnea syndrome: site and mechanism of upper airway obstruction, in Guilleminault C, Dement WC (eds): Sleep Apnea Syndrome. New York, Alan R. Liss, Inc., 1978, pp 235–246

74. Suratt PM, Dee P, Atkinson RL, et al: Fluoroscopic and computed tomographic features of the pharyngeal airway in obstructive sleep apnea. Am Rev Respir Dis 127:487–492, 1983

75. Walsh JK, Katsantonis GP: Somnofluoroscopy as a predictor of upp efficacy. Sleep Res 13:214, 1984

76. Fodor J, Malott JC, Colley D, et al: Somnofluoroscopy in the evaluation of sleep apnea. Radiologic Technol 53:105–109, 1981

77. Cohn M, Hesla PE, Kiel M, Nay KN: Dysfunctional palatomegaly in obstructive sleep apnea syndrome (osas). Chest 88:435, 1985

78. Powell N, Guilleminault C, Riley R, Smith L: Mandibular advancement and obstructive sleep apnea syndrome. Bull europ Physiopath resp 19:607–610, 1983

79. Gulleminault C, Riley R, Powell N: Obstructive sleep apnea and abnormal cephalometric measurements. Chest 86:793–794, 1984

80. Fredberg JJ, Wohl MB, Glass GM, Dorkin HL: Airway area by acoustic reflections measured at the mouth. J Appl Physiol 48:749–758, 1980

81. Rivlin J, Hoffstein V, Kalbfleisch J, et al: Upper airway morphology in patients with idiopathic obstructive sleep apnea. Am Rev Respir Dis 129:355–360, 1984

82. Valero A, Alroy G: Hypoventilation in acquired micrognathia. Arch Int Med 115:307–310, 1965

83. Tammeling GJ, Blokzijl ES, Boonstra S, Sluiter HJ: Micrognathia, hypersomnia and periodic breathing. Bull Physiopath Respir 8:1229–1238, 1972

84. Coccagna G, Donato G, Verucchi P, et al: Arch Neurol 33:769–776, 1976

85. Imes NK, Orr WC, Smith RO, Rogers RM: Retrognathia and sleep apnea. JAMA 237:1596–1597, 1977

86. Conway WA, Bower GC, Barnes ME: Hypersomnolence and intermittent upper airway obstruction. JAMA 237:2740–2742, 1977

87. Davies SF, Iber C: Obstructive sleep apnea associated with adult-acquired micrognathia from rheumatoid arthritis. Am Rev Respir Dis 127:245–247, 1983

88. Kuo PC, West RA, Bloomquist DS, McNiel RW: The effect of mandibular osteotomy in three patients with hypersomnia sleep apnea. Oral Surg 48:385–392, 1979

89. Bear SE, Priest JH: Sleep apnea syndrome: correction with surgical advancement of the mandible. J Oral Surg 38:543–549, 1980

90. Spire JP, Kuo PC, Campbell N: Maxillo-facial surgical approach: an introduction and review of mandibular advancement. Bull europ Physiopath resp 19:604–606, 1983

91. Riley R, Guilleminault C, Herran J, Powell N: Cephalometric analyses and flow-volume loops in obstructive sleep apnea patients. Sleep 6:303–311, 1983

92. Patton TJ,, Thawley SE, Waters RC, et al: Expansion hyoidplasty: a potential surgical procedure designed for selected patients with obstructive sleep apnea syndrome. Experimental canine results. Laryngoscope 93:1387–1396, 1983

93. Kaya N: Sectioning the hyoid bone as a therapeutic approach for obstructive sleep apnea. Sleep 7:77–78, 1984

94. Riley R, Guilleminault C, Powell N, Derman S: Mandibular osteotomy and hyoid bone advancement for obstructive sleep apnea: a case report. Sleep 7:79–82, 1984

95. Browman CP, Sampson MG, Yolles SF, et al: Obstructive sleep apnea and body weight. Chest 85:435–436, 1984

96. Sugerman HJ, Fairman RP, Lindeman AK, et al: Gastroplasty for respiratory insufficiency of obesity. Ann Surg 193:677–685, 1981

97. Victor DW, Sarmiento CF, Yanta M, Halverson JD: Obstructive sleep apnea in the morbidly obese. Arch Surg 119:970–972, 1984

98. Halverson JD, Zuckerman GR, Kochler RE, et al: Gastric bypass for morbid obesity. Ann Surg 194:152–160, 1981

99. Norman S, Cohn MA: Follow-up care at sleep disorders centers: a commitment beyond diagnosis. Sleep 8:71–73, 1985

Eugene C. Fletcher

7

Sleep Apnea Treatment Algorithm

The preceeding two chapters on the medical and surgical treatment of sleep apnea describe numerous modalities available to the clinician in treating apnea patients. However, a unified and logical approach to the treatment of such patients is important, and will be attempted in this brief chapter. It is emphasized that the following approach may not be universally accepted and is based upon the personal experience of the author, experience of colleagues, descriptions in the literature, and opinions expressed at scientific meetings. There may be disagreement with some parts of the algorithm by clinicians experienced with a particular therapy, such as continuous positive airway pressure (CPAP), or who are acquainted with an otolaryngologist achieving good results with uvulopalatopharyngoplasty. Thus, the clinician should read and apply this algorithm within the framework of his or her own practice.

A complete history (Fig. 7-1) should be performed on each patient presenting with complaints that may be related to apnea or a hypoventilation syndrome. Particular points in the history are "How much does hypersomnolence bother or debilitate the patient?" For example, falling asleep while watching TV is one thing, falling asleep while driving on a freeway or in front of the boss is another. It is important to determine the effect of symptoms on the patient's job. Disability may range from mild somnolence during work to impairment of cognitive function that may not be obvious to the patient but may interfere with promotions and jeopardize his or her job. Thus from a subjective standpoint, not only the degree of symptomatology but effect of these symptoms on day to day life will determine the urgency and therefore the type of treatment. Such symptoms as morning headache, although infrequent, may indicate severe hypercarbia or hypoxemia and should influence the therapeutic decision. A complete review of symptoms is important in identifying concomitant diseases such as significant chronic obstructive pulmonary disease and underlying coronary artery disease. In one study, the presence of apnea-related premature ventricular contractions was related to the presence of left ventricular dysfunction and

ABNORMALITIES OF RESPIRATION DURING SLEEP
ISBN 0-8089-1812-5

Copyright © 1986 by Grune & Stratton, Inc.
All rights of reproduction in any form reserved.

Complete History, attention to:

- **Effect of somnolence on lifestyle, job, driving**
- **Cognitive function**
- **Headaches**
- **Presence of heart, lung disease**

Complete Physical Exam, attention to:

- **Presence and degree of obesity**
- **Presence and degree of systemic hypertension**
- **Correctable upper airway pathology**
- **Signs of cardiac, pulmonary disease**
- **Signs of hypothyroidism, acromegaly**
- **Signs of congestive heart failure**

Initial Laboratory Evaluation

- **Electrocardiogram**
- **Chest roentgenogram**
- **Pulmonary function studies in smokers**
- **Resting arteral blood gases (all patients)**
- **Radionuclide right ventricular ejection
  fraction (optional)**

Fig. 7-1.

symptomatic coronary artery disease.[1] Perhaps the patient with such a history may be at greater risk for sudden death (unproven) and perhaps should be treated more aggressively.

Next, a complete physical examination (Fig. 7-1) must be performed with attention to important areas bearing on selection of the proper treatment. The presence and degree of obesity may have important prognostic implications and may influence the physician regarding initial therapy. The presence of systemic hypertension may also influence therapeutic decisions. Correctable pathology in the nose and throat must be looked for. Surgical treatment of a deviated nasal septum or nasal polyps may be an initial treatment approach to the obstructive apnea patient. Enlarged tonsils, a small oro-pharyngeal cavity, or obvious stricture may lead the clinician to suggest a surgical procedure to ameliorate the apnea condition. A chest examination compatible with chronic lung disease should alert the physician to factors such as daytime hypoxemia,[2] which may influence him toward more aggressive approaches in curing the apnea (see Chapter 9). Signs of hypothyroidism or acromegaly should be sought as these findings could strongly influence therapy. The presence of peripheral edema or a cardiac gallop may clue the physician to the presence of right ventricular dysfunction. All of these areas may be further looked at by objective laboratory measures, confirming findings on physical exam. For example, in an older patient who has smoked, pulmonary function studies are indicated to rule out unsuspected chronic obstructive pulmonary disease (COPD). A daytime resting arterial blood gas is critical to determine the presence of awake alveolar hypoventilation. Our laboratory routinely obtains radionuclide studies to evaluate right ventricular function both as a noninvasive measure of the hemodynamic sequelae of the apneic state and as an objective parameter to follow the hemodynamic response to therapy.[3] This is not, however, a standard procedure for many sleep laboratories and it's application to therapy may still be considered research. Other objective measurements of upper airway pathology are reserved until the severity of the apnea is documented and surgical approaches are entertained.

With this information at hand, formal polysomnography (Fig. 7-2) is obtained as outlined in Chapter 1. There are particular parts of the report that are important. First, the number of apneas during the night and apnea index may influence therapeutic decisions. The average nadir saturation during apneas is an important indicator of the severity of hypoxemia, especially if there is a high apnea index. An even better indicator of the end organ hypoxemic effect may be mean nocturnal saturation if available. Since nadir saturation is directly proportional to apnea duration, long duration apneas[4,5] will generally be associated with deeper desaturations. Of paramount importance is the presence of apnea induced arrhythmias, especially com-

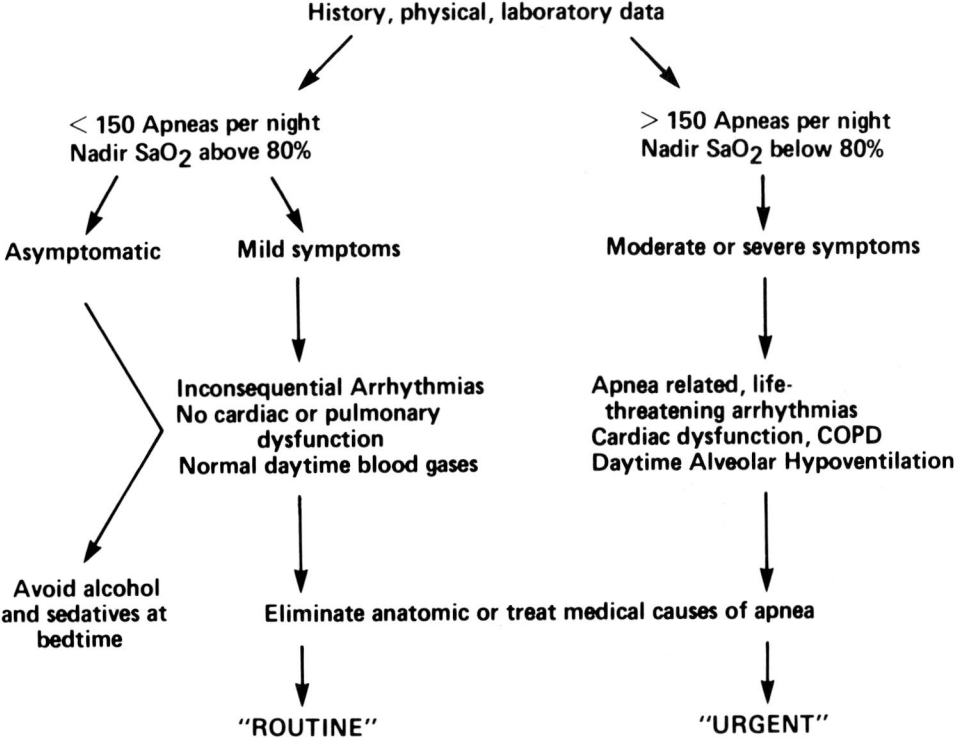

Fig. 7-2.

plex premature ventricular beats, ventricular tachycardia, complete heart block, and asystole. These arrhythmias may reflect insufficient myocardial oxygen supply during apnea and, in theory, may be progenitors of sudden death seen with apnea.[6]

A lack of symptoms in a patient with apnea proven by polysomnography may arouse much discussion among experts dealing with sleep disorders. Perhaps the patient sought medical attention only because the spouse or bed partner complained about snoring; or apnea was discovered incidental to a sexual dysfunction workup. It is hard to improve upon the asymptomatic state and as odds have it, the asymptomatic patient will be the one that suffers a medication side effect or operative complication. A word of caution is in order here. Some stoic patients may deny symptoms. If the apnea index seems high relative to a paucity of symptoms, the clinician must at least confirm the history with the patient's spouse or bed partner or obtain some objective measure of somnolence such as the multiple sleep latency test. An additional objective measure of cognitive function may also be helpful. If the patient has no symptoms or mild hypersomnolence that does not bother him and the physician is satisfied that no detrimental hemodynamic or cardiac sequellae are imminent, consideration should be given either to no therapy or stopping at dietary therapy in the obese subject. The patient should be warned that alcohol or sedatives at bedtime could worsen the apnea bringing about symptoms and other potential sequelae of sleep apnea syndrome. Furthermore, significant weight gain should be avoided for the same reason. If the apnea is position dependent, avoidance of the appropriate position may obviate future problems. The patient should be instructed to warn his surgeon about apnea any time general anesthesia is considered.

At this point, one of the first therapeutic considerations should be correction of obvious anatomic abnormalities such as tonsilar hypertrophy, severe mandibular abnormalities, and perhaps to a lesser degree, nasal septal deviation (correction of apnea with septal straightening is not 100 percent successful; see Chapter 6) or other nasal pathology. Possible causative medical problems such as hypothyroidism and acromegaly should be treated. Having eliminated obvious anatomic or medical causes of apnea, it is helpful to divide the patients into two groups, a "routine" group in which therapy may follow at a more leisurely pace, and a more "urgent" group in whom some mitigating factor may dictate more rapid treatment. Admittedly, the dividing point of 150 apneas per hour and nadir saturation below 80 percent (representing an arterial PaO_2 below 50 torr) is very arbitrary and suggested only to "alert" the clinician that a more serious form of apnea may be present and other factors must be examined closely. More than 150 apneas per night, in and of itself, does not mean that the patient's situation is urgent. The polysomnographic results must be combined with information on the severity of symptoms, concomitant diseases such as coronary artery disease and COPD, signs of end organ effects of hypoxemia such as cor pulmonale, and cardiac arrhythmias during sleep, to help define the two groups. If the patient has signs of end organ damage from repetitive hypoxemic episodes or if he shows evidence of daytime alveolar hypoventilation with awake hypercarbia ($PaCO_2 > 44$ torr) and hypoxemia ($PaO_2 < 55$ torr) immediate therapy should be pursued as objective data has shown that daytime ventilation may improve markedly with either CPAP or tracheostomy[3,7,8] and that pulmonary hypertension may be reduced with cure of the apnea.[3]

The reasons for placing a patient in the "urgent group" (Fig. 7-3) should be discussed with the patient and some initial therapeutic modality that will relieve the

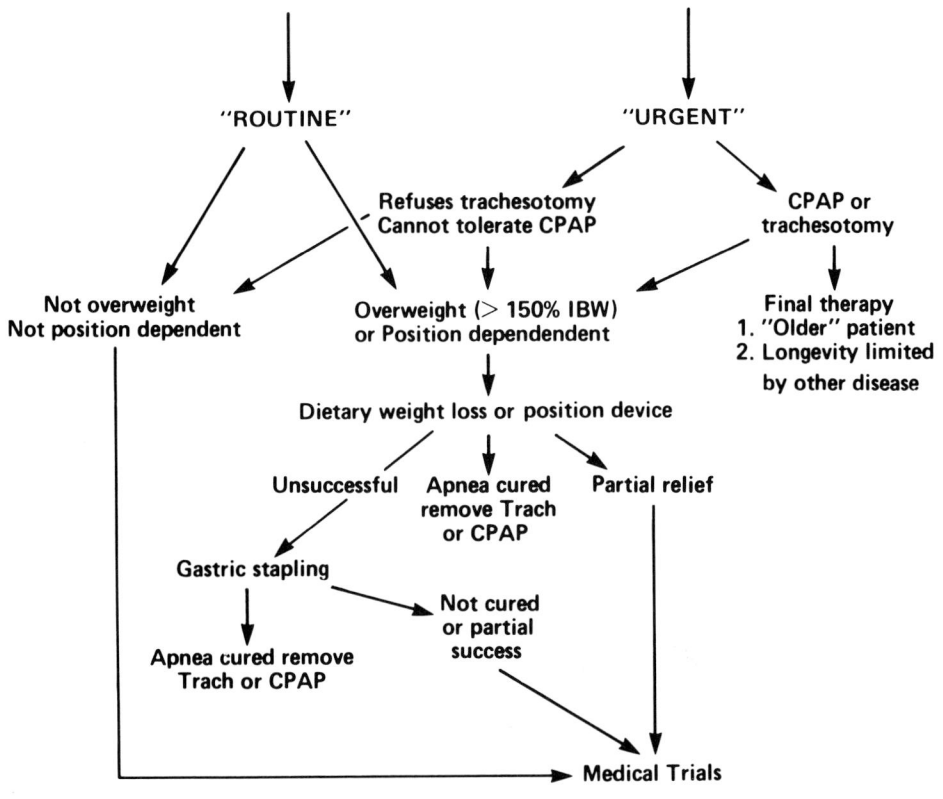

Fig. 7-3.

apnea should be instituted. This will accomplish three goals: to reduce the risk of any adverse cardiovascular catastrophy, to arrest progression of end organ damage to the heart by controlling systemic blood pressure and correcting nocturnal hypoxemia, and to show the patient just how bad he or she has felt by eliminating symptoms so that the patient is strongly motivated to pursue permanent correction of the problem. It is appropriate to warn the patient not to use alcohol, hypnotics, and tranquilizers before sleep.

There are really only two choices for immediate elimination of apnea. CPAP is certainly the least invasive and may be well tolerated, although individual patient compliance may vary. Tracheostomy is a low morbidity, 100 percent curative approach but is plagued by social stigmata and long-term care problems that may be unattractive to the patient. In a patient with severe, life threatening apnea manifesting obvious end organ damage from hypoxia, it is the job of the physician to explain the pros and cons of this procedure carefully and dispell any misconceptions that the patient may have such as "I won't be able to talk if I have one of those." Once the patient has accepted some form of therapy, or if he refuses these choices (but has been sufficiently warned of the danger to himself having refused immediate therapy), the physician should then proceed to other forms of therapy that are aimed at correcting apnea. If the patient refuses tracheostomy or cannot tolerate CPAP, he should enter the usual workup schema with the understanding that he is at risk for continued symptoms, cardiovascular damage, and perhaps sudden death. If the patient accepts tracheostomy or CPAP but is young, middle aged, or actively employed, it is unlikely that they will enthusiastically look forward to 20 to 30 years of tracheostomy care or the nightly use of a CPAP face mask. In this group, further therapeutic measures might subsequently obviate the need for tracheostomy or CPAP and return the patient to a more normal life. In the elderly group (depending on degree of activity, career, and social conditions), those with high risk of cardiovascular and pulmonary complications, and those with decreased longevity due to concomitant disease, other diagnostic and therapeutic interventions (with the possible exception of weight loss) might be unnecessary since expected life span may be more dependent upon these associated diseases. Thus, in the elderly with severe symptoms or hemodynamic abnormalities, tracheostomy or CPAP may be the simplest, safest, and least expensive form of therapy and therefore be a therapeutic endpoint.

As stated in the previous chapters, weight loss in overweight patients is the most benign, most physiologic, and perhaps the least successful form of therapy because of either poor initial compliance or inability to adhere to diet once the weight has been lost. Aggressive dietary management should be directed toward those who give a clear history of worsening of symptoms concomitant with weight gain. Those who are "least likely to succeed" are those with lifelong obesity. The dividing point of >150 percent ideal body weight is arbitrary and is only meant to separate out the massively obese patient since they frequently have more severe apneas, greater desaturations, and may respond less well to drugs and upper airway surgery. While most sleep clinicians still consider weight loss a first line treatment for obstructive sleep apnea syndrome, many would agree that it is the least successful therapy. In my experience, patients who do lose weight and improve, slowly regain the weight and return to their previous symptomatic state. An older observation that has recently regained popularity is the fact that apnea density may be markedly effected by position.[9–12] Apnea index may decrease greatly from the supine to the lateral decubitus position. Patient position during polysomnography should be noted by the technician. If the apnea appears to be position dependent, one older form of therapy is sewing a tennis ball into the back of the patient's night garment[9] and more recently, position training.[10] If position is not a factor and weight loss is unsuccessful, there are no complicating medical conditions that would place the patient at high operative risk (beside obesity), and a surgeon experienced with gastric stapling is available, this procedure may be considered. It may be especially successful in those with lifelong obesity who have failed multiple attempts at dietary control. This procedure has not gained wide spread acceptance for the treatment of obstructive apnea and objective reports are scarce.[13,14] The reasons for this are several. Weight loss is not 100 percent certain to eliminate apneas. The amount of weight lost from these procedures is unpredictable. Surgical risk and the possibility of subsequent medical problems may outweigh the possible benefit from such a noncurative procedure. As an alternative to gastric surgery, one might attempt medical trials for the apnea, but past experience of many clinicians has shown that drug therapy is less likely to be successful in the massively obese individual.

If the patient is not overweight to begin with, loses some weight by diet or surgery but significant apneas continue, or is unsuccessful at dietary weight loss and refuses gastric surgery, one may consider a trial of medical measures (Fig. 7-4) such as protriptyline, progesterone, CPAP (if not already using), oxygen, tongue retaining

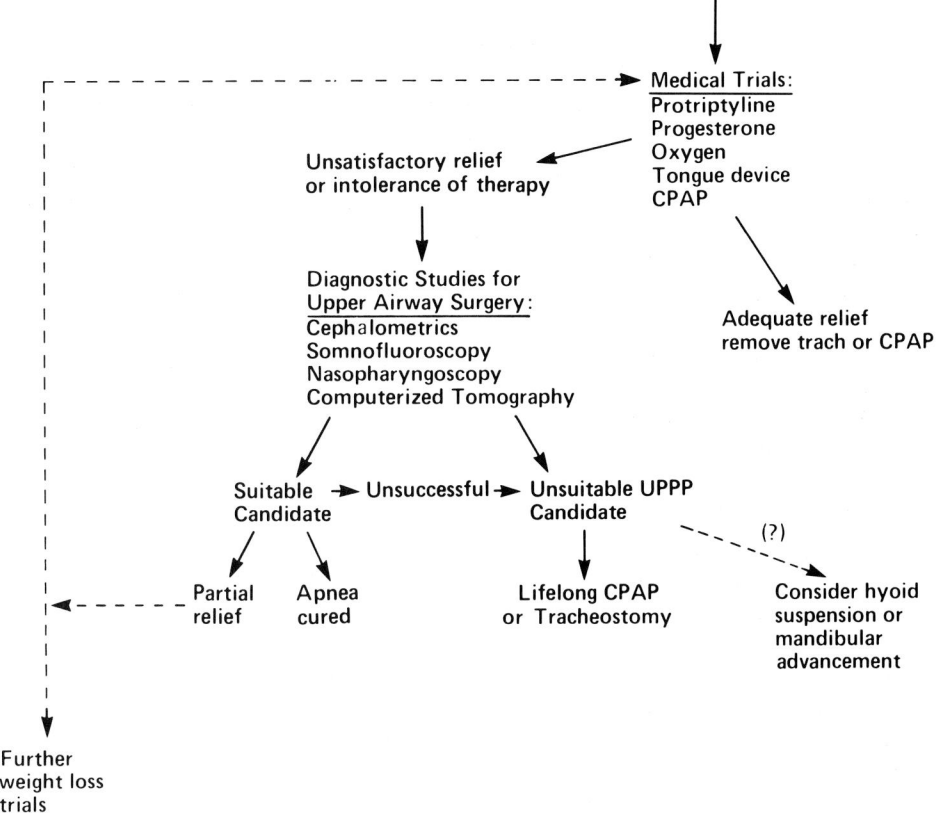

Fig. 7-4.

devices, etc. designed to minimize symptoms and cardiovascular morbidity associated with apnea. Perhaps a combination of therapies such as protriptyline and oxygen may be successful in reducing apnea frequency and oxyhemoglobin desaturation. If the patient was following the "routine" path, the clinician may want to recommend a trial of nasal CPAP that perhaps may only need to be used on an intermittent basis to improve symptoms (keeping in mind that the long-term effect of intermittent CPAP on cardiopulmonary hemodynamics has not been examined).

If medical therapy is tried and found unsatisfactory in terms of relief of symptoms, improvement in apnea frequency, or intolerance of medication side effects, or in the case where the physician or patient do not wish to experiment with different medications (the younger patient may not look forward to lifelong "pill taking"; multiple expensive sleep studies may be required to evaluate success) a surgical approach to the upper airway should be considered (Fig. 7-4). In view of the more or less random success of uvulopalatopharyngoplasty (UPPP) (see Chapter 6), every effort must be made to localize the primary site of obstruction (presuming nasal obstruction and obvious anatomic pathology have already been eliminated). Obstruction may occur in the oropharynx with inward collapse of the soft palate, tonsils, and redundant pharyngeal mucosa during inspiration, or it may occur first in the hypopharynx with genioglossus and posterior-lateral pharyngeal wall collapse.

Conceivably, both areas could be affected at the same time. Various measures of looking at the oro-hypopharyngeal airway have been discussed in Chapter 6. Probably the easiest and most economical to obtain is lateral head and neck films following a swallow of barium to help delineate the tongue and soft palate (cephalometrics). Particular attention is paid to the soft palate and posterior airway size. Fiberoptic examination of the oro-hypopharynx is readily available to most otolaryngology and pulmonary specialists. Somnofluoroscopy is perhaps more accurate since it takes into consideration the pathophysiological changes during sleep and real time motion of the pharynx can be monitored. It may be impractical in some settings since fluoroscopic time can be expensive, the weight of the patient may exceed specifications of the fluoroscopy table (usually 300 lb limit), and the patient may not fall asleep in a reasonable time. In the latter setting, a Mueller maneuver with occluded mouth and nose may simulate the site of "sleep" apnea occlusion. It should be remembered by the reader that although these approaches may improve the chances of successful UPPP, they are untested by prospective studies and this hypothesis awaits confirmation.

Should the patient prove a likely candidate for UPPP but surgery results in only partial relief of apnea and symptoms, one may elect to reapproach weight loss (if overweight) as an additive therapy, or perhaps try ancillary medical therapy again. If the patient is not a likely candidate for UPPP because of a narrow hypopharyngeal airspace, or if the patient has poor results from UPPP, other surgical approaches to widening the hypopharynx such as mandibular advancement and hyoid suspension may be considered. It must be pointed out that the latter surgical approaches are highly specialized, basically untested and unproven, and should probably be reserved for centers having more extensive experience with them. Before considering surgery beyond UPPP, it may be more practical and less expensive to procede with permanent tracheostomy or lifelong nasal CPAP if tolerated.

It should be evident to the reader by now that our present approach to sleep apnea syndrome leaves much to be desired both in terms of diagnostic expense and therapeutic capabilities. It could be said that the efficacy of the various therapies available for a given disease entity is inversely proportional to our understanding of the disease and it's treatment. Obstructive sleep apnea is no exception. However, rapid strides are being made in home monitoring for diagnosis and knowledge of pathophysiologic mechanisms. Hopefully, the next five years will see rapid advancement both in defining the place of our present treatments as well as the appearance of new, more effective therapy.

CASE HISTORIES

The following case histories are those of patients treated by the guidelines outlined above in the treatment algorithm. They point out the varied modes of presentation and how the presenting historical, physical, polysomnogram, and laboratory data should influence the clinician and patient in choosing the appropriate therapy.

Case Number 1:

K.J.I. is a 45-year-old male attorney who presented with excessive daytime sleepiness for the past five years. He also had a history of loud snoring, waking at night with a feeling of choking and dry mouth, and difficulty going back to sleep following these episodes. He had great difficulty staying awake while talking to clients and while driving. He is not a smoker and denied other significant medical illnesses. He had been normal weight most of his life and had gradually gained 22 kgs over the preceding 10 years. He underwent surgical correction of a deviated nasal septum five years ago.

On physical exam his blood pressure was 112/68, pulse 52 and irregular, respiratory rate 18, height 181 cm., and weight 100 kg. (126 percent of ideal body weight). Nasal and oropharyngeal exam were within normal limits. The patient was noted to have mild retroagnathia. The remainder of the physical exam was normal. Laboratory data were all within normal limits except for the electrocardiogram and radionuclide cardiac study. The electrocardiogram showed ventricular bigeminy. The gated wall ventriculogram showed a normal left ventricular ejection fraction of 50 percent with an inferior hypokinetic segment. The right ventricular ejection fraction was abnormal at 38 percent.

Polysomnography revealed 341 episodes of obstructive apnea and an apnea index of 68 per hour. The duration of the longest apnea was 96 seconds and the lowest saturation during an apnea was 67 percent. He had numerous premature ventricular contractions that were also seen on his daytime resting EKG tracings. There were occasional sinus asystoles related to the apneic periods. Afternoon nap studies revealed a shortened sleep onset latency.

Because of the patient's severe symptoms, evidence of right ventricular dysfunction and possible left ventricular disease, early definitive treatment was recommended. A trial of nasal CPAP showed that 10 cm H_2O pressure eliminated the apneas and the patient purchased his own machine, which he continues to use nightly. Dietary weight loss was recommended but the patient's attitude was somewhat negative since previous efforts at weight loss had failed. Lateral head and neck cephalometrics revealed a slightly long (but not grossly enlarged) soft palate and very narrow posterior airspace (see Figure 6B, Chapter 6). Because of this, it was felt that UPPP was not likely to be successful. The patient has returned to an asymptomatic state on nasal CPAP and plans indefinite use of this therapeutic modality.

Analysis. The patient had severe symptoms, evidence of mild right ventricular dysfunction, a hypokinetic area in the left ventricle as well as marked cardiac arrhythmias both during wake and during apneic episodes at night. He was not morbidly obese and had little improvement to expect from weight loss. He was in urgent need of treatment but did not desire surgery. His cephalogram indicated that he would be a poor candidate for UPPP. Nasal CPAP adequately eliminated the apneas and ablated symptoms. He appeared comfortable with that treatment and will likely use it as permanant therapy.

Case Number 2:

L.J.A. is a 38-year-old male truck driver who presented with complaints of daytime hypersomnolence for 10 years but more severe for the past 3 to 4 years. He frequently fell asleep while driving, watching television, or talking to people and was in danger of losing his job because of somnolence. He was not a smoker and had no history of cardiac or pulmonary disease.

Physical examination revealed a slightly obese male with a systemic blood pressure of 130/78. The patient's height was 168 cm and weight was 92 kg (128 percent of ideal body weight). There was no obvious nasal or oropharyngeal pathology. Laboratory data were within normal limits. The right ventricular ejection fraction was 48 percent. His left ventricular ejection fraction was normal at 55 percent.

Polysomnography showed 150 obstructive apneas and numerous desaturating hypopneas. The apnea index was 35 per hour and the average nadir saturation during apneas was 87 percent. The average duration was 51 seconds. The apneas were not position dependent. Other than mild sinus bradycardia-tachycardia, no serious arrhythmias were noted.

Because the patient was modestly overweight, had no apparent cardiovascular sequelae from the apnea, and appeared motivated, dietary therapy was attempted. At the same time, protriptyline was started at bedtime in a progressively increasing dose. The patient reached 25 mgs per day and felt no improvement in his somnolence symptoms. In addition, he experienced undesirable side effects from the protriptyline including dry mouth, dizziness, and complaints of sexual dysfunction. Because of these, the protriptyline was discontinued. He also failed to lose any weight over a 6 month period.

Lateral head and neck films (Fig. 6-6A) showed a grossly enlarged soft palate (length, 45 cm) and patent posterior airspace (20mm wide). A combined tracheostomy and UPPP were performed. Following recovery from these procedures the symptoms abated. Three months after surgery, with the tracheal canula closed at the time of study and for 2 weeks preceding study, repeat polysomnography revealed a total of 39 apneas (apnea index 6 per hour). Decanulation was performed and the patient returned to his usual lifestyle.

Analysis. The patient had moderate symptoms but no evidence of cardiovascular dysfunction and there appeared to be no urgency in treating his problem. Both weight loss and one medical regimen failed. He appeared to be a good UPPP candidate and this therapy was successful in ameliorating both his apnea and symptoms.

Case Number 3:

W.W.A. is a 66-year-old, obese, cigarette smoking male contractor who presented with complaints of excessive daytime somnolence for 10 years and a lifelong history of heavy snoring. Three years previously he had been diagnosed as having sleep apnea by formal polysomnography but refused tracheostomy. He had 4 serious automobile accidents in the 5 years preceeding his present admission. The worst accident, in which the patient suffered a broken wrist and multiple rib fractures, occurred 4 weeks before admission and prompted his seeking further medical care for his apnea. He also suffered from restless sleep and had fallen out of bed numerous times sustaining scalp lacerations and fracturing his clavicle. His wife had moved to a separate bedroom 10 years ago. He had been unable to work for 7 years because he could not drive to work without falling asleep. He had recurrent dependent ankle edema for 10 years. He complained of a chronic productive cough, exertional dyspnea, and smoked one pack of cigarettes per day for 46 years. He recently noted wheezing whenever he got a "cold."

On physical exam his height was 175 cm and weight was 105 kg. (142 percent of ideal body weight). Vital signs were normal. The oropharynx was shallow but no other airway abnormalities were noted. His right arm was casted. He had 4+ pitting ankle edema and stasis skin changes. Electrocardiogram showed "P pulmonale." His chest roentgenogram showed evidence of COPD and pulmonary hypertension. His left ventricular ejection fraction was normal at 57 percent and his right sided fraction was low at 36 percent. Right heart catheterization revealed a pulmonary artery pressure of 43/24 mmHg, a mean pressure of 30.1 mmHg, and pulmonary vascular resistance of 221 dyne/sec/cm^{-5}. Pulmonary function tests revealed an FEV_1 of 1.73 liters (60 percent of predicted) and an FEV1/FVC ratio of 0.70. Arterial blood gases showed a pH of 7.37, a $PaCO_2$ of 49 torr and a PaO_2 of 68 torr.

Polysomnography showed over 400 obstructive and mixed apneas during the night. The apnea index was 80 per hour with an additional 9 obstructive hypopneas per hour. The mean apnea duration was 32 seconds and the mean fall in saturation during apneas was 17.9 percent. Although bradycardia was evident during the apneas, no significant ventricular arrhythmias or heart block were noted.

Since his initial diagnosis 3 years before the present hospitalization, the patient had tried numerous diets and efforts at weight loss were unsuccessful. Therefore, tracheostomy was performed during the present admission with immediate relief of symptoms. Short central apneas of a duration similar to the central portion of his mixed apneas disappeared two to three nights after surgery. Followup studies 2 years after tracheostomy show normalization of blood gases (ph 7.39, $PaCO_2$ 38 torr, and PaO_2 88 torr) and lowering of pulmonary artery pressure to 30/19 mmHg (mean 26.3 mmHg) and a pulmonary vascular resistance of 169 dyne.sec.cm^{-5}. He has had to have operative revision of intratracheal granulation tissue one time but continues to do well otherwise.

Analysis. This patient fits the "urgent" category for apnea treatment. He had severe symptoms that threatened his life through motor vehicle accidents. He had classic pulmonary hypertension and cor pulmonale by all objective criteria. This was probably contributed to by his underlying chronic obstructive pulmonary disease. Dietary therapy had been unsuccessful. Nasal CPAP was not available at the time, and tracheostomy was performed with abolition of his apnea and symptoms. He is presently content with the tracheostomy and will continue with this therapy.

Case Number 4:

K.W.C. is a 60-year-old male with a history of gradually worsening daytime hypersomnia, peripheral edema, and dyspnea on exertion. The patient has a history of heavy snoring for 15 to 17 years, with restlessness and thrashing during sleep for 2 years. He worked as a supervisor in a supermarket and had difficulty staying awake. He fell asleep while driving and watching television and had been having increased irritability for 6 months. He had experienced peripheral ankle and foot edema for 2 years. He was a heavy smoker and had a history compatible with chronic bronchitis.

Physical exam showed a mildly overweight man (114 percent of ideal body weight) with mild respiratory distress. There were no upper airway abnormalities but he had bilateral expiratory wheezes over both lung fields and both ankles were edematous with chronic stasis skin pigmentation.

The patient was initially hypoxemic on admission with a PaO_2 of 38 torr and a $PaCO_2$ of 62 torr. Following therapy with intravenous aminophylline and other bronchodilators his blood gases stabilized at a PaO_2 of 66 and a $PaCO_2$ of 49 torr. Pulmonary function studies during a period of clinical stability showed an FEV_1 of 1.55 L/sec, an FEV_1/FVC ratio of 0.47, and a residual volume 231 percent of predicted. His left ventricular ejection fraction was 70 percent and right ventricular ejection fraction was 41 percent.

On polysomnographic exam the patient had 48 obstructive and mixed apneas per hour. The mean duration was 19.0 seconds and the mean desaturation was 8.1 percent. There were no significant arrhythmias.

Because of the patient's symptoms, daytime hypoxemia and COPD, and signs of cor pulmonale, tracheostomy was recommended but the patient refused. With the use of nocturnal supplemental oxygen and protriptyline, the patient's apnea index was reduced to 7 per hour, mean duration 16.1 seconds and mean fall in saturation of 3.4 percent. He also takes theophylline chronically. He has continued on this regimen for over 2 years, has no hypersomnolence or sleep related complaints, and continues to work full time.

Analysis. This patient had moderate to severe sleep apnea symptoms as well as obvious COPD. He appeared to have cor pulmonale by objective data. Although falling into the urgent category for immediate treatment of apnea, he refused tracheostomy. The patient was only mildly overweight and could expect little improvement from dietary weight loss. However, he had a good response to protriptyline and oxygen with significant reduction in his apneas and has elected to remain on that regimen.

Case Number 5:

W.W. was a 62-year-old male admitted for congestive heart failure. He consulted his family physician 5 years previously for ankle swelling and was told that he had hypertension and heart failure. He also suffered from exertional dyspnea, cough, and wheezing and had a 75 pack per year smoking history. He had been hospitalized in respiratory failure and treated with mechanical ventilation at least two times in the past. Lifelong obesity had been a problem and at the time of admission to this hospital weighed in excess of 136 kg. (163 cm tall and 200 percent of ideal body weight). Daytime hypersomnolence became a problem at about the time the ankle swelling and hypertension was noted. He had a long history of snoring, with restlessness and thrashing during sleep, and on one occasion fell out of bed. He had a history of waking with occipital headaches for 3 months prior to presentation. At one time during the past 2 years the patient managed to lose 23 kg. and noted significant improvement in his symptoms. He had, however, regained the weight and all symptoms returned. His hypersomnolence and dyspnea had caused him to seek medical disability and retire from work.

On physical examination the patient was morbidly obese and had a systemic pressure of 170/100 mmHg. There were no obvious abnormalities of the upper airway. Lung exam showed diffuse expiratory wheezes and the patient had 3+ pitting edema to the knees.

Laboratory data was unremarkable except for the following. His arterial pH was 7.42, PaO_2 was 66 torr, and $PaCO_2$ was 45 torr. Right ventricular ejection fraction by gated wall radionuclide study was 19 percent and the left ventricular ejection fraction was 65 percent. His FEV_1 was 1.25 L/sec and the FEV_1/FVC ratio was 0.53.

The patient had 50 obstructive and mixed apneas per hour of sleep. The mean duration was 18.5 seconds and mean desaturation was 14 percent. Supplemental oxygen only reduced his apnea index to 40 with apnea prolongation to 25 seconds.

Because of the patient's incapacitating symptoms, systemic hypertension, cor pulmonale, and daytime alveolar hypoventilation, and past failure to maintain weight loss, tracheostomy was advised (CPAP was unavailable at that time). He refused surgery but agreed to additional attempts at weight loss and also used supplemental oxygen during sleep. He was also treated with bronchodilators and p.r.n. antibiotics for his COPD. Over a 2 year followup, he failed to lose weight, his hypersomnia symptoms progressively worsened, and he underwent repeated admissions for peripheral edema and respiratory insufficiency. He died in his sleep during one of these admissions. No obvious cause of death was found at autopsy. Death was attributed to cor pulmonale and asphyxia because of viscera congestion and diffuse petechial hemorrhages of the esophageal and tracheal mucosa frequently seen in strangulation.

Analysis. This patient urgently needed correction of his nocturnal hypoxemia and alveolar hypoventilation. He had multiple end organ manifestations of hypoxemia and the complicating factor of COPD. Despite repeated warnings, he refused definitive therapy and diluded himself into thinking that he could lose weight. Nasal CPAP might have been a viable alternative but was not available during the time of treatment of this patient. His early death was almost certainly preventable.

Case Number 6

H.B.J. is a 66-year-old male who was found to have sleep apnea during nocturnal polysomnography performed as part of a sexual dysfunction workup. He admitted to a history of loud snoring and occasional daytime sleepiness when inactive or bored, but denied any difficulty in staying awake during conversations, while watching TV (if interested in the program), while at work, or while driving. Aside from his complaints of decreased sexual drive, he had been in good health. His medical history was remarkable only for mild systemic hypertension for 1 year controlled by dietary salt restriction. The patient did not smoke or drink alcohol.

His nocturnal sleep study showed 295 obstructive and 4 central apneas and the apnea index was 43 per hour. The longest apnea duration was 42 seconds, and the lowest saturation was 85 percent. He was noted to have sinus arrhythmia with occasional, simple premature ventricular contractions. Gated nuclide study revealed a right ventricular ejection fraction of 60 percent, and a left ejection fraction of 71 percent. Wall motion was normal on both sides.

On physical exam, the patient weighed 112 kg. (138 percent IBW) with a systemic pressure of 148/90 and a pulse of 60 per minute. Nasal exam revealed mild septal deviation and oropharyngeal exam revealed a slightly large soft palate. Chest exam was normal.

Weight loss was recommended, but after 6 months he had gained 9 kilograms. Despite the increased weight, he had no complaints of daytime somnolence. Because the patient was basically asymptomatic and had no overt evidence of hemodynamic dysfunction, medical and surgical therapy were not recommended. He has been warned about the effects of alcohol, sleeping pills, and weight gain upon his apnea. He will be followed on a regular basis and will be observed for signs of hemodynamic dysfunction.

Analysis. It would be difficult to improve upon this patient's minimal symptomatic state with surgical or other aggressive therapies. The patient was warned to take precautions about further weight gain and use of sedating medications and will continue to be followed periodically.

Case Number 7

A.E.L. is a 48-year-old plumber with a 25-year history of compensated paranoid schizophrenia, currently treated with haloperidol 1 mg b.i.d. He had a history of excessive daytime somnolence, restless sleep and very loud snoring for 5–10 years prior to presentation. His mother and sister who lived with the patient noted over the preceeding 6 months that he fell asleep during meals, conversations, while driving and indeed spent more time dozing than awake. He had been observed by them to stop breathing for long periods. He smokes 2 packs of cigarettes per day. He drank up to two fifths of liquor a day until 5 years ago. He had a history of systemic hypertension controlled by oral diuretics.

On physical exam, he weighed 135 kilograms (173 percent IBW) and his blood pressure was 160/95 mmHg. He was found to have moderate nasal obstruction despite septoplasty performed in 1979. The remainder of the exam was essentially normal. Gated wall cardiac motion studies showed a right ventricular ejection fraction of 58 percent with a left ejection fraction of 61 percent. Chest roentgenogram showed moderately enlarged pulmonary artery outflow tracts.

Polysomnography revealed 660 obstructive apneas per night. The longest duration was 99 seconds, and the lowest oxygen saturation was less than 30 percent. A mildly accentuated sinus arrhythmia was present during sleep but no serious arrhythmias or conduction defects were noted.

Because of the severe symptoms, marked apneic desaturation, evidence suggestive of pulmonary hypertension, and previous unsuccessful attempts at self weight regulation, early definitive treatment was recommended and a tracheostomy was performed. At the time of hospitalization for the surgery, Mr. L. was found to have glucose intolerance with a blood sugar of 400 mg/dL and was started on insulin, which was later switched to an oral agent.

The patient lives with his mother who does all the cooking. She placed him on the recommended diet for weight loss, and at follow-up 10 months later, he had lost 46 kilograms. He was instructed to plug his tracheostomy tube at night for 3 weeks and a repeat polysomnogram was performed. Apnea frequency was reduced to 24 per night with an index of 4 per hour. Nadir saturation was 86 percent and the longest duration of apnea was 66 seconds. The tracheostomy tube was removed, and the tract was allowed to heal. The danger of weight gain was explained to both the patient and his family.

Analysis. The patient had severe symptoms of daytime hypersomnolence felt to result from his sleep apnea. His family was concerned about recent worsening of symptoms and wanted the problem alleviated. Tracheostomy eliminated the apnea and hypersomnolence, improved his personality and motivation, and probably contributed to his successful weight loss program. Near complete resolution of the apnea resulted from his weight loss and the tracheostomy stoma was successfully closed.

REFERENCES

1. Alford NJ, Fletcher EC, Nickeson D: Effects of acute oxygen in patients with sleep apnea and chronic obstructive lung disease. Chest 89:30–39, 1986

2. Bradley DT, Rutherford R, Grossman RF, et al: Role of daytime hypoxemia in the pathogenesis of right heart failure in obstructive sleep apnea syndrome. Am Rev Respir Dis 131:835–839, 1985

3. Fletcher EC, Schaaf JW, Miller J, Fletcher J: Cardiopulmonary hemodynamics in patients with obstructive sleep apnea and chronic lung disease. Chest 80:545, 1985

4. Strohl KP, Altose MD: Oxygen saturation during breath-holding and during apneas in sleep. Chest 85:181–186, 1984

5. Findley LJ, Ries AL, Tisi GM, Wagner PD: Hypoxemia during apnea in normal subjects: mechanisms and impact of lung volume. J Appl Physiol: Respirat Environ Exercise Physiol 55:1777–1783, 1983

6. Shepard JW Jr, Garrison MW, Grither DA, et al: Relationship of ventricular ectopy to nocturnal O_2 desaturation in patients with obstructive sleep apnea. Chest 88:335–340, 1985

7. Guilleminault C, Cummiskey J: Progressive improvement of apnea index and ventilatory response to CO_2 after tracheostomy in obstructive sleep apnea syndrome. Am Rev Respir Dis 126:14–20, 1982

8. Sullivan CE, Berthon-Jones M, Issa FG: Remission of severe obesity-hypoventilation syndrome after short-term treatment during sleep with nasal continuous positive airway pressure. Am Rev Respir Dis 128:177–181, 1983

9. Kavey NB, Gidro-Frank S, Sewitch DE: The importance of sleeping position in sleep apnea and a simple treatment technique. Sleep Res 11:152, 1982

10. Jackson E, Schmidt H: Modification of sleeping position in the treatment of obstructive sleep apnea. Sleep Res 11:149, 1982

11. Cartwright RD: Effect of sleep position on sleep apnea severity. Sleep 7:110–114, 1984

12. Schmidt HS, Fortin LD: Position effect in obstructive sleep and central sleep apnea. Sleep Res 14:210, 1985

13. Sugerman HJ, Fairman RP, Lindeman AK, et al: Gastroplasty for respiratory insufficiency of obesity. Ann Surg 193:677–685, 1981

14. Peiser J, Lavie P, Ovnat A, et al: Sleep apnea syndrome in the morbidly obese as an indication for weight reduction surgery. Ann Surg 199:112–115, 1984

Eugene C. Fletcher

8

Sleep, Breathing, and Oxyhemoglobin Saturation in Chronic Lung Disease

The extensive investigation of breathing during sleep in normals published by Bulow[1] in the early 1960s heralded a new interest in sleep respiration. This classic monograph provided critical observations of the respiratory pattern during electroencephalographic (EEG) sleep stages and attempted to correlate CO_2 drive with various levels of wakefulness and light sleep. It also summarized polysomnographic techniques that would be used later by other investigators in examining respiration during sleep in various disease states. One of the first of these to undergo investigation was chronic obstructive pulmonary disease (COPD).[2,3] However, because the EEG was slow in being adapted to early studies and a practical method of continuous monitoring of oxyhemoglobin saturation was another 10 to 15 years in coming, it wasn't until the late 1970s that systematic studies began to appear.

There are three major areas of interest to be covered in examining the interaction of breathing, lung disease, and oxyhemoglobin saturation during sleep. First, irregularities of breathing and gas exchange can cause profound decreases in sleeping arterial oxygen saturation. Oxyhemoglobin desaturation is accompanied by reversible elevation of pulmonary artery pressure and vascular resistance. Discovery of this has in turn stimulated interest in the role of nocturnal desaturation in the development of sustained pulmonary hypertension and cor pulmonale. Second, recent observations of sleep architecture (distribution of nocturnal EEG sleep stages) in patients with COPD have shown abnormalities that may reflect the poor sleep quality of which many such patients complain. This may in part be due to hypoxemia, but all COPD patients who complain of poor quality sleep are not hypoxemic at night. Third, several publications have demonstrated irregularities of cardiac rhythm during sleep in COPD patients, again possibly related to hypoxemia. This chapter will provide an in-depth discussion of each of these areas with emphasis on the possible hemodynamic implications of nocturnal hypoxemia.

ABNORMALITIES OF RESPIRATION DURING SLEEP
ISBN 0-8089-1812-5

Copyright © 1986 by Grune & Stratton, Inc.
All rights of reproduction in any form reserved.

OXYHEMOGLOBIN DESATURATION

Because of the sigmoid shape of the oxyhemoglobin dissociation curve, as early as 1958 Robin[4] proposed that depressed ventilation during sleep in COPD patients could cause significant hemodynamic changes. For example, a 10 or 15 torr decrease in arterial PO_2 in normals would cause little change in oxygen carrying capacity and pulmonary artery pressure. But similar decreases in patients with COPD whose resting blood gases were near the shoulder of the oxyhemoglobin dissociation curve would decrease blood oxygen content considerably if alveolar ventilation or gas exchange affected arterial PO_2. Initial studies[2,5-7] were somewhat contradictory, probably because of random sampling of blood gases and inability to monitor sleep stages. One of the earliest studies[2] observed a mean fall in sleeping arterial PO_2 of 7 torr in 19 patients with severe COPD. These values did not differ from those of reported normals, but neither EEG sleep staging nor continuous monitoring of saturation were employed so that larger falls in saturation might have been missed. Two authors[6,7] using random sampling of arterial blood gases in sleeping COPD patients demonstrated significant decreases in arterial PO_2 of a greater degree than that seen in normals. Although these authors disagreed on the magnitude of carbon dioxide retention seen during sleep, both concluded on the basis of alveolar-arterial oxygen gradient widening that gas exchange deteriorated during sleep in such subjects.

The combined use of continuous oxygen saturation monitored by ear oximetry and sleep staging determined by EEG allowed full appreciation of abnormalities of oxygen saturation during sleep in patients with lung disease. An early report[8] of 10 patients with COPD monitored during nap studies revealed 78 episodes of transient desaturation in 6, lasting from 4 to 300 seconds and dropping as much as 16 percent below baseline. Other investigators[9,10] demonstrated larger falls in arterial oxygen saturation.

Another early study employing ear oximetry and EEG monitoring during nocturnal sleep[11] revealed transient drops in oxyhemoglobin saturation of as much as 36 percent beginning at baseline saturations from 73 percent to 94 percent. This article separated desaturation episodes into two types: those associated with abnormalities of breathing such as apnea and hypopnea (accounting for 42 percent of the episodes) and those *not* associated with *obvious* disordered breathing. Those episodes associated with apnea and hypopnea (Fig. 8-1) tended to be short (less than one minute) and showed relatively less desaturation (i.e., a mean of 7.6 percent in this study). Eleven of 83 episodes of arterial oxyhemoglobin desaturation lasted longer than 1 minute (up to 30 minutes) and were associated with profound decreases in oxyhemoglobin saturation (Fig. 8-2). The mean maximum fall in oxygen for these desaturations was 22 percent and all of the episodes lasting longer than 5 minutes occurred during rapid-eye-movement (REM) sleep.

The observation of nocturnal sleep desaturation has now been extended to several disease states associated with either intrinsic abnormalities of the lung, or chest wall abnormalities that are associated with the eventual development of respiratory insufficiency. For example, several reports have associated kyphoscoliosis with nocturnal oxyhemoglobin desaturation.[12,13] Mezon reported five subjects with varying degrees of respiratory impairment from kyphoscoliosis, three of whom (males) showed central apneas with desaturation or Cheyne-Stokes breathing. One female showed mild REM related, nonapneic oxyhemoglobin desaturation. Five

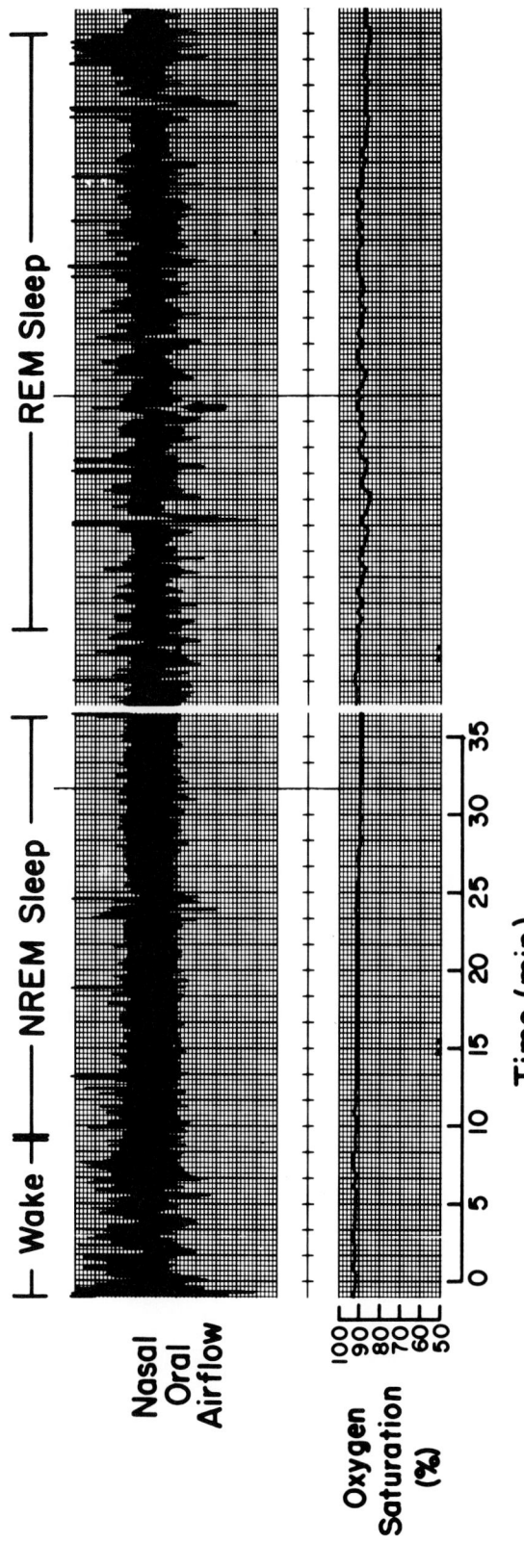

Fig. 8-1. Slow (3mm/min) strip chart recording of nasal thermistor and ear oximeter channels on polysomnogram of a patient with moderately severe COPD. The left panel is taken from the beginning of the night and shows wake, stage 1, and stage 2 sleep. Respiration (expiration represented by sharp 0.2mm spikes) is regular and only a small fall in oxyhemoglobin saturation (about 1 percent) is observed with sleep onset. The right panel shows stage REM sleep. There are repetitive hypopneas represented on the thermistor channel by decreased amplitude of the thermistor deflection (see arrow) and on the saturation channel by a sharp 2–6 percent fall in saturation usually lasting less than one minute. These hypopneas may be obstructive or central in origin (see text).

157

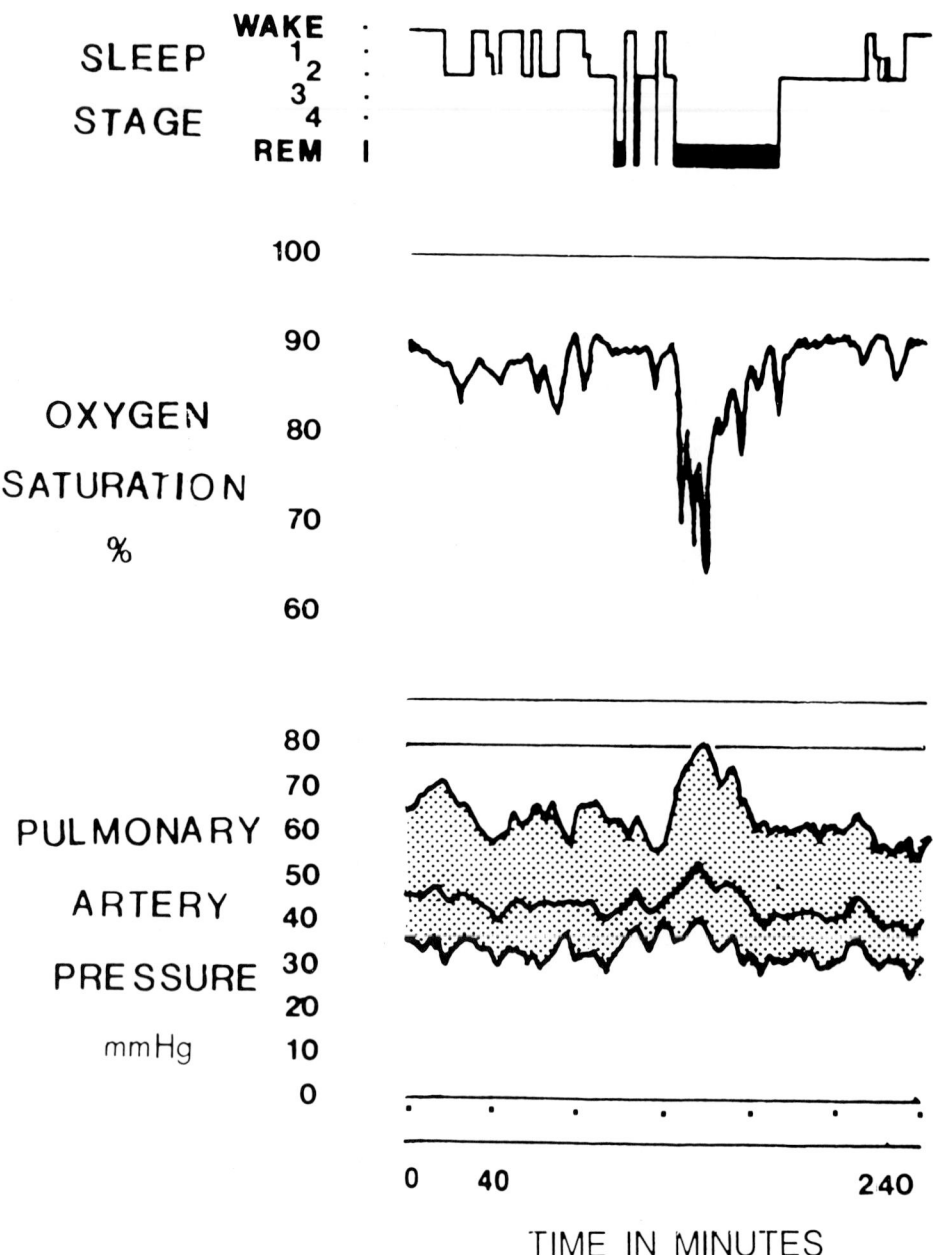

Fig. 8-2. Sleep stage (top), oxyhemoglobin saturation by ear oximetry (middle), and pulmonary artery pressure (bottom) during nocturnal sleep in a single subject breathing room air. Note that the desaturation associated with REM sleep is longer than that associated with apnea or hypopnea (about 30 minutes) and is accompanied by transient elevation in pulmonary artery pressure.

kyphoscoliotics studied by Guilleminault[13] showed obstructive apneas as well as central and obstructive hypopneas. One subject showed a 6 minute hypopnea episode during REM sleep that was reminiscent of REM sleep desaturation seen in COPD. Nocturnal desaturation in young patients with cystic fibrosis has now been reported by several groups.[14–16] Oxygen saturation in cystic fibrosis patients fell 3.5 percent during nonrapid-eye-movement (NREM) sleep compared to 2 percent in controls and 7.4 percent during REM sleep compared to 3 percent in controls.[15] Large decreases in saturation similar to those seen during REM sleep in COPD patients have been seen in patients with severe cystic fibrosis. A recent report[17] has shown REM related desaturations as well as decreases in saturation related to disordered breathing in children with COPD not related to cystic fibrosis. Interstitial lung disease has been reported to be associated with transient falls in SaO_2.[18] As in COPD, desaturations of both the short duration (associated with disordered breathing) and longer (associated with REM sleep) occur. In one patient during REM sleep, a 26 minute period of desaturation running between 80 and 85 percent was observed. Nocturnal desaturation has also been reported in asthmatic children. Smith[19] found a mean maximal decrease of 8.1 percent from baseline, reaching saturations of 88 percent.

Various neuromuscular disorders have been associated with nocturnal decreases in SaO_2 but a detailed discussion is beyond the scope of this chapter, and the reader is referred to Chapter 10. Disordered breathing in the form of apneas has been reported in a few patients with poliomyelitis.[20] Similar abnormalities have also been reported with bilateral diaphragmatic paralysis[21,22] and in patients with myotonic dystrophy.[23]

DISTURBED EEG SLEEP ARCHITECTURE

Physicians caring for patients with COPD frequently hear complaints of poor quality sleep. Objective evidence of disturbed sleep has been demonstrated by several authors.[7,24–27] Leitch reported a sleep efficiency (total sleep time/time in bed) of 71 percent (normal > 90 percent) in 10 patients with severe COPD. These same subjects showed delayed sleep onset, prolonged and frequent periods of wakefulness during the night, and frequency stage shifts (17.1 per hour). Brezinova[26] found the number of intervening arousals to be more frequent in bronchitics than in control subjects. The results of Arand[24] were similar and correlated these findings with subjective complaints of daytime sleepiness when such a history is carefully sought.

There are multiple factors that could account for this disturbed EEG sleep pattern. Retained secretions and increased nocturnal cough, the use of methylxanthines that have a sleep reducing effect similar to caffeine, and hypercapnia/hypoxemia are all potential causes of poor nocturnal sleep. Several studies[28,29] have examined the role of hypoxemia and supplemental oxygen in patients with poor EEG sleep patterns. Fleetham found decreased total sleep time, increased arousals (10/hr), and frequent stage shifts (20.9/hr) similar to the findings of Leitch. They found that arousals (40 percent of total) were related temporally to periods when oxyhemoglobin saturation was below baseline.[29] However, supplemental oxygen that raised saturation to near normal levels did not change any of these parameters. These results differ from other authors. An earlier report by Kearley[28] in which patients slept half of the night breathing room air and half breathing supplemental oxygen (cross-over study) showed a 52 percent sleep efficiency breathing air and an 80% percent efficiency breathing oxygen. Such results must be interpreted with caution since physiologic events occurring during sleep in the first half of the night may not be equivalent to sleep occurring during the second half even though the distribution of stages may be numerically equal. Confirming these findings, Calverly[30] found that 2L/min nasal oxygen during sleep improved mean nocturnal saturation, decreased sleep latency, and increased all stages of sleep including REM and slow wave sleep.

NOCTURNAL CARDIAC ARRHYTHMIAS IN COPD

Several early studies[31,32] noted the incidence of premature supraventricular (PAC's) and ventricular (PVC's) contractions to range from 69 percent to 72 percent in COPD patients during continuous Holter monitoring. Holford noted in his study that "In 6 patients, there was an interesting diurnal variation, the peak incidence of arrhythmia recurring at the same time during each 24-hour period, in most cases during the early hours of the morning." This observation has been confirmed by other authors.[33,34] Flick found PVC's to be twice as common at night, with a peak incidence during 3–5 A.M. and 6–7 A.M. While PVC's occurred 25 percent less frequently during oxygen administration nights in Flick's study, the difference was not statistically significant. However, several episodes of ventricular tachycardia and idioventricular rhythm occurred only on the room air nights. Trilapur was able to abolish ST-T changes, decrease heart rate, and shorten Qtc in patients with type "B" COPD with the administration of nocturnal supplemental oxygen but was unconvinced that these changes were related to *acute* hypoxemia. A recent study presents evidence that hypoxemia may indeed be related to the development of ventricular arrhythmias in some patients with COPD. Shepard et al[35] examined nocturnal oxyhemoglobin saturation and cardiac arrhythmias in 42 clinically stable COPD patients. Premature ventricular complexes occurred in 64 percent of the patients and complex PVC's in 40 percent. There was no relationship between saturation and arrhythmia frequency for the group as a whole. But, in six subjects who experienced profound oxyhemoglobin desaturation (below 80 percent) in stage REM sleep, there was a 150 percent increase in PVC's during these periods (Fig. 8-3). These authors believe that the increase in ventricular irritability was due to a combination of factors including hypoxemia, hypercarbia, elevation of systemic blood pressure with increased myocardial oxygen demands, increased catecholamines, and in one subject, the presence of hypokalemia.

The exact role that cardiac arrhythmias and perhaps myocardial dysfunction during nocturnal hypoxemia play in the morbidity and mortality in COPD remains to be determined. One publication[36] suggests that death in COPD patients during the early morning hours may be accounted for in part by increased myocardial oxygen demands that reach levels similar to those achieved during maximum exercise. These authors measured continuous SaO_2 and systemic blood pressure during sleep and calculated myocardial oxygen consumption in 31 COPD subjects. They found that myocardial oxygen consumption reached its peak at a time when SaO_2 was at its lowest (usually during REM sleep), and systemic systolic blood pressure was at its

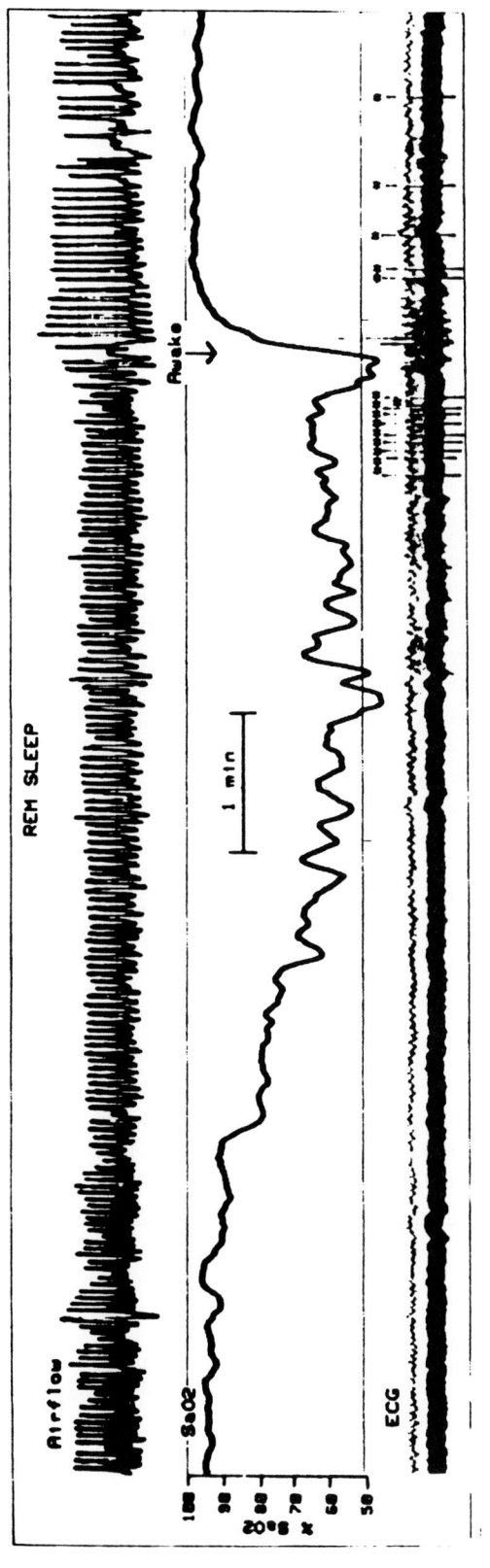

Fig. 8-3. Polysomnographic tracing of a patient with COPD experiencing a REM related decrease in oxyhemoglobin saturation. Multiple premature ventricular complexes (indicated by asterisks) occur at the nadir saturation near the end of the REM period and during the initial part of recovery following hypoxemia. (From Shepard JW Jr, Garrison MW, Grither DA, et al: Am J Med 78:28–34, 1985. With permission.)

161

highest. Perhaps the increased longevity associated with use of continuous home supplemental oxygen[37,38] is due to improvement in basal sleeping oxygen and the amelioration of episodes of transient hypoxemia, which in turn improves myocardial function as well as decreasing electrical irritability.

PATHOPHYSIOLOGY OF DESATURATION: DISORDERED BREATHING, HYPOVENTILATION, AND GAS EXCHANGE

The small fluctuations in SaO_2 of 3–5 percent related to disordered breathing probably do not represent a serious threat to the cardiopulmonary integrity of the COPD patient. These short hypopneas and occasional apneas are either central, reflecting a sudden decrease in central drive to breath, or obstructive, reflecting the inability of inspiratory forces to overcome upper airway resistance. This latter type is most commonly associated with snoring and is considered an "incomplete apnea." Recent studies[24,39] have investigated hypopneic desaturation in COPD subjects. These authors used esophageal pressure balloons to evaluate respiratory effort. Four of seven subjects had hundreds of short episodes of desaturation (both during NREM and REM sleep) associated with snoring and increased amplitude of intrathoracic pressure, evidence of acute partial airway obstruction, probably in the oropharynx.[24] The other three showed similar short (and long) episodes of desaturation associated with decreases in abdominal movement or intrathoracic pressure swings, evidence of decreased central respiratory drive. In the latter group, the hypopneic episodes occurred almost entirely during REM sleep (see Figs. 8-1 and 8-4). The reader should not interpret these data to mean that there is a higher incidence of apnea in patients with COPD. A recent study[40] found no difference in the frequency or duration of apneas and hypopneas among 20 healthy subjects, 7 pink puffers, and 13 (nonoverweight) blue bloaters. In fact 2 of 3 subjects with more than 5 apneas per hour came from the normal group. This does not, however, preclude the possibility that some additional factor such as obesity could predispose to the presence of apneas in COPD patients.

The cause for central hypopnea during REM sleep is unknown but may be related to other forms of periodic breathing (e.g., Cheyne-Stokes) in which the arrhythmia is due to oscillations of blood PO_2 and PCO_2 around a homeostatic "set point." The cause for obstructive hypopnea may be due to a physiologic relaxation of upper airway muscles during REM sleep, a documented phenomenon.[41] This relaxation leads to increased proximal airway resistance and tendency to collapse the oropharynx during inspiration. Such an increase in upper airway resistance during NREM and REM sleep has been demonstrated in normals with the use of intra-airway pressure measurements.[42] An interesting but as yet unexplained observation is that these hypopneas and sometimes apneas are worse during the phasic eye movement of REM sleep (Fig. 8-4).

The origin of the longer, nonapneic REM oxyhemoglobin desaturation is somewhat complex and has been subjected to more investigation than desaturation associated with the short hypopneas. Hypoxemia, whether awake or asleep, is due either to decreased alveolar ventilation or abnormalities of gas exchange (shunt, ventilation perfusion $(\dot{V}/\dot{Q})$ mismatch, or diffusion impairment). Both of these mechanisms are likely contributors to the development of REM hypoxemia.

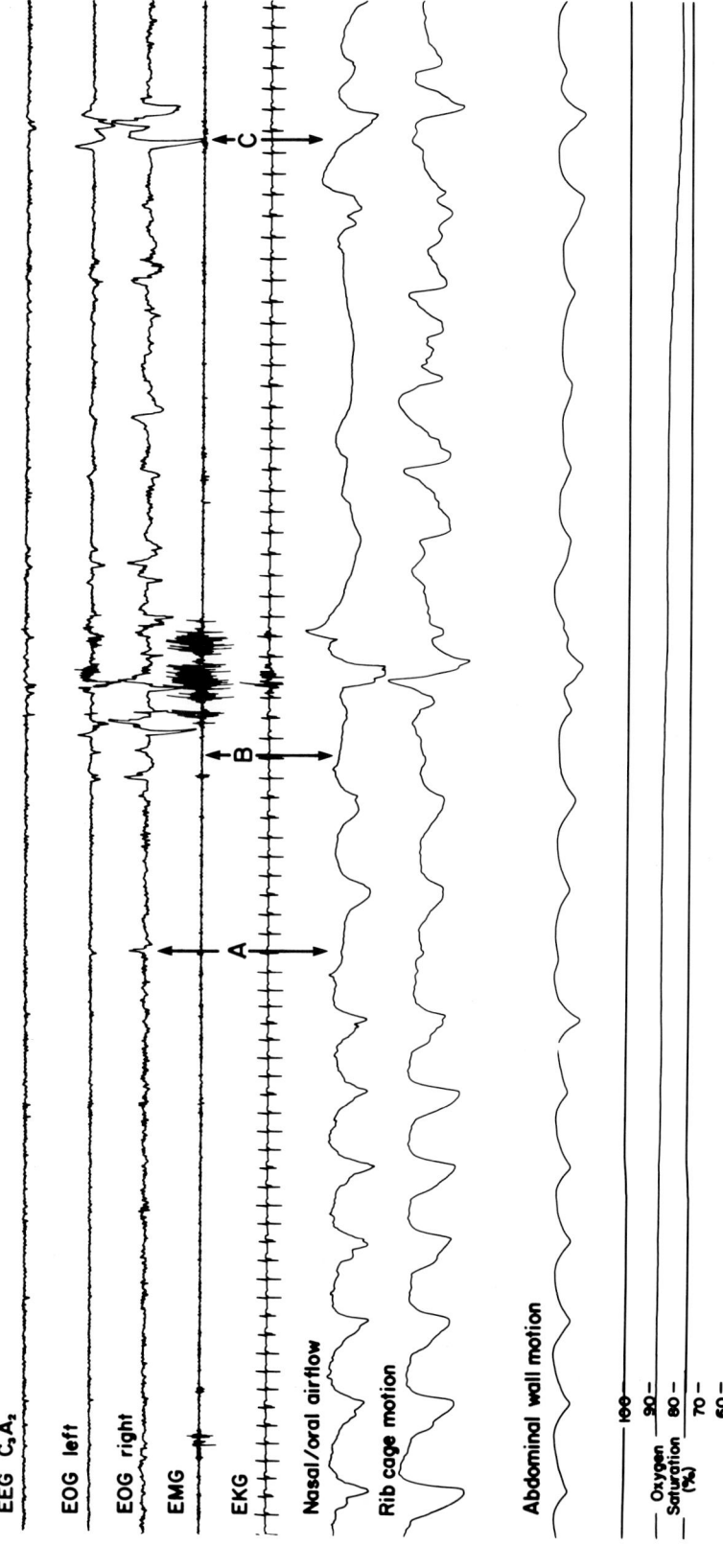

Fig. 8-4. Hypopnea and apnea associated with burst of rapid-eye-movement (phasic eye movement) in REM sleep. Note that although the entire panel represents REM sleep, respiration is regular until first eye movement (A), which is followed by hypopnea. The second burst (B) is followed by an obstructive apnea, which is then followed by further hypopnea after point C. The oxyhemoglobin saturation is abnormal throughout REM sleep and begins to fall further with the first hypopnea.

163

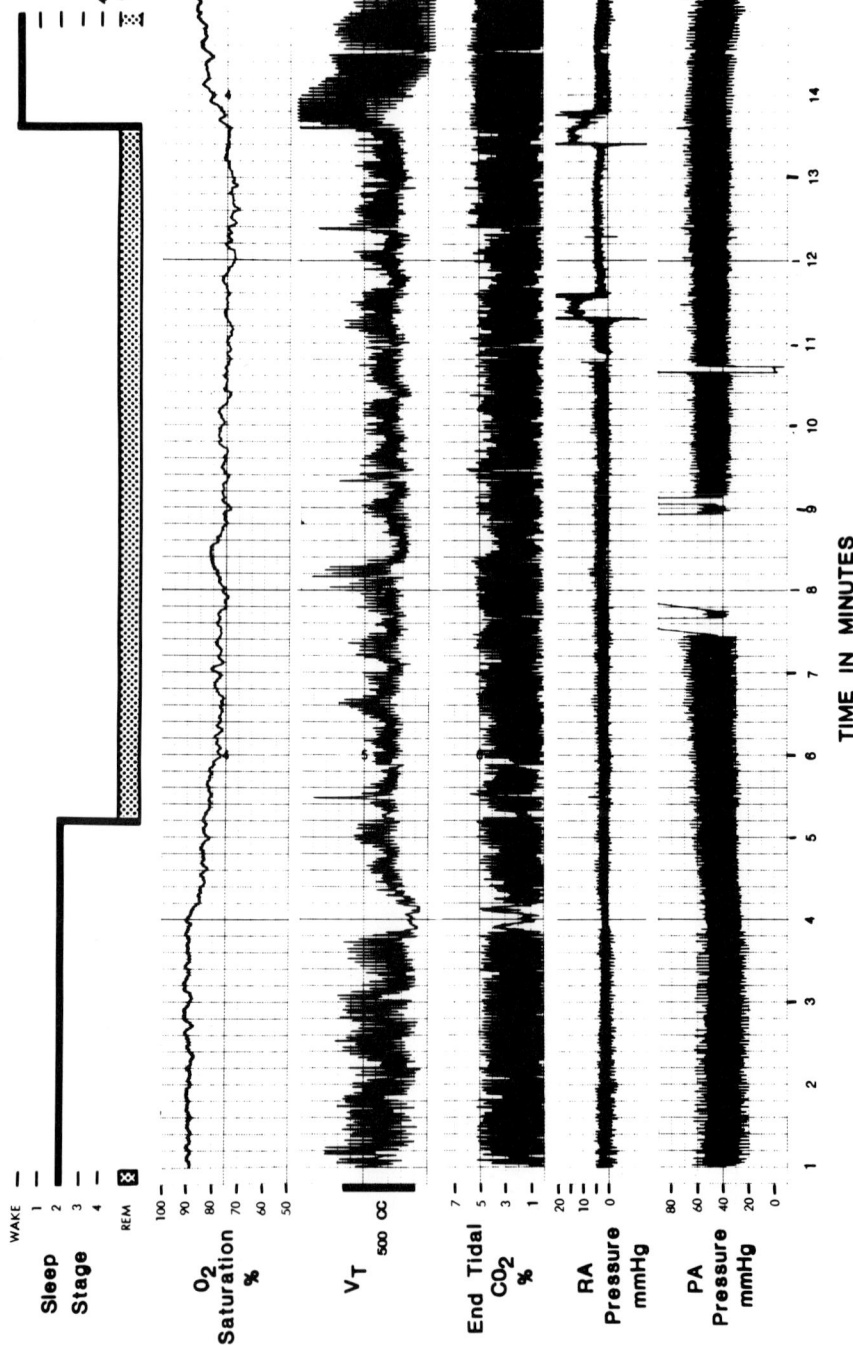

Fig. 8-5. Respiration during REM sleep oxygen desaturation in a patient with COPD. This figure illustrates the contribution to desaturation from hypoventilation. Although the respiratory rate does not change appreciably, overall tidal volume is lower during the REM portion. This appears to result from a decrease in central drive as inspiratory pleural pressure, reflected by negative deflections in right atrial (RA) pressure, decrease during REM sleep and return to normal upon REM termination. (From Fletcher EC, Gray BA, Levin DC: Nonapneic mechanism of arterial oxygen desaturation during rapid-eye-movement sleep. J Appl Physiol Environ Exercise Physiol 54:632–639, 1983. With permission.)

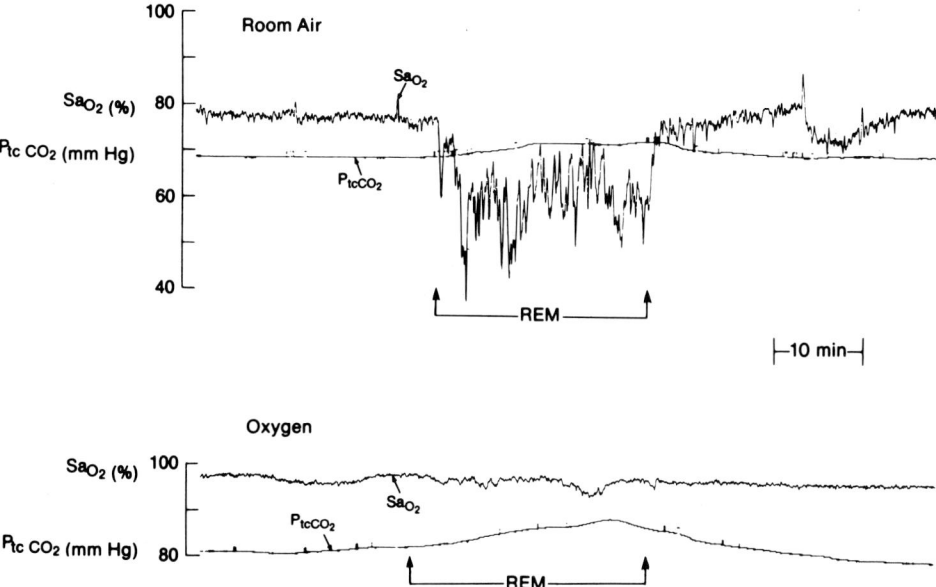

Fig. 8-6. Simultaneous tracings of oxyhemoglobin saturation (SaO_2) and transcutaneous pressure of carbon dioxide ($PtcCO_2$) in a patient with REM desaturation (top). Note the minimal rise in $PtcCO_2$ during the desaturation, which implies mechanisms other than hypoventilation accounting for the desaturation. CO_2 retention is mildly aggravated by the use of supplemental oxygen administered on a subsequent night (lower). (From Goldstein RS, Ramcharan V, Bowes G, et al: Effect of supplemental nocturnal oxygen on gas exchange in patients with severe obstructive lung disease. N Engl J Med 310:425–429, 1984. With permission.)

Semiquantitative measures of minute ventilation including visual observation,[6] nasal thermistor,[11] and pneumographs or related devices[43] have been used to demonstrate alveolar hypoventilation as one cause of hypoxemia during REM sleep. Using a respiratory inductive plethysmograph to measure quantitative changes in ventilation[44] a 25.8 percent decrease in minute ventilation from NREM to REM sleep occurred in 36 episodes of REM sleep observed in 6 COPD subjects with transient, nonapneic, REM desaturation. This was brought about mainly by decreased tidal volume as respiratory rate did not change (Fig. 8-5). A 44 percent fall in inspiratory pleural pressure during these episodes indicates that a central decrease in the respiratory drive (as opposed to airway obstruction) was responsible for this hypoventilation. Using a tightly calibrated respiratory inductance plethysmograph, Hudgel[45] observed similar decreases in minute ventilation and tidal volume in both desaturating (>10 percent) and nondesaturating COPD subjects from NREM to REM sleep. Using the diaphragm EMG as a measure of respiratory effort, decreased drive appeared to be the cause of REM hypoventilation.

In addition to the observation of changes in minute ventilation, increases in arterial carbon dioxide tension (PCO_2) from NREM to REM sleep have been used as direct evidence that alveolar hypoventilation occurs. One author[6] observed a mean increase in $PaCO_2$ of 3 torr from NREM to REM sleep in 6 sleeping hypoxemic COPD patients. The study by Fletcher et al[44] demonstrated a 3.2 torr increase. It can be argued that these increases in PCO_2 are usually not enough to account for the more profound drops in PaO_2 that accompany the "hypoventilation." A good example of this is demonstrated (Fig. 8-6) in a simultaneous tracing of SaO_2 measured by ear oximeter and PCO_2 measured continuously by transcutaneous carbon dioxide analyzer.[46] A 24 minute period of REM desaturation with SaO_2 averaging 50–60 percent is accompanied by only a 4 mmHg percent increase in $PaCO_2$.

Because of the inconsistency of mild hypercapnia but severe desaturation, several early authors[6,7,9] postulated that gas exchange abnormalities contributed to the hypoxemia. Assuming a respiratory quotient (R) of 0.82 to calculate alveolar-arterial oxygen gradient (A-a DO_2) these authors found that in many of the patients, gas exchange appeared to deteriorate between NREM and REM sleep (Fig. 8-7). However, in nonsteady-state ventilation, R varies by virtue of the body's ability to store CO_2 during periods of hypoventilation and the ability of the lungs to eliminate CO_2 in excess of metabolic production during periods of hyperventilation. Since REM sleep respiration is often irregular with periods of hypopnea and hyperpnea, the assump-

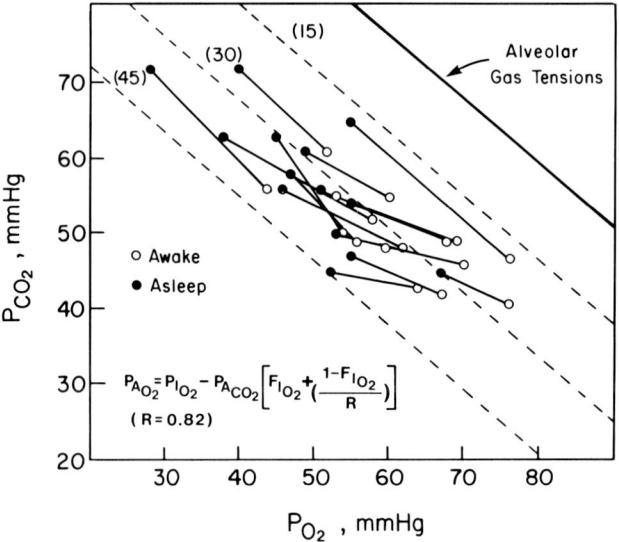

Fig. 8-7. Waking (open circle) and minimal sleeping arterial blood gases (closed circles) plotted on the O2-CO_2 diagram. The heavy solid line represents the alveolar oxygen tension calculated from the alveolar air equation and $PaCO_2$ assuming an R of 0.82. The dashed lines represent isopleths of alveolar-arterial oxygen gradients of 15, 30, and 45 mmHg. Connecting lines between points that have slopes lower than the isopleths represent "a widening of alveolar-arterial oxygen difference during sleep, likely due to areas of worsening ventilation-perfusion mismatch." (From Koo KW, Sax DS, Snider GL: Arterial blood gases and pH during sleep in chronic obstructive pulmonary disease. Am J Med 58:663–670, 1975. With permission.)

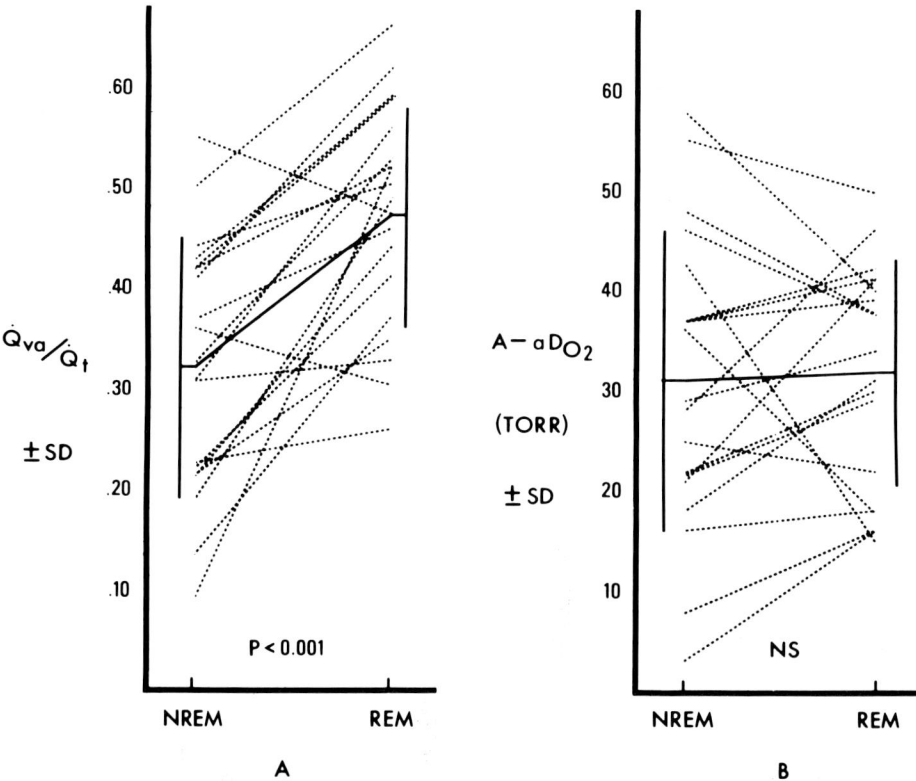

Fig. 8-8. Change in 2 parameters of gas exchange before and during 19 periods of REM sleep in 7 subjects breathing room air. The increase in venous admixture ($\dot{Q}_{va}/\dot{Q}_t$) from nonREM (NREM) to REM sleep is highly significant (A) while the change in alveolar-arterial oxygen gradient is not. This is explained by a change in blood R between NREM and REM sleep. (From Fletcher EC, Gray BA, Levin DC: Nonapneic mechanism of arterial oxygen desaturation during rapid-eye-movement sleep. J Appl Physiol Environ Exercise Physiol 54:632–639, 1983. With permission.)

tion of a constant R may not be valid. To overcome this problem, using a measured blood R calculated from simultaneously drawn arterial and mixed venous blood samples, Fletcher[44] calculated venous admixture ($\dot{Q}_{va}/\dot{Q}_t$) on paired blood specimens from 19 episodes of NREM and REM sleep in six desaturating COPD subjects. This method has an additional advantage over A-a DO_2 for measuring changes in gas exchange in that it uses oxygen content rather than tension in its calculation. This takes into consideration the blood's oxygen carrying ability, which will vary with the subject's position on the oxyhemoglobin dissociation curve. These authors found that $\dot{Q}_{va}/\dot{Q}_t$ increased from a mean NREM value of 0.322 to a REM value of 0.472 (P < 0.001) whereas the change in A-a DO_2 for the same samples (using the calculated blood R) was not significant (Fig. 8-8). Thus, deterioration in gas exchange accounted for about 88 percent of the fall in oxygen seen during REM sleep. Of note is the fact that for any given REM desaturation, hypoventilation or abnormal gas exchange or both could contribute to the hypoxemia.

PATHOPHYSIOLOGY OF DESATURATION:
LUNG MECHANICS

Among the many physiologic accompaniments of REM sleep is active neuronal inhibition of postural muscle activity. Those muscles affected are the intercostals and other accessory muscles of respiration[47] and perhaps some inhibition of tonic activity in the diaphragm.[48,49] This could result in a decrease in tidal volume, fall in functional residual capacity (FRC), and maldistribution of ventilation. In normals this fall in tidal volume may not materialize because the diaphragm is able to increase excursion and make up for the nonfunctioning intercostals.[50,51] Also, any fall in FRC in normals would probably not cause changes in gas exchange as long as thoracic gas volume remains above closing volume. Such falls in FRC have been documented in infants using whole body plethysmography (Henderson-Smart: a 31 percent fall in thoracic gas volume during REM),[50] in normal adults using magnitometers[52] and

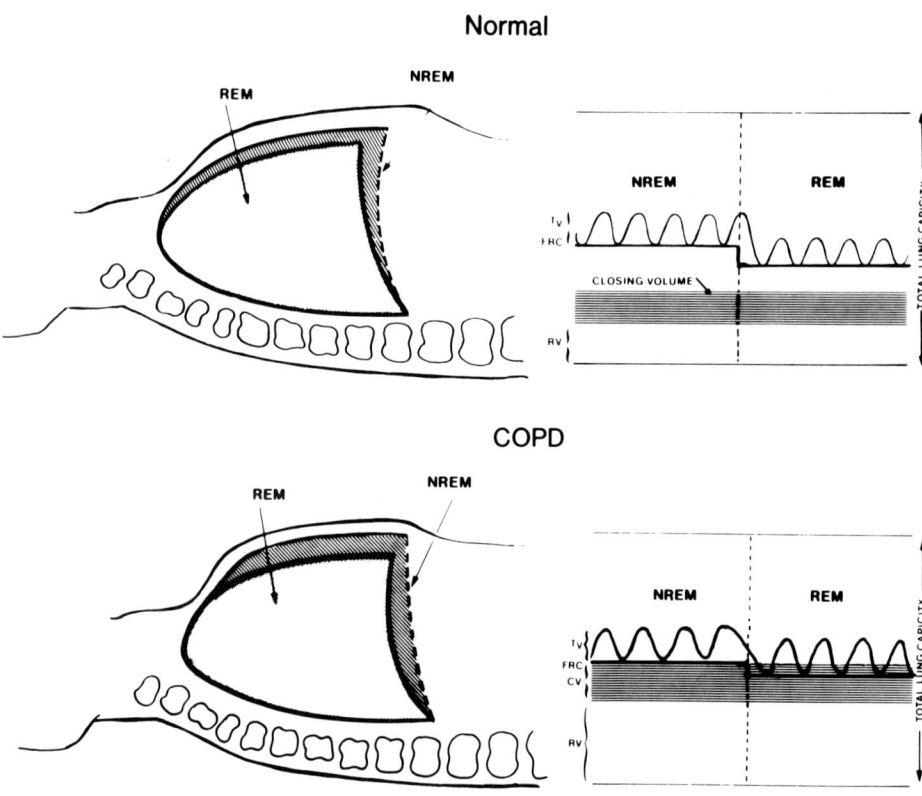

Fig. 8-9. Drawing representing the change in functional residual capacity (FRC) from NREM to REM sleep in a patient with COPD and REM related oxyhemoglobin desaturation. When a subject with normal lung mechanics (top panel) enters REM sleep there is a small drop in FRC which, although bringing the thoracic gas volume closer to closing volume, does not significantly effect gas exchange. When a patient with COPD enters REM sleep (bottom), the fall in FRC places some dependent portions of the lung below closing volume allowing shunting of blood past underventilated or closed alveoli. Uneven distribution of gas throughout the lung may also occur because of ventilation occurring near FRC.

helium dilution,[53] in patients with cystic fibrosis using magnitometers,[15] and in patients with COPD using the respiratory inductive plethysmograph.[42]

In individuals with diseased lungs functioning with abnormal chest wall and diaphragm mechanics as well as pre-existing $\dot{V}/\dot{Q}$ disturbances, a multiplicity of factors may contribute to the development of significant REM-related oxyhemoglobin desaturation as recently summarized by Phillipson.[54] First, since patients with COPD breath at higher than normal thoracic gas volumes with flattened diaphragms, loss of intercostal muscle tone would predictably have a greater effect than in normals. Since the diaphragm is already functioning at a point near maximal contraction,[55] it may be unable to increase excursions to make up for the loss in tidal volume and may subsequently fatigue. Also, a low tidal volume increases the dead space/tidal volume ratio (Vd/Vt) adding to already present wasted ventilation. Second, such patients have higher than normal closing volumes and during awake and NREM respiration may breath just above the level where alveoli begin to close during exhalation. The combination of loss of intercostal muscle tone and inability of the diaphragm to increase thoracic gas volume because of abdominal contents pushing upward may now cause FRC to fall *below* closing volume. This may add to the number of low $\dot{V}/\dot{Q}$ areas already present in diseased lungs by further increasing maldistribution of ventilation or actually creating microatelectatic areas through which blood is shunted (Fig. 8-9). Third, patients with COPD are at a further disadvantage because of their position on the oxyhemoglobin dissociation curve (Fig. 8-10). In normals beginning at a PaO_2 of 95 torr, a fall in PaO_2 of 20 torr due to alveolar hypoventilation would cause a fall of 6 percent in oxyhemoglobin saturation. In a COPD patient already at the shoulder of the curve with a PaO_2 of 55 torr, the same 20 torr drop in PaO_2 will result in a hemoglobin saturation of 65 percent, greatly impair-

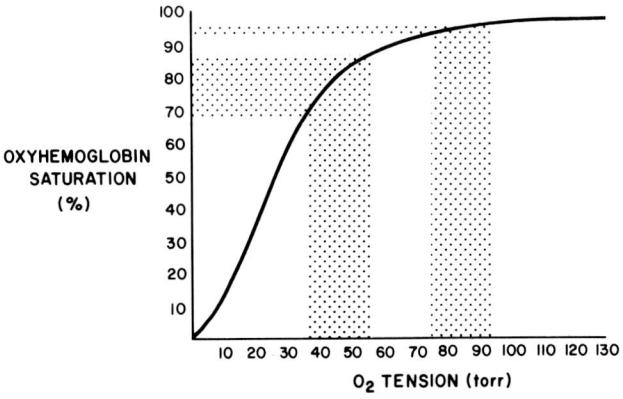

Fig. 8-10. The oxyhemoglobin dissociation curve demonstrates that a 20 torr fall in PaO_2 in normals will cause only a small decrease in oxyhemoglobin desaturation. The same fall in PaO_2 in a patient with COPD beginning at the steep portion of the curve (PaO_2 = 55 torr) causes a much larger fall in saturation.

ing oxygen carrying capacity. Fourth, if the patient is a CO_2 retainer, a small drop in alveolar ventilation will cause a proportionately higher alveolar PCO_2 than the same drop in normals. A higher alveolar CO_2 tension will tend to lower alveolar PO_2, further aggravating the hypoxemia. Fifth, both lower airway resistance in the form of bronchospasm[57] and upper airway resistance in the form of loss of pharyngeal constrictor tone[42] may add to the resistive load and work of breathing during REM sleep. This additional burden may go unnoticed in normals but in patients with impaired lung function, this further deterioration of lung mechanics may add insult to injury. Sixth, depressed cough reflex[58] and mucocilliary clearance may allow pooling of secretions further adding to $\dot{V}/\dot{Q}$ mismatch. Finally, adding to the already depressed hypoxic and hypercarbic ventilatory responses frequently seen in COPD,[59,60] additional depression of chemoresponsiveness during REM sleep[60,61] may further impair their ability to respond to the additional hypoxemia and hypercarbia brought about by the above mentioned factors. Several authors[39,60] have attempted to correlate diminished ventilatory chemosensitivity in COPD subjects with severity of REM related oxyhemoglobin desaturation (see below).

CLINICAL SIGNIFICANCE: DIAGNOSIS AND POTENTIAL CONSEQUENCES

To date, the only method of finding nocturnal oxyhemoglobin desaturation is to study the patient with lung disease in a sleep lab or at minimum, to obtain an oximeter screening study on the patient in the hospital. No daytime parameter of lung mechanics or gas exchange has been shown to reliably predict patients who will develop nocturnal oxyhemoglobin desaturation. Numerous authors have tried to correlate symptoms, age, body weight, sex, pulmonary function studies, blood gases, ventilatory control, and other waking parameters with nocturnal desaturation for purposes of bypassing an expensive sleep study. In general it can be said that the worse the COPD and the lower the awake PaO_2, the more likely the patient is to experience significant nocturnal falls in oxyhemoglobin saturation but this may not be predictive in an individual patient. For example, in one study[6] all 7 subjects whose mean awake, resting daytime PaO_2 was below 60 torr dropped below 50 torr during sleep. Yet in the same study, 7 subjects whose awake PaO_2 was above 60 torr (range 62–76 torr) also fell below 55 torr during sleep. Attempts at correlating pulmonary function with nocturnal desaturation have been unsuccessful.[30,62]

It has become apparent that the bronchitic[63] or type "B" COPD patient (hypercarbic, hypoxemic, history of cor pulmonale, severe dyspnea, bronchitis, and often overweight) is more likely to desaturate than the eucapneic and normoxic "pink puffer."[30,40,43,62,64] Douglas[43] found transient oxyhemoglobin desaturation in all of 10 "blue bloaters" and in neither of two "pink puffers." Flenley[64] found frequent REM related oxygen desaturation in all of 15 "blue bloaters" with pulmonary hypertension and polycythemia (PaO_2 = 42 torr; $PaCO_2$ = 54 torr) whereas eight "pink puffers" had infrequent desaturation (PaO_2 = 72 torr; $PaCO_2$ = 35 torr). DeMarco[62] found a lower baseline oxygen saturation, more frequent episodes of desaturation, and larger falls in saturation in four blue bloaters, (mean fall 29.5 percent) than in six pink puffers (mean fall 4.7 percent). Of note is the fact that the "pink puffer" group had a mean percent ideal body weight of 88 while that of the "blue bloater" group was 110 percent. It may well be that weight correlates with REM desaturation just as it correlates with other forms of sleep disordered breathing and associated desaturation.[65,66]

Blunted ventilatory response to hypercapnea and hypoxia are additional determinants of the "blue and bloated" syndrome[67] and therefore might also be predictive of nocturnal desaturation. Indeed, several publications[39,60,68] have suggested that blunted ventilatory responses to CO_2 and hypoxia may be markers of nocturnal desaturation in patients not clinically classifiable as blue bloaters or pink puffers. Littner[39] found 6 of 9 subjects with COPD who desaturated more than 11 percent from baseline during sleep. They measured hypercapnic and hypoxic responses by ventilation and maximum rate of change of mouth pressure (dP/dt) during transient occlusion of the airway at the beginning of inspiration. The ventilatory and dP/dt responses to hypercapnia and hypoxia were significantly lower in these six desaturators than in three patients who did not desaturate. Fleetham[60] used similar techniques ($P_{0.1}$ instead of dP/dt) to examine ventilatory drive responses in 41 hypoxemic subjects with COPD. He found that the drop in saturation during sleep was negatively correlated with hypercarbic ventilatory drive. Hypoxic ventilatory drive did not correlate with the degree of oxyhemoglobin desaturation. This may have resulted from the fact that all patients in the study were hypoxemic and had blunted hypoxic drives to begin with. In spite of these data, a cause-effect relationship between nocturnal desaturation and decreased waking chemosensitivity has not been proven. Furthermore, chemosensitivity may change during sleep, perhaps making results of waking studies not applicable to the sleep state.

In summary, the nocturnal oxyhemoglobin desaturator will most likely be the male COPD patient with classic chronic bronchitis, hypoxemia, hypercarbia, perhaps mild obesity, and often, previous episodes of cor pulmonale. The hypercarbia may indicate a blunted hypercarbic ventilatory drive further pointing toward nocturnal REM desaturation. Since these patients are already candidates for home supplemental oxygen by virtue of their hypoxemia and cor pulmonale, the diagnosis of desaturation is academic as they will be receiving appropriate treatment. Perhaps it is more important to find the desaturator with a resting daytime PaO_2 above 55–60 torr who cannot yet be classified a "blue bloater." Clinical experience indicates that this will be the bronchitic who is normal or slightly overweight, perhaps has occasional peripheral edema, a borderline or overtly elevated hematocrit, and perhaps large pulmonary arteries on chest roentgenogram. Unfortunately, these are very general criteria and ear oximetry would be needed to confirm the presence or absence of desaturation.

Pulmonary artery pressure during sleep has been observed in a limited number of COPD patients using flow directed pulmonary artery catheters.[10,43,69,70] Douglas[43] observed prolonged elevation of pulmonary artery pressure during a REM related arterial oxygen desaturation episode in a single patient. Coccagna et al[10] showed a mean maximum fall in PaO_2 from the awake state to REM sleep of 15.9 torr that was accompanied by a corresponding rise in mean pulmonary artery pressure from 37 mmHg to 55 mmHg in 13 patients with COPD. All of these subjects had awake resting hypercarbia ($PaCO_2$ = 49–59 torr) and severe hypoxemia ($PaO_2 < 50$ torr). Boysen[69] monitored four patients (mean daytime PaO_2 of 58 torr) with flow directed pulmonary artery catheters in place while breathing room air (first half of the night) and oxygen at 2L/min (second half of the night). They observed transient increases in pulmonary artery pressure associated with arterial oxygen desaturation resulting from both disordered breathing events and REM related desaturations. These falls in saturation and accompanying transient elevations in pulmonary artery pressure were ameliorated with low flow oxygen. In a study examining the acute and chronic effect of supplemental oxygen on pulmonary artery pressure during sleep, Fletcher and Levin[70] demonstrated that oxygen lowered mean sleeping pressure in four subjects who experienced REM sleep under both room air and supplemental oxygen conditions (Fig. 8-11). These authors found that the transient elevations in pulmonary artery pressure were, in the majority of cases (7/13) due to increased pulmonary vascular resistance. Increased cardiac output alone or in combination with increased vascular resistance, also contributed to the elevated pressure.

Both Flenley[71] and Block[72] have proposed that these repetitive transient elevations of pulmonary artery pressure may become sustained through some as yet unknown mechanism leading to chronic pulmonary hypertension and cor pulmonale associated with the "blue bloater" syndrome. Block has stated:

> Those patients with the most severe, prolonged, or frequent episodes of nocturnal desaturation would be most likely to sustain the greatest degree of nocturnal pulmonary hypertension, which might ultimately become irreversible.

The mechanism for the development of sustained pulmonary hypertension is unknown but several authors have demonstrated that repetitive episodes of transient hypoxia in experimental animals can lead to many of the changes seen in chronic

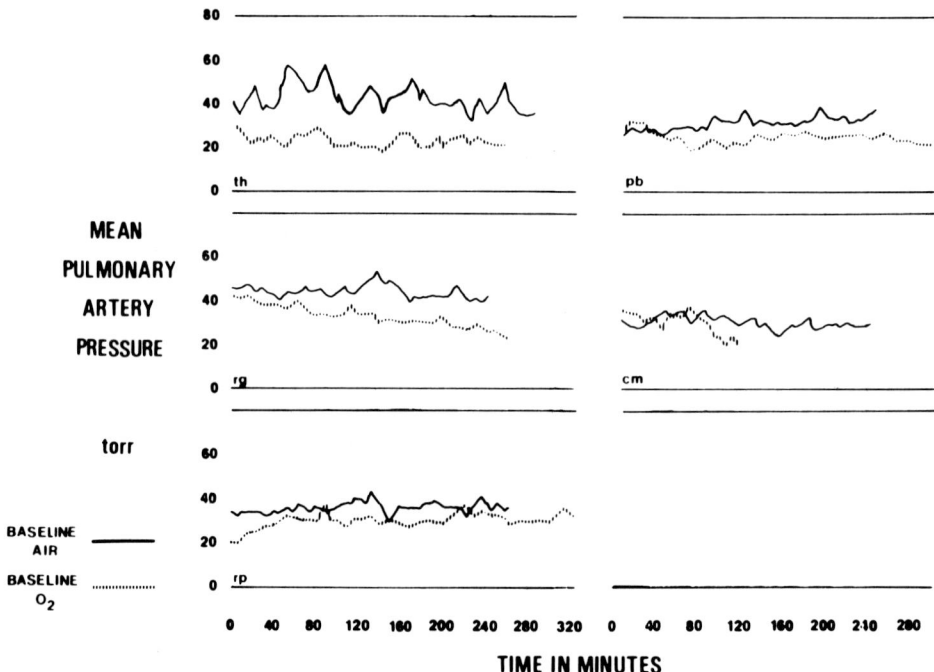

Fig. 8-11. The effect of acutely administered supplemental oxygen on mean pulmonary artery pressure during sleep. The solid line represents pulmonary artery pressure with the patient breathing room air at baseline and the dashed line represents mean pulmonary artery pressure breathing supplemental oxygen at 4 L/min on another night. (From Fletcher EC, Levin DC: Cardiopulmonary hemodynamics during sleep in subjects with chronic obstructive pulmonary disease: The effect of short and long term oxygen. Chest 85:6–14, 1984. With permission.)

pulmonary hypertension. For example, exposing rats to hypoxic gas mixtures (PaO_2 in the range of 55–60 torr) during 8 of 24 hours for 21 days causes elevation of right ventricular systolic pressure and an increase in the ratio of right ventricular weight to body weight.[73] Since the acute administration of 100 percent oxygen to such animals does not relieve the high right ventricular systolic pressure, a mechanism other than hypoxic pulmonary vasoconstriction must be invoked to explain the lasting changes of intermittent hypoxia.[74] Shorter periods of exposure to intermittent hypoxia (4 hours/day, 24 exposures, alveolar PO_2 = 64 torr) have caused increased right ventricular weight (+33 percent) and red cell mass (+44 percent), although 75 exposures were required to demonstrate an elevation of right ventricular systolic pressure.[75] In these animals, the development of smooth muscle fibers in pulmonary vessels usually devoid of muscle may explain the more lasting effect of intermittent hypoxia. Under similar conditions, McGrath[76] has demonstrated that intermittent hypoxic stress caused a higher mortality in older rats. Perhaps intermittent hypoxia could have a greater effect in older humans with lung disease.

Several mechanisms could be operative in inducing chronic changes in pulmonary vascular hemodynamics: (1) increased pulmonary blood flow; (2) pulmonary venous congestion induced by transient left ventricular failure; or (3) lingering biochemical or cellular mediator of pulmonary vascular constriction and muscle cell hypertrophy. One or more of several local effects of transient hypoxia could be postulated. For example, transient hypoxemia in dogs ventilated acutely with hypoxic gases showed that bradykinin converting enzyme activity was reduced to zero at a PaO_2 less than 26 torr and returned to full activity 2 minutes after becoming normoxic.[77] The same and other authors have noted similar changes in angiotensin converting enzyme during induced hypoxia. It is possible that other as yet undiscovered enzymatic or hormonal changes brought about by acute hypoxia lead to hypertrophy of vascular smooth muscle. Another possible mechanism is endothelial cell damage. It is well demonstrated that endothelial cell damage in the systemic circulation causes platelet deposition, which in turn invokes vascular smooth muscle growth through the release of a mitogenic factor.[78] A similar mechanism on a chronic basis could be operative in the lung if vascular endothelium were damaged directly by hypoxemia or indirectly by enzymatic changes. Subsequent deposition of platelets could invoke hypertrophic responses in vascular smooth muscle. Johnson[79] has demonstrated decreased platelet survival in COPD patients with hypoxemia and improvement in survival with supplemental oxygen.

All of these mechanisms are highly theoretical as no direct proof exists that recurrent episodes of transient nocturnal hypoxemia leads to pulmonary hypertension in patients who are not severely hypoxemic (<60 torr) during the day. Likewise, no proof exists that correction of nocturnal hypoxemic episodes in such patients would delay or prevent the onset of such permanent hemodynamic abnormalities. Clinical studies to demonstrate the natural history of such desaturation and the effects of supplemental oxygen are now in progress.

TREATMENT

Thus far, the only effective therapy that has been shown to ameliorate or eliminate nocturnal oxyhemoglobin desaturation and the accompanying transient elevation of pulmonary artery pressure is low flow supplemental oxygen administered during sleep. Oxygen between 2 and 4 L/min has been shown to elevate baseline sleeping saturation, and eliminate or ameliorate both short hypopneic desaturation and longer, REM related desaturation. It has also been shown to prevent transient REM elevation of pulmonary artery pressure[46,69,70] and used chronically, to lower mean sleeping pulmonary artery pressure and pulmonary vascular resistance.[70]

Based upon current knowledge, efforts to correct nocturnal hypoxemia with supplemental oxygen should be directed to the following patients. Those patients with a daytime PaO_2 below 55 torr should be instructed to use nocturnal oxygen compulsively as a large percentage of them will undergo further desaturation at night. Those patients with a daytime PaO_2 above 55–60 torr but with signs of right sided hemodynamic abnormalities such as roentgenographic, electrocardiographic, physical (unexplained peripheral edema), or laboratory (unexplained polycythemia) evidence of pulmonary hypertension and cor pulmonale should undergo some form of nocturnal saturation monitoring to rule out desaturation and assure reversal with supplemental oxygen.

Patients who complain of marked disturbances of sleep with frequent awakening might conceivably benefit from supplemental oxygen although there is great potential for placebo effect. Precedent exists for such treatment in hypoxemic "blue bloaters." Using supplemental oxygen, Calverley[30] demonstrated reduction in sleep onset latency, increased total sleep time, increased stages 2, 3/4, and REM sleep, and reduction in intervening wakefulness in six hypoxemic bronchitics. It is dangerous however, to equate these results to patients without severe daytime hypoxemia. Objective demonstration of the benefit of supplemental oxygen on sleep architecture might be in order before prescribing an expensive drug such as oxygen (especially patients with a daytime PaO_2 above 55 torr) for the purpose of improving sleep quality. Admittedly, the cost of a formal sleep study might deter the collection of such objective evidence. At this point, there is not enough information available to judge the effect of other sleep aids such as hypnotics, on sleep quality. One investigator[80] has demonstrated that the use of hypnotics in nonhypercarbic COPD patients increased the frequency of sleep disordered breathing events, increased frequency of episodes of desaturation, and increased duration and severity of desaturation. While these changes were statistically significant, the author felt that they were of such a small degree that they might not be clinically significant. Sleep time did improve in these subjects with the use of hypnotics.

While at this point, oxygen might appear to be the most effective drug for treatment of nocturnal oxyhemoglobin desaturation, much remains to be learned about its possible adverse effects. For example, while carbon dioxide retention following the application of supplemental oxygen during sleep tends to be minimal (4–6 torr above awake levels) (Fig. 8-6) larger increases may be seen in those COPD patients that have coexistant disordered breathing, especially sleep apnea. Goldstein[46] reported increases in $PaCO_2$ of 15, 20, and 21 torr and morning headaches in 3 COPD patients with concomitant obstructive sleep apnea. Alford et al[81] found similar results in 20 patients with severe sleep apnea and COPD. Although no acute detrimental effect from nocturnal oxygen was demonstrated, significant end apneic respiratory acidosis was induced by supplemental oxygen. The long-term effects of hypercapnea on pulmonary hypertension in the face of improved oxygenation is unknown. The subject of combined COPD and sleep apnea is discussed in greater depth in Chapter 9.

Several respiratory stimulants have been looked at with limited success but none have been shown to reverse the profound REM desaturations. Medroxyprogesterone acetate (MPA) has been shown to have a central stimulatory effect on respiration both in normals and in patients with COPD.[82–84] MPA administered to 17 awake patients with COPD over a 4 week period caused a significant reduction in $PaCO_2$ (51 torr to 42 torr) in 10 of these. This was due to a 15 percent increase in alveolar ventilation. It is postulated that the noncorrectors did not decrease their $PaCO_2$ in spite of improved minute ventilation because of increased CO_2 production. No improvement in gas exchange occurred as alveolar-arterial oxygen difference widened in the correctors from 29 to 36 torr. Also, responders were not separable from nonresponders by any tested clinical parameters including ventilatory chemoresponsiveness. The same authors[83] evaluated sleeping ventilation and $PaCO_2$ in five COPD subjects on and off MPA. MPA significantly decreased NREM $PaCO_2$ from 57 to 49 torr. Mean oxyhemoglobin saturation increased 4 percent during NREM sleep, 6 percent during tonic REM sleep, and 9 percent during phasic REM sleep. A subsequent article[85] examined 19 COPD subjects while asleep and found that nocturnal SaO_2 was *not* improved even though awake saturation *was*. Only five were CO_2 retainers with severe hypoxemia and specific mention of REM desaturation was not made. If alveolar ventilation but not gas exchange is improved, the ability of progesterone to correct REM desaturation might be limited. Also, long-term effects of the drug in maintaining the ventilatory improvement and side effects have not been examined in COPD patients.

Almitrine recently received attention because of it's ability to improve ventilation. It's mechanism of action appears to be improvement in hypoxic ventilatory drive by stimulation of peripheral chemoreceptors. There is some suggestion that pulmonary gas exchange is improved since the change in blood gases appear out of proportion to the small increase in alveolar ventilation. The awake increase in PaO_2 generally ranges from 6–10 torr and the fall in $PaCO_2$ varies from 2–4 torr.[86–88] Connaughton[89] has demonstrated that almitrine improves mean nocturnal oxyhemoglobin saturation (89 percent versus 83 percent) and decreases the degree of desaturation (mean nadir saturation 77 percent versus 65 percent) in bronchitic type COPD patients. The mechanism is probably by improvement in baseline saturation to a higher level on the oxyhemoglobin dissociation curve. There appears to be a major drawback to this drug. It has been well demonstrated to cause acute elevations in pulmonary artery pressure both in animals and in humans with COPD. This effect appears significant as recently reported by MacNee et al.[87] Ten bronchitics treated with almitrine bismesylate increased their mean pulmonary artery pressure at rest from 22 mmHg to 33 mmHg. At 3 months followup of 5 patients treated chronically, resting pulmonary artery pressure increased from 17 to 23 mmHg and 35 to 42 mmHg during exercise.

In spite of tremendous strides in the area of sleep and breathing in the past 10 to 15 years, more questions have been created than answered. Before such drugs as oxygen, MPA, almitrine, and others can be recommended judiciously, the natural history of this disorder must be determined. The theoretical effects of recurrent, transient hypoxemia on pulmonary vascular hemodynamics, left ventricular function, arrhythmias, and sleep quality must be proven. Finally, the effect of therapy on morbidity and mortality must be assessed with long term prospective studies.

REFERENCES

1. Bulow K: Respiration and wakefulness in man. Acta Physiol Scand (Suppl.) 59:1–110, 1963

2. Trask CH, Cree EM: Oximeter studies on patients with chronic obstructive emphysema, awake and during sleep. New Engl J Med 266:639–642, 1962

3. Pierce AK, Jarret CE, Werkle G Jr, Miller WF: Respiratory function during sleep in patients with chronic obstructive lung disease. J Clin Invest 45:631–636, 1966

4. Robin ED: Some interactions between sleep and disease. Arch Intern Med 102:669–675, 1958

5. Interiano B, Perkins PT, Fuleihan F, et al: Changes in arterial blood gases during sleep in patients with cardiopulmonary diseases. Am Rev Respir Dis 105:980, 1972

6. Koo KW, Sax DS, Snider GL: Arterial blood gases and pH during sleep in chronic obstructive pulmonary disease. Am J Med 58:663–670, 1975

7. Leitch AJ, Clancy LJ, Leggett RJ, et al: Arterial blood gas tensions, hydrogen ion, and electroencephalogram during sleep in patients with chronic ventilatory failure. Thorax 31:730–735, 1976

8. Wynne JW, Block AJ, Hunt LA, Flick MR: Disordered breathing and oxygen desaturation during daytime naps. Johns Hopkins Med J 143:3–7, 1978

9. Flick MR, Block AJ: Continuous in vivo monitoring of arterial oxygenation in chronic obstructive lung disease. Ann Intern Med 86:725–730, 1977

10. Coccagna G, Lugaresi E: Arterial blood gases and pulmonary and systemic arterial pressure during sleep in chronic obstructive pulmonary disease. Sleep 1:117–124, 1978

11. Wynne JW, Block AJ, Hemenway J, et al: Disordered breathing and oxygen desaturation during sleep in patients with chronic obstructive lung disease (COLD). Am J Med 66:573–579, 1979

12. Mezon BL, West P, Israels J, Kryger M: Sleep breathing abnormalities in kyphoscoliosis. Am Rev Respir Dis 122:617–621, 1980

13. Guilleminault C, Kurland G, Winkle R, Miles LE: Severe kyphoscoliosis, breathing and sleep. Chest 79:626–630, 1981

14. Francis PWJ, Muller NL, Guiwitx D, et al: Hemoglobin desaturation. Its occurrence during sleep in patients with cystic fibrosis. Am J Dis Child 134:734–740, 1980

15. Muller NL, Francis PW, Gurwitz D, et al: Mechanism of hemoglobin desaturation during rapid-eye-movement sleep in normal subjects and in patients wih cystic fibrosis. Am Rev Respir Dis 121:463–469, 1980

16. Stokes DC, McBride JT, Wall MA, et al: Sleep hypoxemia in young adults with cystic fibrosis. Dis Child 134:741–743, 1980

17. Gaultier C, Praud JP, Clement A, et al: Respiration during sleep in children with COPD. Chest 87:168–173, 1985

18. Bye PT, Issa F, Bethan-Jones M, Sullivan CE: Studies of oxygenation during sleep in patients with interstitial lung disease. Am Rev Respir Dis 129:27–32, 1984

19. Smith TF, Hudgel DW: Arterial oxygen desaturation during sleep in children with asthma and its relation to airway obstruction and ventilatory drive. Pediatrics 66:746–751, 1980

20. Guilleminault C, Motta J: Sleep apnea syndrome as a long term sequela of poliomyelitis, in Guilleminault C, Dement WC (eds): Sleep Apnea Syndromes. New York, Alan R. Liss, 1978, pp 309–315

21. Newsom-Davis J, Goldman M, Loh L, Casson M: Diaphragm function and alveolar hypoventilation. Q J Med 45:87–100, 1975

22. Amis TC, Ciofetta G, Hughes JMB, Loh L: Regional lung function in bilateral diaphragmatic paralysis. Clin Sci 59:485–492, 1980

23. Coccagna G, Mantovani M, Parchi C, et al: Alveolar hypoventilation and hypersomnia in myotonic dystrophy. Neurol Neurosurg Psychiatry 38:977–984, 1975

24. Arand DL, McGinty DJ, Littner MR: Respiratory patterns associated with hemoglobin desaturation during sleep in chronic obstructive pulmonary disease. Chest 80:183–190, 1981

25. Fleetham JA, Mezon B, West P: Chemical control of ventilation and sleep arterial oxygen desaturation in patients with COPD. Am Rev Respir Dis 122:583–589, 1980

26. Brezinova A, Catterall JR, Douglas NJ, et al: Night sleep of patients with chronic ventilatory failure and age matched controls: Number and duration of the EEG episodes of intervening wakefulness and drowsiness. Sleep 5:123–130, 1982

27. Fletcher EC, Martin RJ, Monlux RD: Disturbed EEG sleep patterns in chronic obstructive pulmonary disease. Sleep Res 11:186, 1982

28. Kearley R, Wynne JW, Block AJ, et al: The effect of low flow oxygen on sleep disordered breathing and oxygen desaturation. Chest 78:682–685, 1980

29. Fleetham J, West P, Mezon B, et al: Sleep, arousals, and oxygen desaturation in chronic obstructive pulmonary disease. Am Rev Respir Dis 126:429–433, 1982

30. Calverley PMA, Brezinova V, Douglas NJ, et al: The effect of oxygenation on sleep quality in chronic bronchitis and emphysema. Am Rev Respir Dis 126:206–210, 1982

31. Holford FD, Mithoefer TC: Cardiac arrhythmias in hospitalized patients with chronic obstructive pulmonary disease. Am Rev Respir Dis 108:879–885, 1973

32. Kleiger RE, Senior RM: Longterm electrocardiographic monitoring of ambulatory patients with chronic airway obstruction. Chest 65:483–487, 1974

33. Flick MR, Block AJ: Nocturnal vs diurnal cardiac arrhythmias in patients with chronic obstructive pulmonary disease. Chest 75:8–11, 1979

34. Tirlapur VG, Mir M: Nocturnal hypoxemia and associated electrocardiographic changes in patients with chronic obstructive airway disease. New Engl J Med 306:125–130, 1982

35. Shepard JW Jr, Garrison MW, Grither DA, et al: Relationship of ventricular ectopy to nocturnal oxygen desaturation in patients with chronic obstructive pulmonary disease. Am J Med 78:28–34, 1985

36. Shepard JW Jr, Schweitzer PK, Keller CA, et al: Myocardial stress—exercise versus sleep in patients with COPD. Chest 86:366–374, 1984

37. Nocturnal Oxygen Therapy Trial Group: Continuous or nocturnal oxygen therapy in hypoxemic chronic obstructive lung disease. Ann Intern Med 93:391–398, 1980

38. Medical Research Council Working Party: Long term domiciliary oxygen therapy in chronic hypoxic cor pulmonale complicating chronic bronchitis and emphysema. Lancet 1:681–686, 1981

39. Littner MR, McGinty DJ, Arand DL: Determinants of oxygen desaturation in the course of ventilation during sleep in chronic obstructive pulmonary disease. Am Rev Respir Dis 122:849–857, 1980

40. Catterall JR, Douglas NJ, Calverley PMA, et al: Transient hypoxemia during sleep in chronic obstructive pulmonary disease is not a sleep apnea syndrome. Am Rev Respir Dis 128:24–29, 1983

41. Orem J: Control of the upper airways during sleep and the hypersomnia-sleep apnea syndrome, in Orem J, Barnes CD (eds): Physiology in sleep. New York, Academic Press, 1980, pp 273–313

42. Hudgel DW, Martin RJ, Johnson B, Hill P: Mechanics of the respiratory system and breathing pattern during sleep in normal humans. J Appl Physiol: Respirat Environ Exercise Physiol 56:133–137, 1984

43. Douglas NJ, Calverley PM, Leggett RJ, et al: Transient hypoxemia during sleep in chronic bronchitis and emphysema. Lancet 1:1–4, 1979

44. Fletcher EC, Gray BA, Levin DC: Nonapneic mechanism of arterial oxygen desaturation during rapid-eye-movement sleep. J Appl Physiol Environ Exercise Physiol 54:632–639, 1983

45. Hudgel DW, Martin RJ, Capehart M, Johnson B: Contribution of hypoventilation to sleep oxygen desaturation in chronic obstructive pulmonary disease. J Appl Physiol: Respirat Environ Exercise Physiol 55:669–677, 1983

46. Goldstein RS, Ramcharan V, Bowes G, et al: Effect of supplemental nocturnal oxygen on gas exchange in patients with severe obstructive lung disease. N Engl J Med 310:425–429, 1984

47. Jouvet M: Neurophysiology of the states of sleep. Physiol Rev 47:117–177, 1967

48. Prechtl HFR, Van Eykjern LA, O'Brien JJ: Respiratory muscle EMG in newborns. A nonintrusive method. Early Hum Dev 1:265–283, 1977

49. Muller N, Volgyesi G, Bryan MH: Diaphragmatic muscle tone. J Appl Physiol 47:279–284, 1979

50. Henderson-Smart DJ, Read DJ: Reduced lung volume during behavioral active sleep in the newborn. J Appl Physiol 46:1081–1085, 1979

51. Tabachnik E, Muller NL, Bryan AC, Levison H: Changes in ventilation and chest wall mechanics during sleep in normal adolescents. J Appl Physiol: Environ Exercise Physiol 51:557–564, 1981

52. Tusiewicz K, Moldofsky H, Bryan AC, Bryan MH: Mechanics of the rib cage and diaphragm during sleep. J Appl Physiol 43:600–602, 1977

53. Hudgel DW, Devadatta P: Decrease in functional residual capacity during sleep in normal humans. J Appl Physiol: Respirat Environ Exercise Physiol 57:1319–1322, 1984

54. Phillipson E, Goldstein RS: Breathing during sleep in chronic obstructive pulmonary disease. Chest 85:24S–30S, 1984

55. Phillipson EA, Bowes G: Control of breathing during sleep, in Cherniack NS, Widdicombe JG (eds): Handbook of Physiology (vol II). Control of Breathing. Washington, D.C., Am Physiol Soc 1986

56. O'Connell JM, Campbell AH: Respiratory me-

chanics in airways obstruction associated with inspiratory dyspnoea. Thorax 31:669–677, 1976

57. Hetzel MR, Clark TJH: Does sleep cause nocturnal asthma? Thorax 34:749–754, 1979

58. Phillipson EA: Control of breathing during sleep. Am Rev Respir Dis 118:909–939, 1978

59. Bradley CA, Fleetham JA, Anthonisen NR: Ventilatory control in patients with hypoxemia due to obstructive lung disease. Am Rev Respir Dis 120:21–30, 1979

60. Fleetham JA, Bradley CA, Kryger MH, Anthonisen NR: The effect of low flow oxygen therapy on chemical control of ventilation in patients with hypoxemic COPD. Am Rev Respir Dis 833–840, 1980

61. Berthan-Jones M, Sullivan CE: Ventilatory and arousal responses to hypoxia in sleeping humans. Am Rev Respir Dis 125:632–639, 1982

62. Demarco FJ, Wynne JW, Block AJ, et al: Oxygen desaturation during sleep as a determinant of the "blue and bloated" syndrome. Chest 79:621–625, 1981

63. Burrows B, Kettel LJ, Niden AH, et al: Patterns of cardiovascular dysfunction in chronic obstructive lung disease. New Engl J Med 286:912–918, 1972

64. Flenley DC, Calverly PM, Douglas NJ, et al: Nocturnal hypoxemia and long-term domiciliary oxygen therapy in "blue and bloated" bronchitics. Physiopathologic correlations. Chest 77:305–307, 1980

65. Block AJ, Boysen PG, Wynne JW, Hunt LA: Sleep apnea, hypopnea, and oxygen desaturation in normal subjects. A strong male predominance. New Engl J Med 300:513–517, 1979

66. Harman E, Wynne JW, Block AJ, Malloy-Fischer L: Sleep disordered breathing and oxygen desaturation in obese patients. Chest 79:256–260, 1981

67. Mathews AW: The relationship between central carbon dioxide sensitivity and clinical features in patients with chronic airway obstruction. Q J Med 182:179–195, 1977

68. Goethe B: Effect of chemosensitivity on arterial oxygen saturation during sleep. Am Rev Respir Dis 119:119, 1979

69. Boysen PG, Block JA, Wynne JW, et al: Nocturnal pulmonary hypertension in patients with chronic obstructive pulmonary disease. Chest 76:536–542, 1979

70. Fletcher EC, Levin DC: Cardiopulmonary hemodynamics during sleep in subjects with chronic obstructive pulmonary disease: The effect of short and long term oxygen. Chest 85:6–14, 1984

71. Flenley DC: Clinical hypoxia: causes, consequences, and correction. The Lancet 1:542–546, 1978

72. Block AJ, Boyson PG, Wynne JW: The origins of cor pulmonale, a hypothesis. Chest 75:109, 1979

73. Nattie EE, Bartlett D Jr, Johnson K: Pulmonary hypertension and right ventricular hypertrophy caused by intermittent hypoxia and hypercapnia in the rat. Am Rev Respir Dis 118:653–658, 1978

74. Ressl J, Urbanova D, Widimsky J, et al: Reversibility of pulmonary hypertension and right ventricular hypertrophy induced by intermittent high altitude hypoxia in rats. Respiration 31:38–46, 1974

75. Widimsky J, Urbanova D, Ressl J, et al: Effect of intermittent altitude hypoxia on the myocardium and lesser circulation in the rat. Cardiovasc Res 7:798–808, 1973

76. McGrath JJ, Prochazka J, Pelouch V, Ostadal B: Physiological response of rats to intermittent high altitude stress: effects of age. J Appl Physiol 34:289–293, 1973

77. Stalcup SA, Lipset JS, Legant PM, Mellins RB: Inhibition of converting enzyme activity by acute hypoxia in dogs. J Appl Physiol: Respirat Environ Exercise Physiol 46:227–234, 1979

78. Harker LA, Ross R, Glomset J: Role of the platelet in atherogenesis. Ann N Y Acad Sci 275:321–330, 1976

79. Johnson TS, Ellis JH Jr, Steele PP: Improvement of platelet survival time with oxygen in patients with chronic obstructive airway disease. Am Rev Respir Dis 117:255–257, 1978

80. Block AJ, Dolly FR, Slayton PG: Does flurazepam ingestion affect breathing and oxygenation during sleep in patients with chronic obstructive lung disease? Am Rev Respir Dis 129:230–233, 1984

81. Alford NJ, Fletcher EC, Nickeson D: Effects of acute oxygen in patients with sleep apnea and chronic obstructive lung disease. Chest 89:30–38, 1986

82. Skatrud JF, Dempsey JB, Bhansali P, Irwin C: Determinants of chronic carbon dioxide retention and its correction in humans. J Clin Invest 65:813–821, 1980

83. Skatrud JF, Dempsey JB, Iber C, Berssenbrugge A: Correction of CO_2 retention during sleep in patients with chronic obstructive pulmonary diseases. Am Rev Respir Dis 124:260–268, 1981

84. Tyler JM: The effect of progesterone on the respiration of patients with emphysema and hypercapnia. J Clin Invest 39:34–41, 1960

85. Dolly FR, Block AJ: Medroxyprogesterone and COPD; effect on breathing and oxygenation in sleeping and awake patients. Chest 84:394–398, 1983

86. Mullins RC, Bell RC, West LG, et al: The efficacy of almitrine in hypoxemic patients with COPD. Am Rev Respir Dis 131(2):A65, 1985

87. MacNee W, Connaughton JJ, Hayhurst MD, et al: The effects of almitrine on pulmonary artery pressure and right ventricular performance in chronic bronchitis and emphysema. Respiration 46:157–158, 1984

88. Prefaut C, Bourgouin-Karaouni D, Ramonatxo M, Michel FB: Blood gases and pulmonary haemodynamic followup during a one year double blind bismesilate almitrine therapy in COPD patients. Am Rev Respir Dis 131(2):A71, 1985

89. Connaughton JJ, Douglas NJ, Morgan AD, et al: Almitrine improves oxygenation when both awake and asleep, in patients with hypoxia and CO_2 retention due to chronic bronchitis and emphysema. Am Rev Respir Dis 132:206–210, 1985

Eugene C. Fletcher

9
Chronic Lung Disease in Patients with Sleep Apnea

Occasional reports of the concomitant occurrence of sleep apnea syndrome and chronic pulmonary disease in the same patient have appeared in the literature.[1-5] Several recent studies have focused attention on the possible interaction of these diseases.[6-10] While the prevalence of this combination is unknown, the pathophysiologic and therapeutic implications are important. Both diseases are associated with hypoxemia: episodic at night in the case of apnea, and continuous (but occasionally episodic) in hypoxemic chronic obstructive pulmonary disease (COPD). In the case of hypoxemic patients with COPD, the nadir oxyhemoglobin saturation associated with apnea may be lower since the level of desaturation is dependent upon the saturation at the beginning of the apnea.[11] This accentuation of desaturation during sleep, combined with a resting daytime hypoxemia resulting from COPD or obesity-hypoventilation syndrome are likely to lead to the earlier development of hypoxemia associated clinical sequelae. These include deterioration of cardiopulmonary hemodynamics with pulmonary hypertension and cor pulmonale, polycythemia, and perhaps worse hypersomnolence and impaired cognitive function.

The reader should understand that at the present time there does not appear to be a causal association between obstructive sleep apnea and chronic lung disease. There is little reason to believe that COPD leads to disorders of breathing or respiratory control during sleep that would predispose to obstructive apnea. This point has been discussed by Catterall[12] who examined the occurrence of apnea and disordered breathing during sleep in 13 nonobese "blue bloaters" compared to that in 20 normal subjects. Apnea was rare in both populations and obstructive apnea was actually seen only in the "normals." The influence of obesity in this setting will be discussed.

Until recently, most reports concerning combined sleep apnea and chronic lung disease were anecdotal.[1-5] The earliest report[1] of a patient with this combination of diseases describes a morbidly obese, middle aged male with recurrent respiratory failure and cor pulmonale responding to intubation, mechanical ventilation, and diuresis. The FEV1 deteriorated from 2.0L/sec to 0.6L/sec over a 10 year period.

ABNORMALITIES OF RESPIRATION DURING SLEEP
ISBN 0-8089-1812-5

Copyright © 1986 by Grune & Stratton, Inc.
All rights of reproduction in any form reserved.

Severe obstructive sleep apnea was discovered on polysomnography. Aubert-Tulkens et al[2] reported a patient with severe sleep apnea and chronic bronchitis who improved both symptomatically and hemodynamically following tracheostomy. While examining the effect of oxygen on sleep disordered breathing in 11 COPD patients, Kearley[3] mentioned 1 obese subject with 73 obstructive apneas per night. In a similar study, Goldstein[4] discovered from 16 to 24 obstructive apneas per hour in 3 patients.

Guilleminault was the first to call specific attention to the combined occurrence of COPD and sleep apnea.[6] He accumulated 26 cases over a 5 year period at a major sleep disorders referral center (almost certainly reflecting a skewed population). The spectrum of COPD was wide, ranging from mild disease consisting of small airways obstruction in a quarter of the subjects to severe obstruction with FEV1/FVC ratios below 50 percent in some. Also, the spectrum of apnea was wide, ranging from 1 apnea per night to as many as 100 apneas and hypopneas per hour. No attempt was made to correlate severity of clinical symptoms and cardiovascular sequelae with severity of obstructive airway disease or apnea. A recent study[7] systematically examined the effect of supplemental oxygen on apnea duration, blood gases, and cardiac arrhythmias in 20 apnea patients with COPD accumulated over an 18 month period from the medical service of a public teaching hospital. As with the Stanford group, there was a wide spectrum of intrinsic lung disease with FEV1/FVC ratios ranging from 76 to 42 percent. All patients had severe apnea with apnea plus hypopnea indices from 58 to 152 per hour.

THEORETICAL IMPACT OF COMBINED APNEA AND LUNG DISEASE

These two causually unrelated diseases have great potential to interact detrimentally, producing end organ effects in the brain, hematopoetic tissue, and cardiovascular system through the mechanism of hypoxemia. Both COPD and obstructive sleep apnea are known to cause acute and chronic hypoxic vasoconstriction. Allowed sufficient time, right ventricular hypertrophy, strain, and decompensation can occur. Cor pulmonale has been reported as a late complication of both diseases.[13–16] It is logical to assume that the additive effect of both diseases occurring together would hasten the onset of cor pulmonale such that cardiac decompensation might be unexpected for the degree of severity of either disease alone. For example, of the 20 patients in Alford's study,[7] 15 had cor pulmonale documented by right ventricular gated wall ejection fractions and right heart catheterization data. Their mean FEV1 was 1.96 ± 0.53 and the FEV1/FVC ratio was 64.8 ± 10.0 percent. In comparison, the mean FEV1 at the time of initial diagnosis of cor pulmonale in a group of patients with COPD alone using the same diagnostic techniques and criteria was 0.90 ± 0.53 and the FEV1/FVC ratio was 45.0 ± 14.0 percent.[16] Thus, it is important to diagnose this combination so that aggressive therapy can forstall such serious hemodynamic consequences. Indeed, one study proposes that cor pulmonale does not occur in sleep apnea unless associated with daytime hypoxemia and expiratory airflow abnormalities from underlying lung disease.[8] These authors found that only 6 of 50 consecutive patients with obstructive sleep apnea syndrome had cor pulmonale. The two features that separated these six from an age, weight equivalent group of eight severe apneics without cor pulmonale was the presence of daytime hypoxemia (PaO_2: 52 versus 73 torr respectively) and expiratory airflow limitation (FEV1 percent predicted: 57 percent versus 105 percent respectively).

Table 9-1 compares objective measures of right sided cardiopulmonary function in two groups of patients with severe sleep apnea syndrome studied in our laboratory. The subjects were selected on the basis of equivalent age, percent of ideal body weight and apnea severity (greater than 30 apneas per hour of sleep). The first group had sleep apnea alone with COPD ruled out by clinical history, physical exam, and pulmonary function studies. The second group had severe apnea with COPD diagnosed by the same criteria. Patients with COPD and apnea had a significantly higher mean diastolic and mean pulmonary artery pressure (mean 35.4 mmHg versus 21.0 mmHg; $p < 0.05$) than the patients with apnea alone. Mean pulmonary vascular resistance appeared higher in the COPD-apnea patients (286 versus 110 dynes/sec/cm-5) but the difference did not reach statistical significance. Right and left ventricular ejection fractions measured by pooled, gated wall motion studies did not differ significantly between groups. While all subjects had severe apnea, the group without COPD actually had somewhat more severe apnea (considering apnea index) than the apnea-COPD subjects yet had a milder degree of cardiopulmonary hemodynamic dysfunction. Similar to the findings in Bradley's[8] study, apnea patients

Table 9-1

Cardiopulmonary Hemodynamics in Apnea Patients with and without COPD

Subj. Num	Age (yrs)	%IBW	Apnea Index (#/hr)	Awake PaO_2 (torr)	Awake $PaCO_2$ (torr)	PAP (mmHg) sys/dia	MEAN PAP (mmHg)	PVR*	RVEF (%)	LVEF (%)
				Group A Sleep Apnea Alone						
1	56	184	76	80	36	25/15	18.3	60	66	56
2	59	194	80	57	42	31/26	27.7	133	32	57
3	45	149	110	88	42	25/12	16.3	120	44	71
4	52	160	98	69	47	38/20	26.0	167	30	61
5	46	138	88	70	38	29/10	16.6	100	52	71
mean	51.6	165	90	73	41	30/17	21.0	116	45	63
s.d.	6.1	23	14	12	4	5/6	5.4	40	15	7
				Group B Sleep Apnea Plus COPD						
1	51	135	95	73	41	40/42	34.7	506	45	55
2	52	177	58	66	54	68/38	48.0	241	39	58
3	60	157	34	39	60	80/43	55.3	536	24	50
4	54	186	36	63	45	45/23	30.3	223	19	53
5	58	167	58	59	52	33/18	24.6	159	35	64
6	55	144	73	61	45	34/21	25.7	108	37	55
7	65	174	130	66	43	35/27	29.3	230	40	50
mean	56.4	163	69	61	49	48/30†	35.4†	286	34	55
s.d.	4.9	18	34	11	7	18/10	11.7	167	9	5

* Dyne/sec/cm-5.

† $P < 0.05$ Comparing means of group A with group B by T test for unpaired data.

Abbreviations: %IBW = percent ideal body weight, PaO_2 and $PaCO_2$ = arterial oxygen and carbon dioxide tension respectively, PAP = pulmonary artery pressure, PVR = pulmonary vascular resistance, RVEF and LVEF = right and left ventricular evection fraction respectively.

with COPD tended to have more severe hypoxemia (61 torr versus 73 torr respectively) and hypercarbia (49 versus 41 torr respectively) than the apnea patients without lung disease.

A graphic example of the interaction of intrinsic lung disease and sleep apnea may be seen in Figures 9-1 and 9-2. A segment of the nocturnal polysomnogram of a 64-year-old obese man with severe sleep apnea but no lung disease displays three mixed apneas, each approximately one minute in duration. A flow directed pulmonary artery catheter with a fiberoptic bundle continuously reads mixed venous oxygen saturation showing 4–6 percent falls in central venous oxygen saturation with each 20 percent fall in arterial oxygen saturation. Using the same recording parameters, Figure 9-2 demonstrates central venous oxygen saturation in another 66-year-old obese man with sleep apnea and severe COPD. In this subject, with a slightly lower baseline arterial saturation than patient one (93 percent versus 89 percent) and markedly lower venous saturation (62 percent versus 38 percent), note the severe fall in central venous oxygen saturation to as low as 15 percent during apneas of equivalent duration.

PATHOPHYSIOLOGY

Beside the obvious chronic hypoxemia resulting from COPD, there are several possible ways that obstructive sleep apnea and chronic lung disease could interact

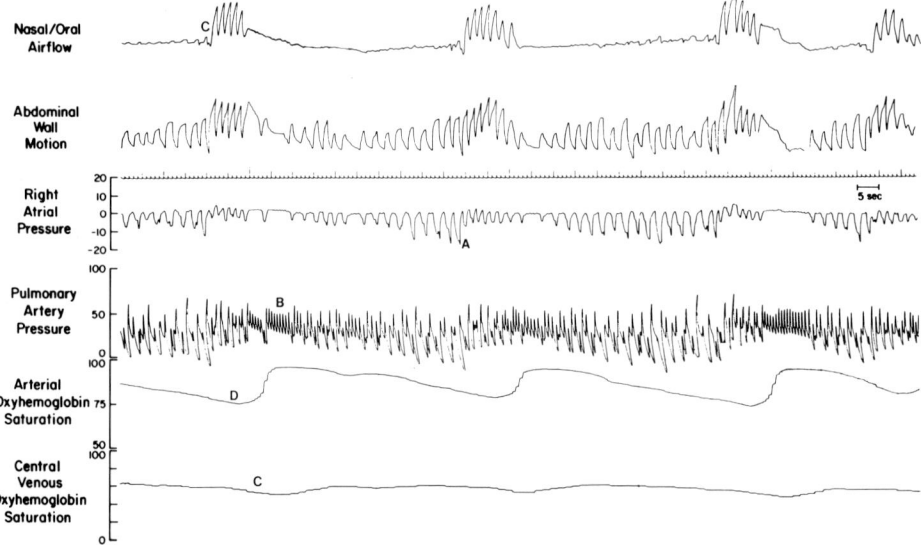

Fig. 9-1. Polysomnographic tracing in a 64-year-old man with severe sleep apnea. The various parameters are labeled at the left. Inspiratory effort is clearly reflected in the right atrial pressure trace by negative deflections that increase with the duration of the apnea (A). Small increases in pulmonary artery pressure are best seen during the central portion of the mixed apnea (B). Small decreases in central venous oxygen saturation (C) are seen coinciding (but slightly following) the marked drops in arterial saturation (D). The nadir saturation follows the termination of apnea because of electronic delays in the monitoring equipment and the fact that the areas of the body being monitored require some circulation time for the desaturated blood to reach the probe.

ARTERIAL (TOP) AND MIXED VENOUS (BOTTOM) SATURATION DURING
REPETITIVE OBSTRUCTIVE APNEAS

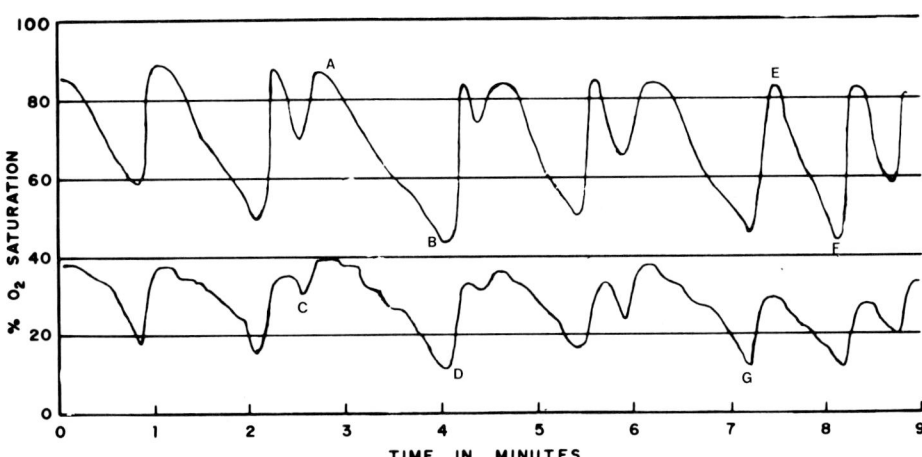

Fig. 9-2. Tracings of arterial (top) and central venous (bottom) continuous oxyhemoglobin saturation in a 66-year-old male with rapidly repetitive sleep apneas and COPD. The central venous trace has been moved to the left to fall directly under the corresponding arterial desaturation. These desaturations result from apneas of about 1 minute duration during REM sleep (note time scale is different from Fig. 9-1). Baseline (nonapneic) arterial saturation is only about 4 percent below that of the previous patient in Figure 9-1, but both arterial and venous saturations fall much further in patient 2. Note that the slope of the fall in arterial saturation (SaO_2/dt) A—B is shallower than the SaO_2/dt of E—F. This may in part be due to the fact that SvO_2 is lower (G) at the beginning of the apnea causing E—F desaturation than SvO_2 (C) near the beginning of the apnea causing the A—B desaturation.

to produce disturbances in pulmonary hemodynamics out of proportion to the severity of either disease alone. First, ventilation/perfusion ($\dot{V}/\dot{Q}$) abnormalities from the underlying lung disease could theoretically lead to worse apneic desaturation as well as aggravation of daytime hypoxemia.[11,17,18] Second, obesity, which appears to be a common accompanying factor, may further lower functional residual capacity (FRC), contributing additional $\dot{V}/\dot{Q}$ mismatch and hypoxemia both while awake and asleep.[19–23] Third, COPD and obesity may predispose to respiratory muscle fatigue because of disadvantaged chest wall mechanics and poor inspiratory muscle reserve acting against upper airway obstruction.[24–30] Additionally, the high airway resistance of COPD combined with the increase in upper airway resistance seen in apnea patients during nonobstructed breathing must certainly add to the inspiratory muscle burden and fatigue. Finally, obesity, obesity-apnea, and COPD may be accompanied by decreased respiratory center chemosensitivity to hypoxemia and hypercarbia allowing more extreme fluctuations in these parameters both while awake and during sleep.[19,27,28,29,31–36]

Understanding the possible interaction of apnea, COPD, and obesity upon oxyhemoglobin desaturation may require rethinking the mechanism of apnea desaturation, as our current concept may be oversimplified. It is generally believed that arterial hypoxemia from apnea results from simple alveolar hypoventilation similar to that during voluntary breath holding. Since no alveolar ventilation occurs, alveolar oxygen tension decreases as oxygen is removed by reduced hemoglobin, and alveolar carbon dioxide tension increases as CO_2 is delivered. The ultimate degree of desaturation will be determined by the duration of the breath hold and volume of the lung (hence, alveolar volume) at onset. The larger the thoracic gas volume at onset and the higher the alveolar PO_2, the longer the oxygen supply will last. Strohl[11] has shown that the rate of fall oxyhemoglobin saturation during apnea is linearly related to the level of saturation at the beginning of the apnea. Most likely, this is a reflection of the store of alveolar oxygen at the onset of the apnea. Figure 9-3 demonstrates the amount of oxygen stored in the lung at various volumes and degrees of hypercarbia. In humans, the lung continues to supply oxygen only during the first 40 seconds of a breath hold beginning at functional residual capacity but 2 minutes beginning at total lung capacity.[17] Findley[18] demonstrated that the degree of desaturation during a 30 second breath hold was proportional to the starting volume of the hold. Healthy young males did not desaturate in 30 seconds when they began the breath hold at total lung capacity. Moderate desaturation occurred from a breath hold at FRC, and more marked desaturation occurred starting at residual volume plus 200 cc's. The effect of initial lung volume on the rate of fall of arterial saturation is well demonstrated in a normal male volunteer, holding his breath at various consecutive lung volumes (Fig. 9-4). The rate of fall of arterial saturation (SaO_2/dt) is much greater for a breath hold begun at residual volume as opposed to total lung capacity. During sleep, the FRC at apnea onset and the alveolar PO_2 should be fairly constant for a

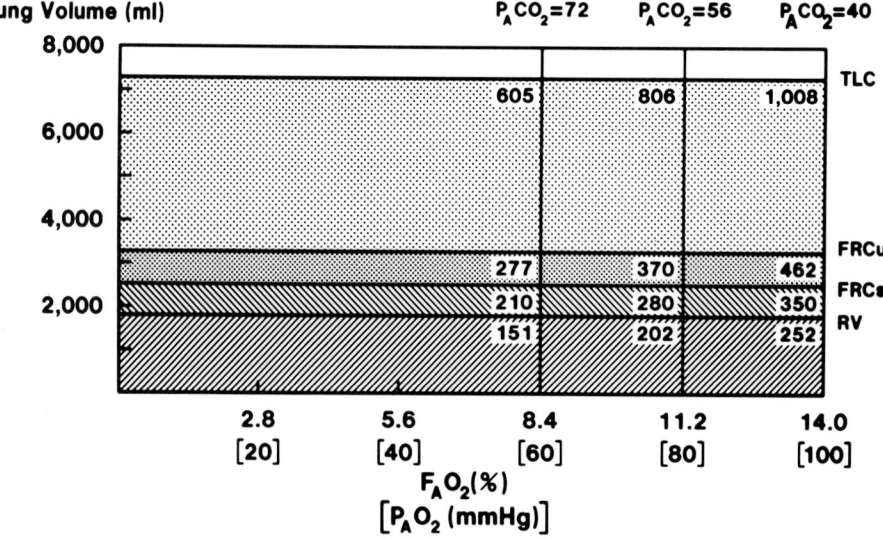

Fig. 9-3. Amount of oxygen in milliliters contained in the lung as alveolar gas based upon lung volume (Y axis) and fractional alveolar oxygen content (X axis) and the degree of hypercarbia. Apnea beginning at supine functional residual capacity (FRCs = supine; FRCu = upright) in a patient with CO_2 retention will contain lower stores of oxygen than apnea beginning above FRC or in a patient without CO_2 retention. Figure courtesy of John W. Shepard Jr., M.D.

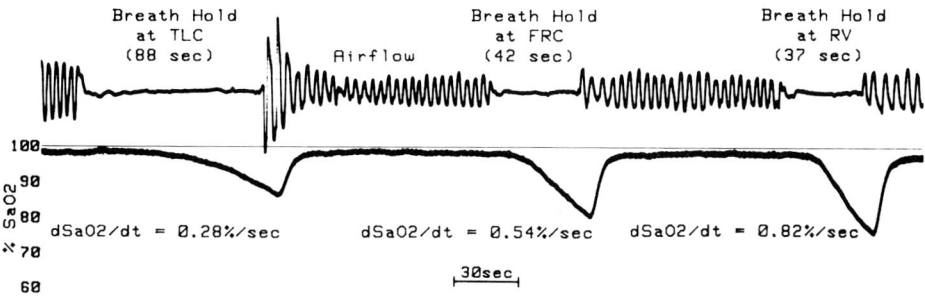

Fig. 9-4. Effect of various lung volumes on the rate of arterial oxyhemoglobin desaturation (SaO$_2$/dt) in the same subject. Figure courtesy of John W. Shepard Jr., M.D.

given individual but may vary between individuals, especially in the presence of obesity or lung disease with hypoxemia (see below).

While Findley demonstrated that breath holding (hypoventilation) accounts for arterial oxygen desaturation during the first 30 seconds of apnea, his data show that an additional mechanism may be operative at low lung volumes and after the first 30 seconds of apnea. Using the Kelman digital computer algorithm[37,38] and expired alveolar oxygen tension to estimate pulmonary capillary oxyhemoglobin saturation, he compared the predicted with the actual nadir oxyhemoglobin saturation measured by an ear oximeter. If the lung behaved as a one compartment model, and alveolar hypoventilation were the only factor influencing arterial oxygenation, both saturations should have agreed at the end of the breath hold period. The predicted and actual saturations agreed at all but the lowest lung volumes. At these low volumes, the predicted fall in oxygen saturation underestimated the measured (oximeter) fall indicating that the expired concentration of alveolar oxygen was higher than expected for the one-compartment lung (Fig. 9-5). This could be explained by the existence of alveoli that were depleted of gas (atelectatic) allowing mixed venous blood to be shunted while they contributed little to end tidal alveolar oxygen tension upon resumption of breathing. Such atelectatic areas could exist at low lung volumes as dependent alveoli fall below closing volume.

The lung volume at which apneic patients begin their breath hold has not been measured but is probably near FRC. For an individual on a given night, this is likely to be fairly constant. A major factor that is known to lower FRC is obesity, and its effect upon lung volumes as well as gas exchange has been well studied. Emirgil[19] observed that FRC and FRC/TLC ratio increased in four obese individuals following significant weight reduction through starvation. Venous admixture ($\dot{Q}_{va}/\dot{Q}_t$) estimated prior to study was abnormal in three and improved after weight loss. Similar observations on gas exchange and obesity have been made by other authors.[20–22] Holey[23] has used [133]xenon to examine regional distribution of ventilation and perfusion in the lungs of obese subjects. He found that there is less ventilation to the well perfused, dependent lobes of severely obese subjects with low functional residual capacities. While the thoracic gas volume of patients with COPD is traditionally thought of as being higher than that of normals this would not argue against the interaction of gas exchange abnormalities and apneic desaturation since closing capacity is also proportionately higher in such patients.

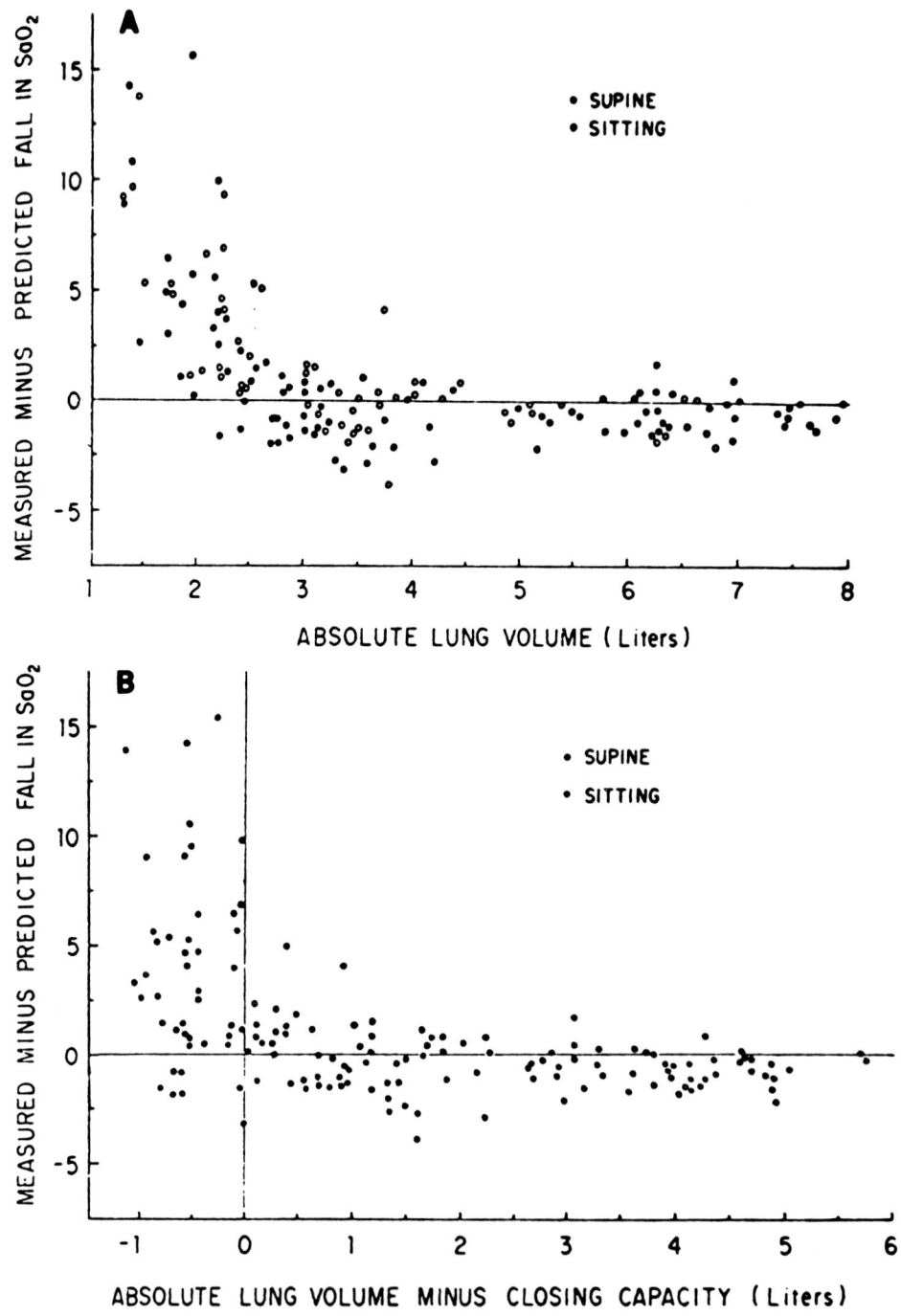

Fig. 9-5. Initial lung volume of apnea and fall in measured minus predicted arterial oxygen saturation during repeated 30 s apneas in 7 normal subjects. "A" shows absolute lung volume plotted against ear oximeter measured saturation minus value predicted by Kelman equation using expired alveolar gas. "B" shows lung volume as absolute minus closing capacity. (From Findley LJ, Ries AL, Tisi GM, Wagner PD: Hypoxemia during apnea in normal subjects: Mechanisms and impact of lung volume. J Applied Physiology 55:1777–1783, 1983. With permission.)

If gas exchange abnormalities do play a role in oxygen desaturation of prolonged apneas or those begun at low lung volumes, the interaction of COPD and obesity with apnea desaturation follows. The lungs of the patient with COPD would already have areas of low ventilation/perfusion and shunt causing decreased alveolar oxygen stores at apnea onset and increasing the severity or rapidity of apnea desaturation. The chest wall load created by the added factor of obesity could further decrease thoracic gas volume at the start of the apnea placing more alveolar units below closing volume, worsening the desaturation. The baseline, nonapneic arterial oxygen saturation of the apnea-COPD patient may already be low because of preexisting ventilation perfusion mismatch, which would further increase the rate of apnea desaturation.

One does not often think of inspiratory muscle fatigue during such a restful activity as sleep, but this may actually be the most stressful activity that patients with combined sleep apnea and COPD can engage in. Patients with COPD breath at a mechanical disadvantage using accessory inspiratory muscles and perhaps with impaired diaphragmatic motion. Asynchronous abdominal and chest wall motion are not uncommonly seen in the severely impaired patient.[24,25,39] Respiratory muscle efficiency is decreased since both the work and energy cost of breathing are increased.[40] The presence of hypoxemia during sleep caused by hypoventilation and abnormal gas exchange might further impair inspiratory muscle function.[26] Obesity alone and obesity-hypoventilation are also associated with either inspiratory muscle impairment or function at a much higher output than normal, allowing less reserve.[27,40] Inspiratory occlusion pressure ($P_{0.1}$) in response to hypercarbic and hypoxemic loads has shown diminished response in obese obstructive apnea patients with abnormal blood gases while awake.[28,29] High inspiratory muscle loads in COPD patients with elevated lower airway resistance may be added to by increased upper airway resistance (pharyngeal relaxation?) seen during "nonoccluded" breaths in normals[41,42] and in apnea patients.[43] With this information, logic would indicate that the obese patient with obstructive apnea and COPD would nightly stress his inspiratory muscles to maximum capacity and the slightest precipitating factor such as an upper airway infection may lead to respiratory failure. Staats[30] has observed asynchronous chest wall-abdominal motion in patients during repetitive apneas implying the presence of transient respiratory muscle failure.

Another area of pathophysiologic interaction between disease states may be the blunted chemosensitivity common to these disorders. Reduced respiratory muscle output (neural or mechanical) in response to hypoxemia and hypercarbia has been demonstrated in obesity,[19] obesity with hypoventilation,[27,31] obstructive sleep apnea,[28,29,32] and bronchitic type COPD patients.[33–35] It is uncertain whether these disorders cause blunted chemosensitivity directly, or if a genetic predisposition[36] allows hypercarbia and hypoxemia to become manifest as these diseases progress. Nevertheless, if multiple diseases combine in limiting the body's ability to respond to hypoxia and hypercarbia, the effect may be more pronounced despite lessor degrees of either disease. For example, the more blunted the hypoxic and hypercarbic drive, the more delayed apnea arousal may be, the more prolonged the apnea, and the greater the desaturation. The improvement in blood gases and respiratory drive following weight loss[19,27] in obese patients and in some apneic patients following tracheostomy[6,32,44] may secondarily reflect improvement of underlying gas exchange abnormalities or could be a primary factor in improving ventilation. This interaction will be discussed further under therapeutic alternatives.

A mechanism that may further affect the rate of fall of arterial oxyhemoglobin saturation is cardiac output and mixed venous oxygen ($S\bar{v}O_2$). In many patients, profound bradycardia occurs during the apnea. This may lead to a fall in cardiac output which would in turn lead to a further fall in $S\bar{v}O_2$ assuming no decrease in peripheral oxygen utilization.[45] With blood containing a lower mixed venous oxygen returning to the pulmonary capillaries of the apneic lung, a more rapid rate of fall of arterial saturation might be expected. This interaction of $S\bar{v}O_2$ and SaO_2 in patients with COPD is described in detail elsewhere.[46] Figure 9-2 shows an example of this interaction in a COPD subject with closely repetitive apneas, apneic bradycardia, and a demonstrated fall in cardiac output on the average of 1 L/min from beginning to end of his apneas. The SaO_2/dt (slope) of arterial desaturation A-B is less than the SaO_2/dt of desaturation E-F. This may be accounted for by the higher $S\bar{v}O_2$ (point C), which preceded the A-B desaturation as opposed to the lower $S\bar{v}O_2$ (point G), which preceded the E-F desaturation.

CLINICAL PRESENTATION

There is not an extensive body of literature describing the presenting characteristics of patients with apnea and COPD. Such characteristics might be worth considering. They may assist in the recognition of, as well as a better understanding of, the pathophysiology of these combined disorders. The following clinical data are taken from the presenting history and physical examination of the twenty cases of Alford et al.[7]

The manner of initial clinical presentation was as follows. Ten patients presented in acute exacerbation of COPD with shortness of breath, hypoxemia, and peripheral edema. Five of these required nasotracheal intubation and mechanical ventilation for respiratory failure. Two patients were admitted for treatment of congestive heart failure and severe peripheral edema. Seven were referred by the house staff for evaluation of possible sleep apnea due to the clinical picture of obesity, peripheral edema, and excessive daytime somnolence. The single subject who denied hypersomnolence (but had severe snoring and restless sleep) was discovered to have apnea while undergoing polysomnography as part of a workup for impotence.

The mean age of the group was 56.8 years (range 39 to 67). All subjects were above ideal body weight (IBW) with a mean percent IBW of 162 (range 114 to 194). All 20 subjects were heavy cigarette smokers, having smoked on the average 71.3 pack years per patient. Nearly all suffered from chronic cough and wheezing, symptoms expected of most COPD patients. Thirteen of 20 admitted to having cough with phlegm production fulfilling criteria for chronic bronchitis. The mean duration of pulmonary symptoms prior to presentation was 6.5 years (range 1–13). Pulmonary function studies, performed during periods of clinical stability while patients were receiving oral bronchodilators varied in the severity of dysfunction. Twelve of the 18 clearly had large airway expiratory flow limitation with FEV1/FVC ratios below 70 percent (mean 57 ± 8.2 percent, N = 12). Seven of the remaining 8 had an FEV1 below 80 percent of predicted but concomitant reduction in FVC produced FEV1/FVC ratios between 70 and 76 percent (restrictive component). All seven of these had impairment of maximal mid-expiratory flow (mean 49 ± 6 percent of predicted N = 7) and air trapping with elevated residual volumes (mean 160 ± 27 percent predicted N = 7). Since none of the subjects exceeded height-weight ratios of 0.87, it is unlikely that the increase in residual volume was due to obesity alone as described in massively obese subjects with ratios greater than 1.0.[47] One subject who was stable and receiving oral bronchodilators, failed to show expiratory airflow obstruction by standard criteria but had marked air trapping with a residual volume 190 percent of predicted. His original presentation was one of wheezing, productive cough, respiratory failure, acidosis, and CO_2 narcosis requiring three days of mechanical ventilation, intravenous bronchodilators and corticosteroids.

Carbon dioxide retention defined as the mean of 3 separate arterial CO_2 tensions 44 torr or above was observed in 12 of the 20 patients (mean 49 ± 5 torr N = 12). Hypoxemia with a PaO_2 below 70 torr was present in 16 (mean 62 ± 4 torr N = 16). These blood gas derangements are more severe than those described by Guilliminault in 26 subjects, only 8 of whom had hypercarbia and 14 of whom had hypoxemia below a PaO_2 of 70 torr.

Excessive daytime sleepiness was almost uniform, present in 19 of the 20 subjects. Hypersomnolence was present for a mean of 5.5 years (range 0.5 to 15 years) prior to presentation. A single subject with 68 episodes of apnea per hour of sleep steadfastly denied excessive somnolence but did admit to restless sleep and snoring. All of the subjects had severe apnea as defined by objective criteria of polysomnography. The mean disordered breathing event index (apnea plus hypopneas) for the group was 88.2 per hour ranging from 58 to 152. The mean apnex index (excluding hypopneas) was 60, with a range of 11 to 130 per hour.

Eighteen of the 20 had strong histories of chronic or recurrent peripheral edema for at least 6 months before the diagnosis of apnea. Using objective criteria of physical exam, EKG changes, chest roentgenogram, pooled gated wall motion studies (right ventricular ejection fraction <45 percent), and in 11 patients, direct measurement of pulmonary artery pressures, 18 subjects had definite right heart failure at the time of or shortly after presentation. Since 3 of these also had reduced left ventricular ejection fractions, the diagnosis of cor pulmonale could be made in only 15 subjects. Using a hemoglobin of 17.5 g/dl as upper limit of normal, four patients had polycythemia.

TREATMENT

Once both diagnoses are established in the same patient, the primary goal of the physician is to provide therapy aimed at correcting hypoxemia. While bronchodilators and corticosteroids play an important role in improving air-flow, COPD is not a curable disease and obstructive sleep apnea is. Therefore, when hemodynamic dysfunction is present, the emphasis in therapy should be aimed at *curing* the apnea. As in any obese patient with sleep apnea, dietary weight loss in a motivated individual will often be the most benign and potentially effective therapy.[48] Unfortunately, experience shows that a cigarette abusing, overweight patient is unlikely to stop smoking, lose weight, and maintain the weight loss. In addition, the clinical situation (e.g., cor pulmonale) may not allow the luxury of slow, medically controlled weight loss. The role of intestinal surgery designed to reduce weight must be questioned if clinically significant COPD is present because of potential perioperative complications in obese patients with lung disease. Based upon personal experience, traditional drugs (protriptyline, medroxyprogesterone) used to treat apnea are unlikely to be helpful in this setting. While successful in ameliorating apnea in some patients, they seldom eliminate it, and cure must remain a goal. One form of medical therapy that shows promise is nasal continuous positive airway pressure (CPAP). Patients with obstructive sleep apnea have been followed up to 30 months with successful elimination of apnea and correction of oxygen desaturation.[49,50] No reports on the chronic application of CPAP to patients with both diseases have appeared in the literature. Since CPAP requires a tight fitting nasal mask, patient compliance might be a significant problem as COPD patients may experience a feeling of suffocation. Furthermore, there are no reports in the medical literature verifying hemodynamic improvement with the long term use of nasal CPAP although there is no reason to doubt its effectiveness in improving pulmonary hemodynamics with continuous nightly use.

The use of supplemental oxygen for the treatment of obstructive apnea in the presence of COPD remains somewhat controversial.[6,50] One of the apparent factors motivating the report by Guilliminault[6] was their belief that supplemental oxygen therapy could be harmful to patients with combined disease by virtue of its apnea prolonging effect. These authors, administering 3L/min of supplemental oxygen over a 5 minute period to 4 of their 26 patients, noted a mean increase in apnea duration from 21 to 42 seconds during nonrapid-eye-movement (NREM) sleep and 37 to 73 seconds during rapid-eye-movement (REM) sleep. In one subject, sinus bradyarrhythmia and atrio-ventricular block developed with the use of oxygen, and supplemental oxygen was deemed potentially hazardous. Attempting to clarify this situation, Alford[7] administered 4L/min supplemental oxygen during sleep to 20 severe apnea patients with COPD over an entire night's sleep. Data on apnea prolongation, respiratory acidosis, and cardiac arrhythmias from the oxygen night were compared to data collected in the same subjects on a sham night. Mean whole night oxyhemoglobin saturation improved from 87.7 to 94.6 percent while mean apnea duration increased from 24.8 to 31.8 seconds on oxygen. "End apneic" hypercarbia and respiratory acidosis worsened using oxygen. The mean "end apneic" pH and PCO_2 breathing room air were 7.34 and 52.5 torr respectively and 7.28 and 62.3 torr breathing supplemental oxygen. Three subjects showed a small increase in the number of premature ventricular arrhythmias per hour but complex ventricular extrasystoles and atrio-ventricular block either did not change or improve with oxygen use. Thus, significant improvement in oxygenation was achieved without obvious worsening of cardiac arrhythmias.

The majority of studies on the use of oxygen in apnea have found no immediate complications.[3,51-53] On the contrary, all have shown improvement in mean nocturnal saturation (despite evidence of apnea prolongation), a general reduction in apnea frequency, and mean time spent in apnea during sleep.[51,52] The next important question to be answered is the long term effect of oxygen on cardiopulmonary hemodynamics and mortality in such patients.

Based upon clinical experience, the author's choice of therapy for apnea in the setting of combined obstructive sleep apnea and COPD is tracheostomy. Very little data is available on the natural history of such patients and chronic follow-up with objective measures of cardiopulmonary function is available in only a few selected patients. The following treatment data from the Houston Veterans Administration Medical Center has been collected on 19 patients with combined sleep apnea and COPD and 5 apnea patients without COPD followed prospectively 17 to 46 months.[44]

Table 9-2
Clinical Characteristics of all Subjects

Subject	Age (years)	%IBW	Duration Apnea Symptoms (years)	Duration Pulmonary Symptoms (years)	Apneas per hour	Mean Apnea Duration (sec)	Mean Apnea Desaturation (%)	FEV1 % pred	FEV1 FVC (%)	Pulmonary Diagnosis	Treatment Code*
					GROUP I APNEA, COPD, TRACHEOSTOMY						
1	39	180	2	3	78	32.9	17.4	63	59	COPD	T
2	62	140	10	9	60	21.3	18.4	57	71	COPD, RESTRICT‡	T,O
3	66	142	11	10	80	32.0	18.6	60	71	COPD, RESTRICT	T
4	65	141	0.5	4	28	20.7	24.1	55	72	COPD, RESTRICT	T
5	51	135	3	4	95	28.2	29.0	62	73	COPD, RESTRICT	T
6	65	174	6	6	130	17.7	17.9	55	72	COPD, RESTRICT	T,O
7	52	177	3	4	58	14.9	14.2	31	42	COPD	T,O
8	60	157	7	3	34	30.8	7.0	35	49	COPD	T,O
9	63	124	2	2	20	26.3	6.6	73	70	COPD	T,O
MEAN	59.1	152	4.9	5.0	64.8	25.0	17.7†	54.6	64.3		
STD DEV	(9.0)	(20.5)	(3.7)	(2.8)	(35)	(6.6)	(7.2)	(13)	(12)		
					GROUP II APNEA, COPD, NONTRACHEOSTOMY						
1	54	186	6	7	36	28.6	11.8	54	50	COPD	O,U
2	64	150	12	15	69	33.5	11.0	39	60	COPD	O
3	67	170	1.5	4	50	18.5	17.9	47	53	COPD	O
4	58	167	7	7	58	35.3	24.9	53	69	COPD	O
5	61	184	3	5	40	28.4	11.4	74	68	COPD	O,U
6	57	133	1.5	4	47	17.5	6.1	62	57	COPD	O,V

(continued)

Table 9-2 (*continued*)

Subject	Age (years)	%IBW	Duration Apnea Symptoms (years)	Duration Pulmonary Symptoms (years)	Apneas per hour	Mean Apnea Duration (sec)	Mean Apnea Desaturation (%)	FEV1 % pred	FEV1 FVC (%)	Pulmonary Diagnosis	Treatment Code*
7	55	144	15	13	73	33.4	8.9	67	57	COPD	O,V
8	60	114	2	4	48	19.0	8.1	45	47	COPD	O,V
9	51	186	6	10	50	24.5	7.4	66	76	COPD, RESTRICT	O
10	65	127	0	4	42	31.6	5.0	53	54	COPD	V
MEAN	59.2	156	5.4	7.3	51.3	27.0	11.3	56.0	59.1		
STD DEV	(5.2)	(26.7)	(4.9)	(4.1)	(12)	(6.8)	(6.0)	(11)	(9)		
GROUP III APNEA, TRACHEOSTOMY											
1	56	184	4	0	76	26.0	11.4	77	76	NORMAL	T
2	59	194	2	0	114	17.1	8.6	91	81	NORMAL	T
3	45	149	1	0	110	21.9	7.9	81	81	NORMAL	T
4	52	160	0.5	0	98	19.1	7.0	86	91	NORMAL	T
5	46	138	5	0	88	37.1	10.8	110	78	NORMAL	T
MEAN	51.6	165	2.5	0*	97.2§	24.2	9.1	89*	81*		
STD DEV	(6.1)	(23.5)	(1.9)		(16)	(7.9)	(1.7)	(13)	(6)		

* Group I value varies from groups II and III by p < 0.05.
† Group III values vary from groups I and II by p < 0.05 to < 0.001.
‡ RESTRICT = patients with combined restrictive and obstructive pattern on pulmonary function studies.
§ Group III value varies from groups II by p < 0.01.
Treatment code: T = tracheostomy; O = oxygen; U = uvulopalatopharyngoplasty; V = vivactil.

194

As CPAP was unavailable to this population at the time, the primary form of therapy recommended for apnea was tracheostomy. Cardiopulmonary hemodynamic function was evaluated at baseline and 12 month intervals using pulmonary function studies, right and left ventricular gated wall ejection fractions, and in 15 of the 24 patients, repeated right heart catheterization.

The groups were divided according to their acceptance or rejection of tracheostomy (tracheostomy was recommended to *all* subjects) as the primary mode of apnea therapy, thus the subjects were not randomized. Group I consists of nine subjects with apnea and COPD who received tracheostomy. Five subjects in this group also received nocturnal supplemental oxygen because of nonapneic REM desaturation during polysomnography following tracheostomy.[10] Group II consists of 10 subjects with apnea and COPD who refused tracheostomy but consented to other forms of therapy (Table 9-2). Ten of the 11 in group II used nocturnal supplemental oxygen, 2 received uvulopalatopharyngoplasty (UPPP) (apneas per hour pre-UPPP 36 and 40, post-UPPP 28 and 12), and 4 took protriptyline chronically. Both groups received the usual medical treatment for COPD including bronchodilators, corticosteroids, and antibiotics as clinically indicated. Group III consisted of five subjects with severe apnea without any clinical or pulmonary function evidence of chronic lung disease who accepted tracheostomy as treatment for apnea.

The groups were not statistically different (analysis of variance, Fisher exact test) with regard to age, percent ideal body weight, duration of apnea symptoms, and mean apnea duration. Group III apnea patients actually had more severe apnea with a mean apnea index of 97 versus groups I and II with indices of 65 and 51 respectively ($p < 0.05$). The two lung disease groups did not vary with regard to severity of pulmonary dysfunction or blood gas abnormalities. No patient lost substantial weight during the follow-up period and group mean weight at follow-up was actually higher at the end than at the beginning of the study. Cor pulmonale, based upon clinical criteria[15] as well as objective hemodynamic and nuclear medicine studies, was judged present in 9/9 group I patients, 7/10 group II and 2/5 of group III subjects.

The following data compare baseline with last obtained followup (mean 27.2 months, range 17 to 46 months following recruitment). Statistical analysis is performed using T test for paired data since each subject acted as his own control. There was a dramatic post-operative improvement in resting daytime awake arterial blood gases in group I while groups II and III showed no significant change (Fig. 9-6). Mean PaO_2 in group I increased from 60 ± 10 to 73 ± 9 torr ($p < 0.005$) at last followup whereas $PaCO_2$ fell from 49 ± 6 to 41 ± 3 torr ($p < 0.001$). Such improvements in arterial blood gases following tracheostomy or CPAP have been noted by previous authors.[2,6,32,54] There was no significant change in left ventricular ejection fraction in any of the groups, but group I (apnea + COPD + tracheostomy) showed a significant improvement in right ventricular ejection fraction (30.6 percent to 41.5 percent $p < 0.005$) at followup (Fig. 9-7). Pulmonary vascular resistance fell significantly in both groups treated by tracheostomy (Fig. 9-8). Mean resting pulmonary artery pressure in group I decreased from 36.4 mmHg to 25.3 mmHg at last follow-up ($p = 0.05$). Thus, it appears that tracheostomy in patients with severe apnea and COPD provided the means to improve resting awake arterial blood gases as well as objective right-sided hemodynamic function, while those patients who received only oxygen, bronchodi-

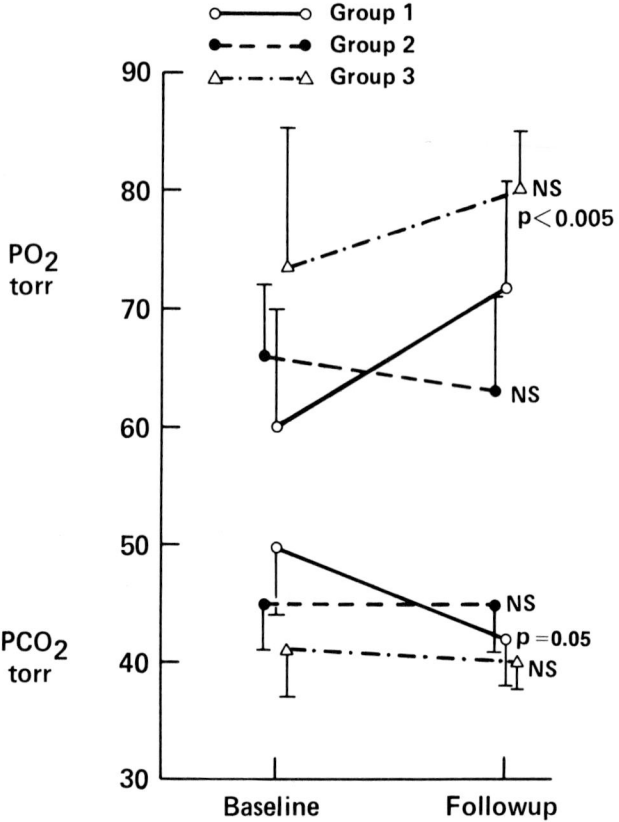

Fig. 9-6. Awake, resting arterial blood gas values from three groups of patients followed prospectively for a mean of 27.2 months. Group I had COPD and sleep apnea and received tracheostomy. Their arterial oxygen tension (PO_2) increased and their arterial CO_2 tension decreased significantly at one year follow-up. Group II (COPD plus apnea but no tracheostomy) showed no significant change in either parameter. Group III (apnea, no COPD, tracheostomy) also did not show significant improvement in these parameters.

lators, and incomplete treatment of the apnea showed no improvement in cardiovascular dysfunction. The group with apnea alone had only borderline hemodynamic dysfunction to begin with (pulmonary artery pressure 30/17, mean 21.0 mmHg, mean RVEF 45 percent) and therefore had less room for improvement.

Four patients died during follow-up. One patient in group I died of adenocarcinoma of the lung with cerebral metastasis. Three patients in group II died and all had autopsies. One expired with dilated cardiomyopathy, one of acute myocardial infarction, and one expired during sleep while in the hospital for acute cor pulmonale and respiratory insufficiency. No specific cause of death was found in the latter case, but contributing factors listed by the pathologist included visceral congestion (liver, spleen, intestine) and diffuse mucosal petechiae in the esophagus and trachea

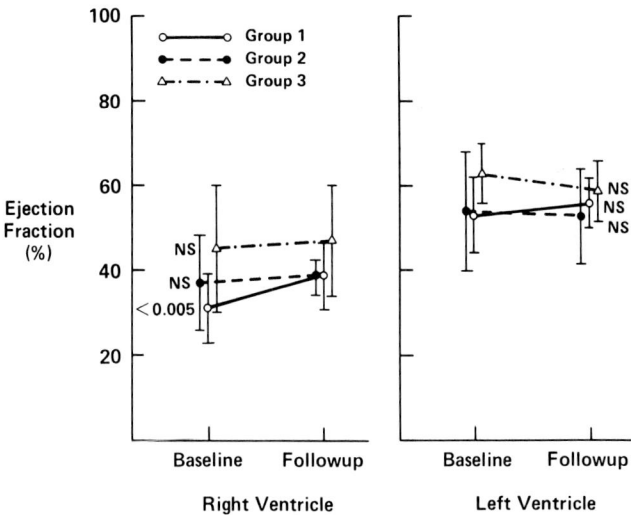

Fig. 9-7. Mean, resting, pooled gated wall right and left ventricular ejection fractions for all 24 subjects in groups I, II, and III. The only group that showed any significant improvement in ejection fraction was group I with COPD and apnea who received tracheostomy.

typical of acute asphyxia. While most patients tolerated the tracheostomy well, there were several chronic problems that accompanied tracheostomy. Although all tracheostomy patients quit smoking, persistent and profuse tracheal secretions made stoma care difficult. This situation subsequently improved with empirical use of inhaled (via the tracheostomy site) beclomethasone diproprionate. In addition, 5 of the 19 apnea/COPD patients have required a total of 8 surgical procedures to revise internal tracheal granulation tissue at the stoma sight. The possible role of nasal CPAP in this setting remains speculative but would, of course, eliminate these complications.

One peculiarity of treating apnea patients with COPD has been published recently.[10] Eleven obese males (including those described above) with coexistent sleep apnea and COPD received tracheostomies for treatment of the apnea. Repeat polysomnography following surgery revealed more than an eight percent fall in saturation below baseline during sleep. The desaturations were identical to those described in Chapter 8 in that the episodes usually lasted five minutes or longer, occurred almost uniformly during REM sleep, were associated with irregular respiration characterized by alternating periods of hypopnea and hyperpnea, and were ameliorated or eliminated by low flow supplemental nasal oxygen administration (Figure 9-9). This probably represents the appearance of two causally unrelated diseases in the same patient. Once the apnea is cured by tracheostomy, one is left with an obese patient with COPD, most likely of the bronchitic or "blue bloater" variety in whom nocturnal REM desaturation has most often been described.

In summary, the interaction of COPD with obstructive sleep apnea, while not deriving importance because of shear numbers of such patients, must still be consid-

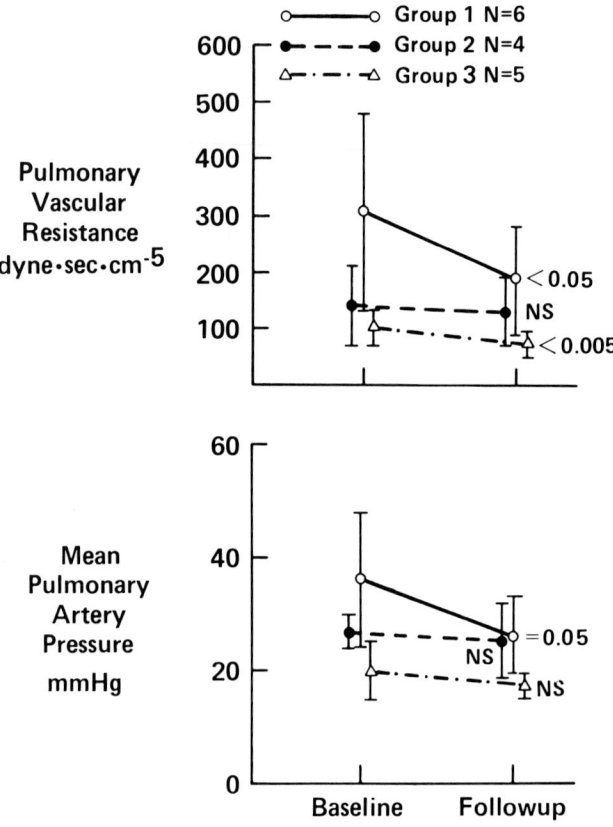

Fig. 9-8. Mean, awake, supine pulmonary vascular parameters in 15/24 subjects (6/9 group I; 4/10 group II; 5/5 group III). Pulmonary vascular resistance decreased significantly in both groups receiving tracheostomy. Mean pulmonary artery pressure following tracheostomy improved in Group I but not in the other groups.

ered because of its bearing on treatment and prognosis in a segment of the apnea population. As the importance of this interaction is realized and abnormal pulmonary function is searched for in patients with obstructive sleep apnea or vice versa, an increase in the recognition of these diseases occurring together will undoubtedly occur. Based upon experience to date, the typical patient may appear as follows. He (the majority will be men) will most often present with complaints of severe exertional dyspnea or other symptoms of COPD and will complain (if questioned carefully) of daytime hypersomnolence and nocturnal sleep disturbances including snoring. He will usually have a heavy cigarette smoking history. Obesity and peripheral edema will likely be found along with the expiratory wheezes and cyanosis often seen with bronchitic COPD patients. He may have a history of a recent episode of respiratory failure requiring ventilator assistance. Most important, the findings on history and physical may be out of proportion to pulmonary dysfunction on objective testing. Once such a patient comes to clinical attention, a formal sleep study is

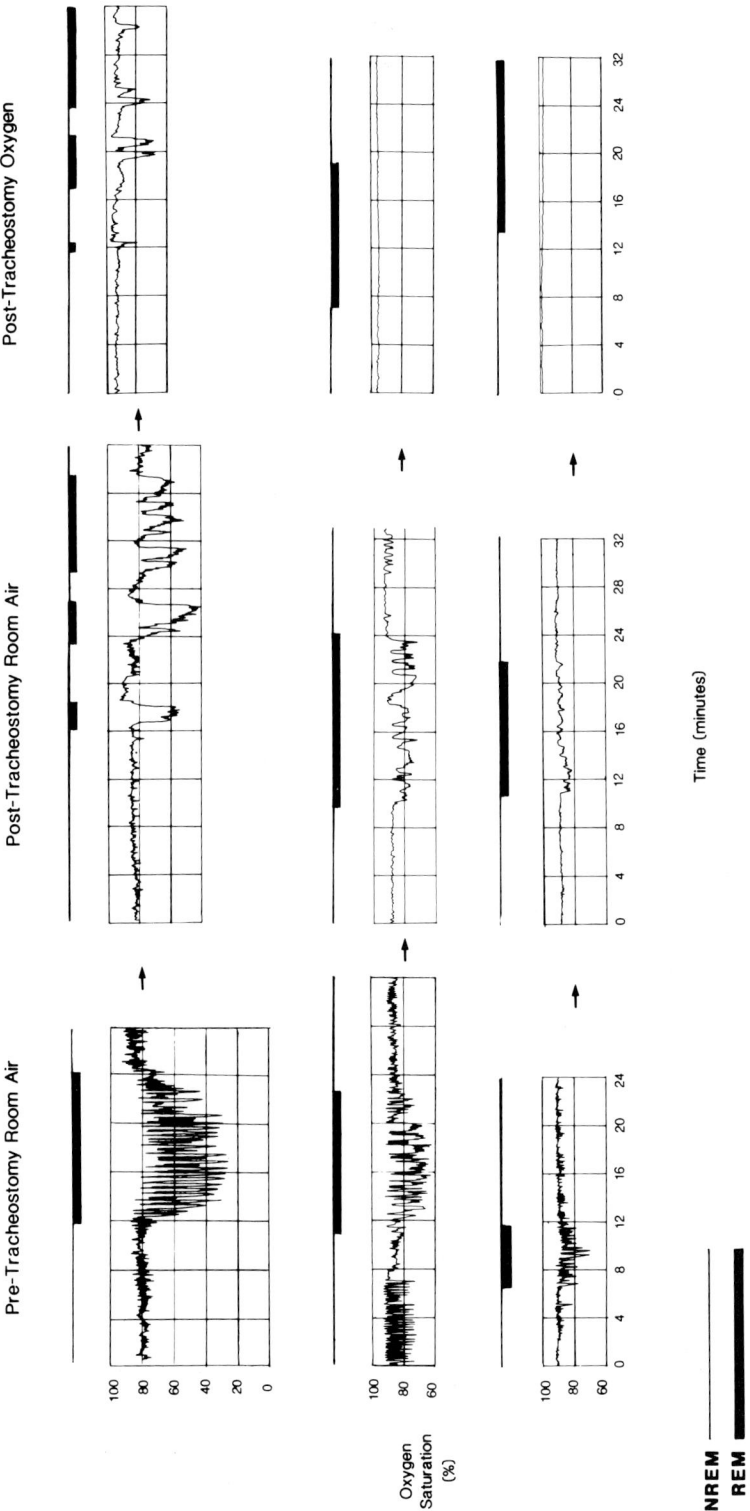

Fig. 9-9. Whole night, slow speed, arterial oxyhemoglobin saturation tracings taken by ear oximeter on three subjects with combined COPD and sleep apnea receiving tracheostomy for sleep apnea. The left panel shows the subjects asleep during baseline monitoring. Sharp, rapid, repetitive desaturations of apnea are observed during REM and nonREM sleep. In the middle panel, the subjects are breathing room air through open tracheostomy tubes and, although no apneic desaturations are noted, there are falls in saturation of 8 percent or more below baseline, mostly during REM sleep. With the use of 4L/min supplemental oxygen over the tracheal stoma, most desaturations are corrected (right panel). (From Fletcher EC, Brown D: Nocturnal oxyhemoglobin desaturation following tracheostomy for obstructive sleep apnea. Am J Med 79:35–42, 1985. With permission.)

important to determine if apnea is present and its severity. Therapy should be aimed at eliminating apnea and correcting hypoxemia. Nasal continuous positive airway pressure may prove to be an effective treatment, but in the face of moderate or severe apnea and evidence of cor pulmonale, tracheostomy must be seriously considered. The success of home supplemental oxygen in the absence of apnea correction remains unproven.

REFERENCES

1. Hensley MJ, Read DJC: Intermittent obstruction of the upper airway during sleep causing profound hypoxemia. A neglected mechanism excerbation chronic respiratory failure. Aust N Z J Med 6:481–486, 1976
2. Aubert-Tulkens G, Willems B, Veriter C et al: Increase in ventilatory response to CO_2 following tracheostomy in obstructive sleep apnea. Bull Eur Physiopathol Respir 16:587–593, 1980
3. Kearley R, Wynne JW, Block AJ, et al: The effect of low flow oxygen on sleep disordered breathing and oxygen desaturation. Chest 78:682–685, 1980
4. Goldstein RS, Ramcharan V, Bowes G, et al: Effect of supplemental nocturnal oxygen on gas exchange in patients with severe obstructive lung disease. N Engl J Med 310:425–429, 1984
5. Sullivan CE, Berthon-Jones M, Issa FG: Remission of severe obesity-hypoventilation syndrome after short-term treatment during sleep with nasal continuous positive airway pressure. Am Rev Respir Dis 128:177–181, 1983
6. Guilleminault C, Cummiskey J, Motta J: Chronic obstructive airflow disease and sleep studies. Am Rev Respir Dis 122:397–406, 1980
7. Alford NJ, Fletcher EC, Nickeson D: Effects of acute oxygen in patients with sleep apnea and chronic obstructive lung disease. Chest 89:30–38, 1986
8. Bradley TD, Rutherford R, Grossman RF, et al: Role of daytime hypoxemia in the pathogenesis of right heart failure in the obstructive sleep apnea syndrome. Am Rev Respir Dis 131:835–839, 1985
9. Onal E, Leech JA, Lopata M: Relationship between pulmonary function and sleep-induced respiratory abnormalities. Chest 87:437–441, 1985
10. Fletcher EC, Brown D: Nocturnal oxyhemoglobin desaturation following tracheostomy for obstructive sleep apnea. Am J Med 79:35–42, 1985
11. Strohl KP, Altose MD: Oxygen saturation during breath-holding and during apneas in sleep. Chest 85:181–186, 1984
12. Catterall JR, Douglas NJ, Calverley PMA, et al: Transient hypoxemia during sleep in chronic obstructive pulmonary disease is not a sleep apnea syndrome. Am Rev Respir Dis 128:24–29, 1983
13. Sackner MA, Landa J, Forrest T, Greeneltch D: Periodic sleep apnea: Chronic sleep deprivation related to intermittent upper airway obstruction and central nervous system disturbance. Chest 67:164–171, 1975
14. Schroeder JS, Motta J, Guilleminault C: Hemodynamic studies in sleep apnea, in Guilleminault C, Dement WC (eds): Sleep Apnea Syndromes. New York, Alan R. Liss, 1978, pp 177–196
15. Fishman AP: Chronic cor pulmonale: According to antecedent disorders, in Fishman AP (ed): Pulmonary Diseases and Disorders. New York, McGraw-Hill Book Company, 1980, pp 863–882
16. Ashutosh K, Mead G, Dunsky M: Early effects of oxygen administration and prognosis in chronic obstructive pulmonary disease and cor pulmonale. Am Rev Respir Dis 127:399–404, 1983
17. Hong SK, Lin YC, Lally DA, et al: Alveolar gas exchanges and cardiovascular functions during breath holding with air. J Appl Physiol 30:540–547, 1971
18. Findley LJ, Ries AL, Tisi GM, Wagner PD: Hypoxemia during apnea in normal subjects: Mechanisms and impact of lung volume. J Appl Physiol: Respirat Environ Exercise Physiol 55:1777–1783, 1983
19. Emirgil C, Sobol BJ: The effects of weight reduction on pulmonary function and the sensitivity of the respiratory center in obesity. Am Rev Respir Dis 108:831–842, 1973
20. Said SI: Abnormalities of pulmonary gas exchange in obesity. Ann Intern Med, 1960; 53:1121–29.
21. Barrera F, Hillyer P, Ascanio G, et al: The distribution of ventilation diffusion and blood

flow in obese patients with normal and abnormal blood gases. Am Rev Respir Dis 108:819–830, 1973

22. Vaughan RW, Cork RC, Hollander D: The effect of massive weight loss on arterial oxygenation and pulmonary function tests. Anesthesiology 54:325–328, 1981

23. Holley HS, Milic-Emili J, Becklake MR, et al: Regional distribution of pulmonary ventilation and perfusion in obesity. J Clin Invest 46:475–481, 1967

24. O'Connell JM, Campbell AH: Respiratory mechanics in airways obstruction associated with inspiratory dyspnoea. Thorax 31:669–677, 1976

25. Rochester DF, Braun NMT, Arora NS: Respiratory muscle strength in chronic obstructive pulmonary disease. Am Rev Respir Dis 119:151–154 (symp), 1979

26. Jardim J, Farkas G, Prefaut C, et al: The failing inspiratory muscles under normoxic and hypoxic conditions. Am Rev Respir Dis 124:274–279, 1981

27. Rochester DF, Enson Y: Current concepts in the pathogenesis of the obesity-hypoventilation syndrome. Am J Med 57:402–420, 1974

28. Garay SM, Rapoport D, Sorkin B, et al: Regulation of ventilation in the obstructive sleep apnea syndrome. Am Rev Respir Dis 124:451–457, 1981

29. Lopata M, Onal E: Mass loading, sleep apnea, and the pathogenesis of obesity hypoventilation. Am Rev Respir Dis 126:640–645, 1982

30. Staats BA, Bonekat HW, Harris CD, Offord KP: Chest wall motion in sleep apnea. Am Rev Respir Dis 130:59–60, 1984

31. Zwillich C, Sutton F, Pierson, et al: Decreased hypoxic ventilatory drive in the obesity-hypoventilatio syndrome. Am J Med 59:343–348, 1975

32. Sullivan CE, Issa FG: Pathophysiological mechanisms in obstructive sleep apnea. Sleep 3:235–246, 1980

33. Lorenco RV, Miranda JM: Drive and performance of the ventilatory apparatus in chronic obstructive lung disease. N Engl J Med 279:53–59, 1968

34. Sorli J, Grassino A, Lorange G, Milic-Emili J: Control of breathing in patients with chronic obstructive lung disease. Clin Sci and Molec Medicine 54:295–304, 1978

35. Altose MD, McCauley WC, Kelsen SG, Cherniack NS: Effects of hypercapnia and inspiratory flow-resistive loading on respiratory activity in chronic airways obstruction. J Clin Invest 59:500–507, 1977

36. Mountain R, Zwillich C, Weil J: Hypoventilation in obstructive lung disease. N Engl J Med 298:521–525, 1978

37. Kelman GR: Digital computer subroutine for the conversion of oxygen tension into saturation. J Appl Physiol 21:1375–1376, 1966

38. Kelman GR, Nunn JF, Prys-Roberts C, Greenbaum R: The influence of cardiac output on arterial oxygenation: a theoretical study. Brit J Anaesth 39:450–457, 1967

39. Ashutosh K, Gilbert R, Auchincloss JH Jr, Peppi D: Asynchronous breathing movements in patients with chronic obstructive pulmonary disease. Chest 67:553–557, 1975

40. Fritts HW Jr, Filler J, Fishman AP, Cournand A: The efficiency of ventilation during voluntary hyperpnea: Studies in normal subjects and in dyspneic patients with either chronic pulmonary emphysema or obesity. J Clin Invest 38:1339–1348, 1959

41. Lopes JM, Tabachnik E, Muller NL, et al: Total airway resistance and respiratory muscle activity during sleep. J Appl Physiol: Respirat Environ Exercise Physiol 54:773–777, 1983

42. Hudgel DW, Martin RJ, Johnson B, Hill P: Mechanics of the respiratory system and breathing pattern during sleep in normal humans. J Appl Physio: Respirat Environ Exercise Physiol 56:133–137, 1984

43. Anch AM, Remmers JE, Bunce H: Supraglottic airway resistance in normal subjects and patients with occlusive sleep apnea. J Appl Physiol: Respirat Environ Exercise Physiol 53:1158–1163, 1982

44. Fletcher EC, Schaaf JW, Miller J, Fletcher JG: Long-term cariopulmonary sequellae in patients with sleep apnea and chronic lung disease. Chest 88:545, 1985

45. Fletcher EC: Cardiac output and mixed venous oxygen during obstructive apnea. Clin Res 33(1):77A, 1985

46. Mithoefer JC, Ramirez C, Cook W: The effect of mixed venous oxygenation on arterial blood in chronic obstructive pulmonary disease. Am Rev Respir Dis 117:259–264, 1978

47. Ray CS, Sue DY, Bray G, et al: Effects of obesity on respiratory function. Am Rev Respir Dis 128:501–506, 1983

48. Browman CP, Sampson MG, Yolles SF, et al: Obstructive sleep apnea and body weight. Chest 7:79–82, 1984

49. Firth RW, Cant BR: Severe obstructive sleep apnoea treated with long term nasal continuous positive airway pressure. Thorax 40:45–50, 1985

50. Sullivan CE, Issa FG, Berthon-Jones FM, et al: Home treatment of obstructive sleep apnoea

with CPAP applied through a nose mask. Bull europ Physiopath resp 20:49–54, 1984

51. Mota J, Guilleminault C: Effects of oxygen administration in sleep-induce apneas, in Guilleminault C, Dement WC (eds): Sleep Apnea Syndromes. New York, Alan R. Liss, 1978, pp 137–144

52. Martin RJ, Sanders MH, Gray BA, Pennock BE: Acute and long-term ventilatory effects of hy-

peroxia in the adult sleep apnea syndrome. Am Rev Respir Dis 125:175–180, 1982

53. Smith PL, Haponik EF, Bleeker ER: The effects of oxygen in patients with sleep apna. Am Rev Respir Dis 130:958–963, 1984

54. Guilleminault C, Simmons FB, Motta J, et al: Obstructive sleep apnea syndrome and tracheostomy. Arch Intern Med 141:985–988, 1981

Eugene C. Fletcher
J. Warren Schaaf

10
Breathing Disorders During Sleep in Other Medical Diseases

Disturbances of breathing during sleep including apnea, hypopnea, prolonged hypoventilation, and abnormalities of gas exchange may accompany a variety of systemic diseases. Many of these sleep disordered breathing events are similar or identical to those described previously in uncomplicated sleep apnea or intrinsic lung disease. Their existence is important to discuss because knowledge of the pathophysiology of disturbed nocturnal breathing in relation to lung, thoracic cage, neurologic, neuromuscular, and hormonal abnormalities leads to a better understanding of normal and pathologic respiratory mechanics and control. Clinicians must understand how sleep-related breathing disorders may undermine the clinical well-being of these patients and interact with the basic disease to hasten cardiovascular deterioration. This knowledge should prompt physicians to search for nocturnal breathing abnormalities when such signs and symptoms appear, and take appropriate corrective measures to eliminate or minimize complications from this additional burden on the cardiovascular system.

DISEASES OF THE LUNG AND RESPIRATORY APPARATUS

Intrinsic Lung Disease

Chronic Obstructive Pulmonary Disease

Nocturnal abnormalities of breathing, oxygenation, and gas exchange associated with chronic obstructive pulmonary disease have been discussed in detail in Chapter 8, and the reader is referred to that chapter.

ABNORMALITIES OF RESPIRATION DURING SLEEP
ISBN 0-8089-1812-5

Copyright © 1986 by Grune & Stratton, Inc.
All rights of reproduction in any form reserved.

Interstitial Lung Disease

Bye et al[1] have reported 13 patients with interstitial lung disease studied during nocturnal sleep. Four of the subjects were snorers, and two had "unequivocal upper airway obstructive sleep apnea syndrome," although apnea frequency was not given. A second group of six non-snorers showed only minimal desaturation during non-rapid-eye-movement (NREM) sleep but developed nonsustained (mean duration 28 seconds) falls in saturation that occupied 16 percent of rapid-eye-movement (REM) sleep and were related to phasic eye movement. One non-snorer developed a sustained reduction in oxyhemoglobin saturation from an awake baseline value of 91 percent to values ranging from 80 to 85 percent during a 26 minute episode of REM sleep. The extent of desaturation varied from patient to patient, and no correlation between awake blood gas values or lung function was found. As in chronic obstructive pulmonary disease (COPD), nocturnal hypoxemia theoretically could contribute to pulmonary hypertension. Sleep studies should be considered in patients with interstitial lung disease if there is evidence of cor pulmonale when daytime blood gases are not as low as would be expected to produce right-sided cardiac decompensation.

Cystic Fibrosis

Polysomnographic sleep studies in patients with cystic fibrosis reveal several types of nocturnal respiratory disorders.[2-6] Less commonly, disordered breathing in the form of apneas and hypopneas are seen. Spier et al[6] report 2 of 10 cystic fibrosis patients who had 33 and 21 obstructive apneas and hypopneas per hour with an average apnea-related fall in saturation of 8 percent per event.

Nonapneic, REM sleep related falls in saturation are more commonly reported in cystic fibrosis and relate to the severity of the lung disease. For example, among his 10 subjects, Spier and others[6] reported a progressive fall in arterial oxyhemoglobin saturation from 89 percent awake, to 83 percent during stage 2 sleep, and 79 percent during REM sleep. Minute ventilation was quite variable between patients, but a significant fall from stage 3–4 sleep to REM sleep was observed. In spite of the observed fall in minute ventilation, transcutaneous PCO_2 only changed from 55.9 mmHg (stage 2 sleep) and 55.8 mmHg (stage 3–4 sleep) to 56.0 mmHg (REM sleep). While the change was statistically significant, the increases in PCO_2 were considered too small to account for the large decreases in mean oxyhemoglobin saturation (from 89 percent to 79 percent). Decreases in lung volume and accumulation of copious secretions resulting in a decrement in ventilation/perfusion matching were offered as explanations for the hypoxemia. Sleep quality was impaired by frequent movement arousals and bouts of coughing. Similar results are reported by Muller[4] who showed an average fall in saturation of 7.4 percent during REM sleep among 20 cystic fibrosis subjects compared to 2 percent for 5 normal subjects. In this study, oxyhemoglobin saturation in 1 subject was reported to drop to 34 percent during REM sleep (without associated apneas) from an awake saturation of 77 percent. A decrease in baseline position of the rib cage and abdomen (observed with the use of magnitometers) in conjunction with loss of intercostal and diaphragm tonic muscle activity (measured using surface electrodes) implied a decrease in functional residual capacity during REM sleep. Other authors believe that hypoventilation may contribute to this hypoxemia. Tepper et al[5] found a reduction in minute ventilation from awake to NREM sleep of 22 percent and from awake to REM sleep of 30 percent. Similar to the findings of Muller, changes in saturation were found to occur mainly during phasic REM sleep. As in patients with COPD, the initial position of the patient's saturation on the oxyhemoglobin desaturation curve (steep portion) may increase the likelihood of nocturnal desaturation.

Nocturnal low flow oxygen therapy has been successfully used to ameliorate oxyhemoglobin desaturation during sleep in cystic fibrosis patients. In the study by Spier,[6] 2 L/min of low flow supplemental oxygen raised the minimal saturation from 79.4 percent to 92.7 percent. Sleep related hypercapnia increased by 5.1 mmHg with the addition of low flow oxygen and was not considered a problem. Clinical studies have been proposed to see if nocturnal low flow oxygen can prevent the development of pulmonary hypertension and eventual cor pulmonale.

Asthma

Much of the information on respiratory disorders during sleep in relation to various medical diseases centers on apneas, hypoventilation, and deterioration of gas exchange. Asthma typifies a disease in which the basic problem, bronchospasm, appears to be exacerbated by or during sleep.

Interest in the phenomenon of nocturnal worsening of asthma was, in part, brought about by the suggestion that sudden "unexpected" death in asthma may be linked to nocturnal decrements in airflow. For example, Ghannam et al[7] found that 11 of 20 hospital deaths related to asthma occurred between midnight and 9 A.M. Cochrane and Clark[8] examined the case records of 38 young people who died of acute asthma. Thirteen of 19 who died in a hospital died between midnight and 8 A.M. In addition, 15 of these had also received sedation. Hetzel et al[9] examined complications among 1169 consecutive hospital admissions for acute asthma. Eight of ten acute respiratory "crises" occurred between midnight and 6 A.M., three resulting in death. Peak flow charts available in nine cases show a greater than 50 percent fluctuation in peak flow throughout the day, frequently lowest during the early morning hours. In both studies, the deaths or "crises" occurred on a general medical ward when more specialized treatment facilities were available, implying that the deaths and respiratory arrests were unexpected. Leeder et al[10] examined 22 outpatient deaths from asthma, and found that 9 were "unexpected" in that the acute attack occurred only minutes before death or the patient's attack was judged as mild or improving. Seven of these nine died between 11:30 P.M. and 8:00 A.M.

Autopsy findings in many patients dying of asthma show the typical changes of extensive mucous plugging, intraluminal inflammatory cells, and airway smooth muscle hypertrophy, implying a chronicity to the disease.[11–13] On the other hand, there is a small group of patients who die from asthma in whom extensive mucous plugging is not present, and in whom severe, reversible bronchoconstriction would appear to account for the acute demise.[12,14,15] It is postulated that this is the group with "unexpected" nocturnal death and that perhaps there is some abnormality of sleep arousal that fails to warn the patient or lead them to seek medical attention.[16,17]

Diurnal variation in expiratory airflow in asthmatics has been of interest to pulmonary physicians for many years. Expiratory airflow reaches a nadir around 2 A.M. in children.[18,19] There is greater variability in adults, with a decrement often developing slowly after midnight and the nadir occurring around 6 A.M.[19–22] Those with profound falls of 25 percent to 50 percent in peak flow[22,23] in the early morning have been labeled "morning dippers",[19] but a portion of patients show a bimodal fall in airflow with nadirs in the morning and evening. Connolly[22] examined peak expiratory flow rates every four hours among 350 patients with some form of airflow obstruction. About $\frac{2}{3}$ of patients with pure asthma (n = 115) showed a morning dip with half of these also demonstrating a bimodal, morning and evening dip. Only one quarter of "wheezy bronchitis" patients (n = 91) showed a morning dip. There was less diurnal variation among patients with less hyperreactive airways such as chronic bronchitis and emphysema patients. Morning dipping appears to follow three patterns.[24] It may be a stable pattern over many years (Fig. 10-1), it may precede a worsening or acute exacerbation of chronic asthma, or it may appear during intensive therapy following an acute exacerbation of asthma (Fig. 10-2).

Normal subjects exhibit a small, early morning decrement in FEV1 that is relative to solar time and irrespective of sleep cycle.[25] The morning dip in expiratory airflow in asthmatics does not appear to be a simple exaggeration of this phenomenon. Clark and Hetzel[16] studied 10 hospitalized asthmatic patients to examine the effect of recumbency and sleep shift changes on morning dipping. They found that the decrement in peak flow was independent of position or the presence of atopy. Temporal readjustment of the morning or "waking" decrement in peak flow occurred within the first sleep cycle upon changing the sleep period to another part of the day, implying that the decrement was sleep related. In a later study[21] the same authors examined the role of sleep versus nocturnal awakening (2 A.M.) and exercise in 21 patients with nocturnal asthma. Seven patients were awakened and exercised on three consecutive nights, yet the overnight fall in peak flow rate remained comparable to the control night. Awakening and exercising five subjects one hour before their established nadir decrement in peak flow also failed to inhibit the fall. Keeping eleven patients awake until 3 A.M. followed by sleep gave variable results. Half

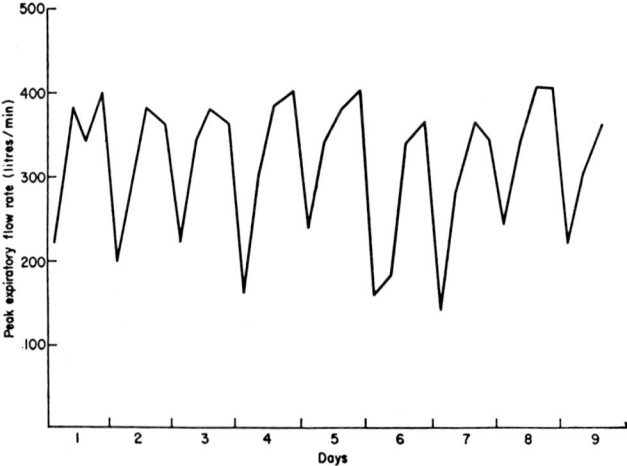

Fig. 10-1. Peak expiratory flow curve measured over a nine day period in a patient with morning "dips." Note that flow returns to normal values during the day, either spontaneously or after bronchodilator therapy. (From Turner-Warwick M: On observing patterns of airflow obstruction in chronic asthma. Br J Dis Chest 71:73–86, 1977. With permission.)

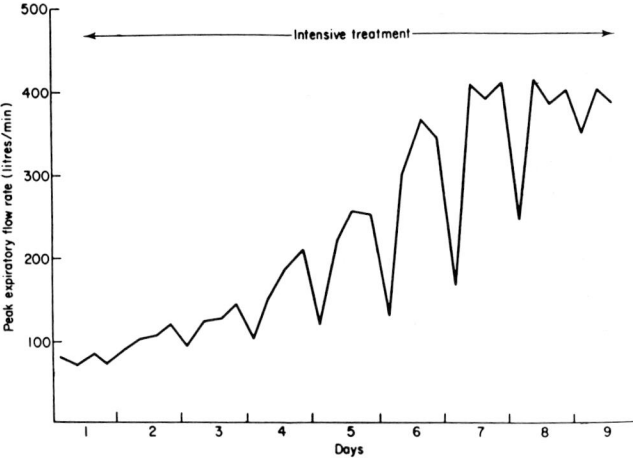

Fig. 10-2. Peak expiratory flow curve measured over a nine day period in a patient recovering from a severe exacerbation of asthma. Note the gradual appearance of "morning dips" as flow returns to normal in spite of intensive bronchodilator therapy.

sustained their usual fall in peak flow and half did not show a decrement until they were allowed to sleep.[21] Since none of the methods of awakening prevented the early morning dip, it appeared that the fall was independent of sleep.

Several studies have investigated the relationship between symptomatic awakenings and sleep stage among asthmatics. Kales[26] was unable to find a relationship between sleep stage and symptomatic awakenings (not tested objectively with air flow measurements) due to asthma in 12 asthmatic adults studied during 35 nights of EEG monitored sleep. Attacks during sleep were infrequent in the first hour then appeared to be distributed evenly throughout stages 1, 2, 3, and REM sleep with infrequent occurrence in stage 4. Sleep stage distribution was similar to controls but total sleep time was reduced among asthmatics because of the frequent awakenings. A later study in 10 asthmatic children studied during 25 nights by Kales[18] revealed that few attacks of nocturnal asthma occur in stage 3 and 4 sleep, and most occur after the first third of the night. Again, the asthmatic children had more frequent awakenings and less total sleep time than normal controls. Montplasir[27] found similar results in adults with an even distribution of attacks between stage 2 and REM sleep adjusted for time spent in each stage. Of interest in this study are the comments on apnea and oxyhemoglobin saturation. The frequency of apneas comparing asthmatic patients and normal controls was not different. However, only asthmatic patients experienced oxyhemoglobin desaturation (mean fall of 4 to 7.2 percent depending upon sleep stage). Nine episodes were related to apnea and only two were related to asthmatic attacks. Catterall[28] has published similar findings.

An allergic etiology has been found in a minority of patients with nocturnal exacerbations of asthma and should be considered in atopic individuals with nocturnal exacerbations. Barnes et al[29] have demonstrated elevated histamine levels coinciding with the nadir value of peak expiratory flow. Turner-Warwick has observed patients in whom control of environmental antigens has improved nocturnal asthma.[19] However, since the majority of patients with nocturnal asthma have been studied while hospitalized and hospital bedding has been shown to be relatively antigen free,[19,30] this is an unlikely explanation for most cases. A delayed hypersensitivity to various antigens has also been demonstrated to account for a few cases of nocturnal asthma, especially in occupation related disease.[19,31–33]

Physical factors such as airway cooling, pooled secretions, and gastroesophageal reflux have been implicated as etiologic in some cases of nocturnal exacerbations of asthma. Chen and Chai[34] demonstrated that warm, humidified air administered in conjunction with regular evening medications eliminated nocturnal asthma in eight patients. The same humidified air administered without medication did not prevent but did reduce the severity of bronchoconstriction. Martin[35] describes a case in which treatment of nocturnal nasal secretions with inhaled steroids improved nocturnal sleep and expiratory airflow. Pooling of lower airway secretions could also play a role in nocturnal bronchospasm but this is unproven.

Several reports have linked nocturnal exacerbation of asthma with symptoms of esophageal reflux. In these reports, surgical correction of hiatal hernias and improvement in reflux symptoms were associated with a subjective improvement in nocturnal asthma symptoms.[36–38] In one study, a statistical comparison between 29 asthmatic patients and 468 nonasthmatic, hospitalized patients showed a higher incidence of reflux and hiatal hernia among the asthmatics.[39] Forty-six percent of the asthmatics had demonstrable reflux and 64 percent had hiatal hernias on upper gastrointestinal radiographic exam. Five percent of controls had reflux and 19 percent had hiatal hernias. No evidence of reflux could be found in only 5 of the 29 asthmatics. An alternative explanation for this relationship is that patients with asthma cough more than controls, and perhaps chronic coughing contributes to the development hiatal hernias and reflux. A double-blind, crossover study using cimetidine demonstrated improvement in symptoms and objective measures of esophageal reflux in 18 patients with both reflux and nocturnal asthma.[40] Fourteen of these patients also noted improvement in their asthma symptoms during the cimetidine use. The mechanism linking gastro-esophageal reflux with nocturnal bronchospasm is most likely increased vagal output brought about by stimulation of esophageal receptors.[41,42]

Because many endogenous hormones are secreted with a circadian rhythm, there have been numerous attempts to link secreted hormones such as cortisol, catecholamines, and histamine with changes in nocturnal airway tone. Plasma cortisol levels are found to be highest in the early morning and thus do not correlate with the decrement in expiratory airflow.[29,43] It could be argued that since there is a several hour lag in therapeutic effect from corticosteroids, the four to six hour lag between nadir cortisol and nadir peak expiratory flow could be causal. However, one author infused low levels of hydrocortisone (sub-therapeutic) to disrupt the diurnal variation in cortisol and noted no effect on expiratory airflow in five of six asthmatics.[20] However, in one subject, the morning dip did appear to be blocked.

Soutar et al[43] examined diurnal variation in urinary epinephrine and norepinephrine every two hours in seven asthmatics over a 24 hour period. Peak expiratory airflow correlated with peak catecholamine levels for the group, but not in all subjects. Barnes et al[29] examined the relationship between plasma epinephrine, cortisol, cyclic AMP, histamine, and peak flow at four hourly intervals in five asthmatics and five controls. They found that the nadir of plasma epinephrine, cyclic AMP, and peak flow occurred at 4 A.M. with peak elevation in plasma histamine at the same time. No such variation in histamine levels was seen in controls. Infusion of low dose epinephrine for 10 minutes at 4 P.M., 4 A.M., and 9 A.M. minimized the 4 A.M. spike in histamine and eliminated the nadir drop in peak flow. However, peak expiratory flow improved at 4 A.M. with a higher epinephrine infusion level even while plasma histamine remained elevated. The authors interpreted these findings to mean that the fall in plasma catecholamines during sleep had a permissive effect upon mast cells that released histamine or other mediators resulting in bronchospasm. Several studies have shown that plasma histamine levels correlate with the degree of bronchospasm.[44,45] It is of note that infused histamine does not cause airway constriction in humans although inhaled histamine can.[46]

Treatment of nocturnal asthma can be quite difficult and requires an integrated, investigative approach. As mentioned above, the possibility of antigenic factors should be explored, especially in the occupational setting. Symptoms of esophageal reflux should be searched for and appropriate diagnostic studies instituted. Since upper gastrointestinal radiography may not be adequately sensitive or specific, the use of esophageal pH metering during sleep may bring additional objectivity to this diagnosis. Treatment with slow release aminophylline and salbutamol has been shown to improve nocturnal asthma and should be titrated to produce an adequate therapeutic blood level in the early morning to maximize effectiveness.[47–50]

Diseases Affecting the Respiratory Apparatus

Bilateral Diaphragmatic Paralysis

Bilateral paralysis of the diaphragm associated with generalized neuromuscular disorders may result in alveolar hypoventilation. These patients compensate well with the help of gravity while awake, but often have dyspnea and paradoxical respiratory movements while supine. Several reports have documented disturbances of alveolar ventilation during sleep with CO_2 retention, oxygen desaturation, daytime somnolence, morning headache, and confusion, and in some cases, cor pulmonale.[51–53] In one patient with limb girdle muscular dystrophy[52] and in one with adult-onset spinal muscular atrophy,[53] polysomnography demonstrated that oxyhemoglobin desaturation and hypoventilation were clearly worse during REM sleep. The desaturation has been linked to intercostal and accessory respiratory muscle inhibition during REM sleep and agrees with previous observations of desaturation in COPD, interstitial lung disease, and cystic fibrosis. The lack of inspiratory stabilization of the rib cage during REM sleep would greatly predispose to hypoventilation as well as decreased lung volume in the absence of diaphragmatic contraction with otherwise normal lungs.

The incidence of nocturnal desaturation in disorders of diaphragmatic motion is unknown. One author found alveolar hypoventilation during sleep in six of eight subjects with diaphragmatic weakness.[54] These subjects had morning headache and daytime fatigue associated with their alveolar hypoventilation. The author strongly recommends the use of magnetometry and transdiaphragmatic pressures to accurately assess and diagnose this condition as fluoroscopy was unable to detect diaphragmatic weakness in six of the eight subjects.[54]

Low flow nocturnal oxygen therapy has met with little success in improving nocturnal oxygenation, and indeed, worsened hypercarbia and morning headache in one subject.[52] The use of a Cuirass ventilator[52–54] or rocking bed[51] appears to be a successful form of therapy. Not only are symptoms of daytime somnolence and morning headache reversed, but daytime blood gases have improved as well.[53] These authors propose that daytime alveolar hypoventilation results from an accumulation of bicarbonate leading to decreased respiratory center sensitivity.

Kyphoscoliosis

Kyphoscoliosis refers to dorsal and lateral deformities of the thoracic spine. As the extent of the deformity increases, cardiorespiratory abnormalities related to impairment of the thoracic breathing apparatus become more common. Lung volumes may be reduced, significant ventilation/perfusion abnormalities may develop and carbon dioxide sensitivity may be reduced, leading to increased $PaCO_2$ levels.[55,56] Patients with more severe scoliosis are at increased risk for sleep apnea syndrome and nocturnal oxygen desaturation than normals, especially during REM sleep, when intercostal muscle tone is decreased.[57,58]

Groups of five patients each have been studied by two authors.[57,58] Although the study sizes are small, there appears to be agreement as to the existence of respiratory abnormalities during sleep. Mezon et al[57] found episodes of central apnea in two of five subjects. In one of these, 77 percent of REM sleep time was spent in apnea. Two subjects displayed a Cheyne-Stokes breathing pattern that was associated with little change in saturation except during REM sleep. Two subjects had no apneas but one of these exhibited prolonged, nonapneic REM desaturation relative to awake saturation. Guilleminault et al[58] observed from 11 to 68 apneas plus hypopneas per hour of sleep in 5 kyphoscoliotic patients, 3 of whom were referred for sleep complaints. In this report, daytime sleep complaints correlated with objective measures of nocturnal disordered breathing. Both reports agree that the respiratory abnormalities are worse during REM sleep. Mezon was unable to relate the degree of thoracic wall deformity, pulmonary function, PCO_2 or chemosensitivity with the presence of sleep disordered breathing. However, those with the most severe sleep-breathing abnormalities showed the greatest degree of polycythemia and cor pulmonale.[57] The use of Cuirass ventilators was not helpful in correcting the obstructive apneas.[58]

Myasthenia Gravis

Neurologic diseases that affect muscle strength, especially cranial muscles, have the potential to induce oxyhemoglobin desaturation during sleep. One such neurologic disease is myasthenia gravis, which has the propensity to effect facial and pharyngeal muscles leading to dysphagia, dysarthria, and possibly, upper airway obstruction. In spite of this potential, reports of sleep disordered breathing are rare.

Spire et al[59] studied eight myasthenic patients during formal polysomnography. Two of these reportedly had apnea indices greater than ten per hour, but the type of apnea was not specified. Other abnormalities included abnormal intrusions of alpha activity during slow wave sleep, short REM latencies, and a lack of chin muscle hypotonia during REM sleep. Martin[60] also mentions a patient with myasthenia who had daytime hypersomnolence and 10 upper airway obstructive apneas per hour with oxyhemoglobin desaturation to the mid 70 percent range.

Muscular Dystrophy

Muscular dystrophy is composed of a group of myopathies having strong genetic predisposition with usual onset of the disease from the first to third decade of life. Respiratory muscle function in muscular dystrophy patients is often significantly reduced, particularly in the supine position. This is explained by diaphragmatic weakness or paralysis, which may not be noticeable in the upright position because of the effect of gravity on the diaphragm and abdominal contents. In the supine position, the force of abdominal contents pushing cephalad and inability of the diaphragm to generate downward motion forces the rib cage to be the dominant source of tidal volume movement. This may result in paradoxic movement of the rib cage and abdomen and is tested for by measuring trans-diaphragmatic pressure, discussed above under diaphragmatic paralysis. With increasing weakness, daytime hypoxemia and hypercarbia may result eventually leading to polycythemia and pulmonary hypertension. More extensive deterioration of blood gases may occur during sleep when non-awake mechanisms of respiratory control take over and there is further loss of muscle tone, particularly during REM sleep.

Several authors have reported daytime hypersomnolence along with severe, nonapneic oxyhemoglobin desaturation during REM sleep in patients with muscular dystrophy.[52,54] Martin et al[61] describe a patient with acid maltase deficiency in whom polysomnography showed prolonged periods of hypoventilation resulting in oxyhemoglobin desaturation to as low as 54 percent. Desaturation was noted during both NREM and REM sleep but as in other reports, was worse in REM sleep. Inspiratory muscle training resulted in significant improvement in nocturnal saturation as well as daytime symptoms. Buchsbaum et al[62] reported two patients with muscular dystrophy having both daytime and nocturnal hypoventilation. In one case, a Curass ventilator was used to improve daytime symptoms and reduce pulmonary hypertension.

Myotonic Dystrophy

Myotonic dystrophy is a rare, genetically transmitted, neuromuscular disease characterized by myotonia, atrophy of the muscles of the face, neck, and upper forearms, cataracts, frontal baldness, testicular atrophy, hypersomnolence, cardiac dysfunction, and respiratory insufficiency leading to death. Cardiac dysfunction is usually associated with disturbed impulse formation and conduction since the myocardium itself is rarely involved to any significant degree.[63] Sudden death during sleep has been reported and may be of cardiac or respiratory origin.[64] Myotonic dystrophy merits special attention because mechanisms other than primary respiratory muscle weakness may contribute to respiratory insufficiency during sleep.

The presence of cyanosis, hypersomnolence, and lethargy was recognized early in myotonic patients[65–67] and has been attributed to respiratory insufficiency and hypercarbia[68] of both central, neural origin as well as peripheral muscular weakness.[69,70] Central chemosensitivity is believed to be depressed.[71] However, some evidence suggests that studies showing low chemosensitivity could be artifactual because of unrecognized respiratory muscle weakness. Peak inspiratory pressures may be a more accurate way of assessing ventilatory response to hypercarbia.[72] Prolonged respiratory depression results from general anesthesia[73,74] and small doses of anesthesia induce exaggerated responses in myotonic patients even with minimal daytime respiratory dysfunction.[75]

The association of myotonic dystrophy and disturbances of respiration during sleep was first reported in 1975. Coccagna et al[76] describe a 50-year-old male with nearly lifelong hypersomnolence who had a strong personal and family history of myotonic dystrophy but only recent onset of myotonia and weakness. During sleep there was worsening of the blood gas values associated with both central apneas (average duration 20 s) and other, longer periods of hypoventilation. This was most notable during REM sleep when pulmonary artery pressure climbed from 72/40 mmHg to 96/53 mmHg. In addition, the patient exhibited several episodes of REM onset sleep following prolonged awakenings (confirmed by other authors). Treatment for one week with nocturnal positive pressure breathing improved both the daytime blood gases and pulmonary hypertension but failed to eliminate the hypersomnolence. Cummiskey et al[77] have also reported the presence of obstructive and mixed apnea (apnea indices 16 and 36) in 2 of 6 patients with myotonic dystrophy and daytime hypersomnolence studied in the Stanford sleep laboratory. Of note in this study is the fact that while awake these six patients all had mild degrees of muscular dysfunction, minimal pulmonary abnormalities, and virtually normal blood gases (PaO_2 awake, supine = 84–95 mmHg and $PaCO_2$ = 36–43 mmHg). However, significant decrement in arterial PO_2 occurred during sleep, especially REM sleep (range 40–75 mmHg). In addition, there was not a good correlation between the severity of the muscular disease or pulmonary dysfunction and the presence of hypersomnolence and apnea.

One study has reported the use of dichlorphenamide (a carbonic anhydrase inhibitor) in the treatment of sleep related oxyhemoglobin desaturation of myotonic patients (Martin). In sleep studies before the use of this drug, 3 female patients showed from 49 to 140 nonapneic and 5 to 91 apneic desaturations during sleep. Following the drug, nonapneic desaturations decreased to 0 to 25 and apneic desaturation decreased to 3 to 15. Two of the three patients sustained improvement in symptoms after one year of followup.

While exact etiologies of the nonapneic and apnea desaturations in relation to the muscular disease and central neurologic dysfunction are poorly understood, the implications of these reports are important. Therapy of sleep related breathing disorders in patients with minimal muscular dysfunction may improve daytime blood gases, delay the onset of pulmonary hypertension and cardiovascular demise, and perhaps minimize symptoms related to respiratory insufficiency.

DISEASES OF THE CENTRAL AND PERIPHERAL NERVOUS SYSTEM

Cerebral Cortex

The earliest known and most widely recognized disturbance of breathing during sleep associated with cerebral disease is Cheyne-Stokes respiration. Frequently reported in patients with congestive heart failure, this respiratory arrhythmia is also seen during wake and sleep in patients with bilateral basal ganglia lesions or with damage deep in the cerebral hemispheres.[78] An early report of Cheyne-Stokes breathing during sleep shows this type of breathing irregularity occurring in drowsy states in healthy subjects.[79] The pattern consists of a crescendo-decrescendo change in tidal volume and rate separated by a respiratory pause or apnea. The tidal volume changes are accompanied by parallel changes in markers of respiratory effort (e.g., chest-abdomen movement, esophageal pressure).

While Cheyne-Stokes breathing is seen commonly, reports of symptoms resulting from this breathing arrhythmia are rare in the medical literature. Power et al[80] report a 63-year-old woman complaining of difficulty with sleep onset and maintenance for 10 years, beginning after a cerebral infarct. A Cheyne-Stokes breathing pattern was seen throughout NREM sleep, but REM sleep was grossly normal. The changes in oxygen saturation were minimal (fluctuations between 88 and 95 percent) compared to that seen with obstructive sleep apnea. However, frequent arousals during stage 1 and 2 sleep occurred and were temporally related to the respiratory dysrhythmia. Such arousals may have led to her sleep complaints. This report is also of interest because the respiratory arrhythmia virtually disappeared during REM sleep, the opposite of that seen in patients with sleep apnea. This gives further credence to the theory that different respiratory control mechanisms are active during NREM and REM sleep.

The development of sleep apnea, especially central apnea, is not uncommon following strokes. However, it is unlikely that cerebral cortical infarct alone could precipitate the sleep apnea syndrome. It is more likely that the development of apnea following a stroke is due to damage to the brainstem with loss of normal respiratory control (resulting in central apnea) or loss of coordinated function of the pharyngeal, palatal, or glottal muscles (resulting in obstructive apnea).

Tumors of the central nervous system are a rare but reported cause of sleep abnormalities. Blood clots, abscesses, or neoplasms causing increased pressure can alter normal sleep patterns. Tumors infiltrating the pons have been reported to change REM sleep, causing loss of the usual muscular atonia. Tumors in the posterior hypothalamus have been associated with hypersomnolence.[81] Increased intracranial pressure in such syndromes as the Arnold-Chiari syndrome or the Dandy-Walker syndrome has caused respiratory abnormalities in infants. The dysfunction is often favorably influenced by placement of a surgical shunt to reduce pressure.[81]

Alzheimer's disease is characterized by diffuse cerebral atrophy, enlargement of the third and lateral ventricles, neurofibrillary degeneration, granulovacuolar neuronal degeneration, and senile plaques. It has been reported to affect chemosensitive ventilatory response[82] as well as sleep achitecture. For example, Alzheimer patients have less stage 3 and 4 sleep, very little REM sleep, and have frequent awakenings with more sleep fragmentation than age-matched normals.[83] It has been postulated that sleep apnea might be more prevalent among Alzheimer patients or that sleep apnea could be worsened because of disruption of neural or chemical control of breathing.

Smallwood et al[84] studied 11 males and 4 females with Alzheimer's disease. They found no significant increase in sleep apnea in comparison to age, sex, and weight matched controls. However, Smirne[85] studied 8 male and 15 female patients with Alzheimer's disease and found that 3 of the males and 5 of the females had an apnea index ranging from 11 to 60 per hour. None were obese nor had upper airway abnormalities. Seven had predominantly obstructive apnea while 1 had predominantly central apneas. There was no correlation between apnea index and the severity of the dementia. Another study of 23 Alzheimer patients[86] found no excess apnea in males but did find an increase among females compared to controls. There was a significant correlation between apnea index and severity ratings of dementia. Moldofsky et al[87] suggested that "variability in respiratory function during sleep from night-to-night might account for day-to-day fluctuations in behavioral state. . . ." In six patients with Alzheimer's dementia, overnight changes on the Mental Status Questionnaire and Simon test were found to correlate with several parameters of nocturnal respiratory function. Larger numbers of patients will need to be studied to clarify the frequency of sleep apnea and any effect upon daytime function in dementia patients.

Alveolar hypoventilation following encephalitis has been reported.[88] White et al[89] reported a case of sleep apnea and nocturnal hypoventilation that occurred in a 17-year-old male following Western Equine Encephalitis infection. After several months the patient's daytime respiration improved and blood gas values off the ventilator normalized. However, polysomnography continued to show central apneas, hypoventilation, and hypercarbia. The patient was treated with nocturnal oxygen and a Cuirass ventilator. Over three month's time, nocturnal ventilation improved, and ventilatory response to hypercapnia and hypoxia normalized.

Brainstem and Spinal Cord

As mentioned above, it is unlikely that cortical stroke alone results in sleep apnea. However, respiratory failure and central apnea have been reported following bilateral medullary infarct[90] as well as unilateral medullary infarct.[91] In such cases, the mechanism of apnea is postulated to be destruction of automatic respiratory centers. A recent report describes severe, symptomatic obstructive sleep apnea following unilateral medullary infarct.[92] The authors attributed airway obstruction to weakness of the pharyngeal and palatal muscles.

Similar mechanisms have been proposed to account for both central and obstructive apnea developing in poliomyelitis patients long after the acute infection.[93–97] Guilleminault and Motta[93] reported five patients with previous bulbar poliomyelitis and recovery (with some residual gait disability due to extremity weakness) who developed excessive daytime somnolence up to 20 years after their acute polio infection. Polysomnography revealed central (52 percent), mixed (32 percent), and obstructive (16 percent) apneas. The mean apnea index was 96 (range 80–104). The authors emphasize that apneas were worse (longest duration and lowest saturations) during REM sleep.

Hill et al[98] report the case of a 27-year-old male who developed respiratory insufficiency and cor pulmonale 20 years after an acute poliomyelitis infection. They recorded numerous central hypopneas with severe oxyhemoglobin desaturation as well as obstructive apneas during nocturnal polysomnography. They attribute respiratory failure in this patient to multiple mechanisms. The acute infection 20 years previously may have caused severe neuronal damage that only became manifest with further age associated neuronal degeneration or the later appearance of additional mechanical factors that stressed the respiratory system. Such factors include the development of mild kyphoscoliosis and the fact that intercostal muscles were nonfunctional causing the patient to rely mainly on diaphragmatic function. This in turn made the patient more susceptible to decreases in thoracic gas volume both while awake and during sleep (especially REM sleep). This patient also displayed decreased chemoreceptor ventilatory response and the presence of paradoxical rib cage—abdominal wall motion "regardless of posture or state of consciousness."

Cuirass ventilators have been used to correct some of the nocturnal hypoventilation in these patients.[93] One consequence of improved thoracic expansion and airflow that is not coordinated with inspiratory pharyngeal muscle contraction is upper airway obstruction that could cause additional apneas and desaturation. A depressed arousal system in these patients may make mechanical failure of the ventilator a life threatening situation. Diaphragmatic pacing has also been suggested[93] as well as nocturnal supplemental oxygen therapy. Nocturnal oxygen administration does not stop the sleep disordered breathing but has prevented or reduced the desaturations. Medroxyprogesterone therapy appears unsuccessful.[98]

Knowing that poliomyelitis is associated with nocturnal sleep disturbances, one would not be surprised to see breathing abnormalities during sleep in amyotrophic lateral sclerosis (ALS). ALS typically presents with motor neuron degeneration of the spinal cord and brainstem, involvement of the hypoglossal nucleus causing dysarthria, and pseudobulbar palsy associated with bilateral corticobulbar tract disease. These lesions can affect tone of the upper airway muscles and tongue, perhaps predisposing to upper airway obstruction during sleep. Minz et al[99] describes 12 patients with ALS, 3 of whom had increased central as well as obstructive apneas. However, it is difficult to determine the frequency of apneas in these subjects from this report.

Surgical destruction of spinothalamic pathways is sometimes used to treat intractible pain. Since respiratory neurons may be located in close proximity to or intermingled with these tracts, surgical damage to the spinothalamic neurons can result in impaired diaphragmatic breathing. Sleep apnea following cervical cordotomy is well documented.[100–102] Because of this complication, bilateral cordotomies are usually done in two steps to reduce the risks of acute, possibly fatal sleep apnea. The respiratory changes are reflected by an attenuation of CO_2 response, decreased tidal volume (with sectioning of the ventral quadrant) and an increased incidence of central sleep apnea. These findings are generally limited to a period of several days to several weeks following surgery.

Autonomic Nervous System

Nocturnal disturbances of breathing have been described in several disorders affecting the autonomic nervous system. Sleep disordered breathing has been demonstrated in acquired and familial dysautonomia, Shy-Drager syndrome, and diabetes mellitus associated with neuropathy. In most cases, these disorders have been linked with the sleep apnea of both the central and obstructive variety but marked hypopnea with desaturation has also been seen. Precisely how autonomic dysfunction may relate to nocturnal respiration is unknown. At least two mechanisms could account for this association. The same process that damages autonomic neurons could also damage sensory or motor neurons to the upper airway, impairing the ability to maintain pharyngeal airway patency. In Shy-Drager syndrome, obstruction has also been blamed on laryngeal abductor paralysis.[103,104] Alternatively, the autonomic nervous system is an important link in the respiratory control loop, providing continuity between the peripheral chemoreceptors and mechanoreceptors and the medullary respiratory controllers. The brainstem metabolic control system that moni-tors blood gas homeostasis and acid-base balance is an important part of the auto-nomic nervous system regulating the respiratory pattern during NREM sleep. Distur-bance of this feedback mechanism may alter respiratory control and arousal mechanisms, predisposing to central apneas and hypopneas. These patients usually have normal daytime respiratory patterns. However, ventilatory control testing may disclose defects in the chemosensitivity seen as a lack of ventilatory response to hypoxic and hypercarbic responses.[105–107] Ventilation is more noticeably affected during slow wave sleep, a time when respiratory control is dependent upon brain-stem metabolic control and usually very regular. Histologic examination of brain tissue in patients with autonomic insufficiency have demonstrated degenerative le-sions in the medullary and pontine autonomic systems as well as some spinal pathways, lending support to this proposed mechanism.[104,108]

Unexplained cardiorespiratory arrest and death may occur in diabetic patients, frequently during anesthesia or respiratory infections, and usually in association with peripheral neuropathy. Fifty percent of diabetic patients die within 2.5 years of the development of neuropathy.[109] About one-third of these deaths are sudden, unex-plained, and probably not associated with arrhythmias.[110–112] As a result of these findings, several investigators have examined nocturnal polysomnograms in patients with diabetic autonomic neuropathy, attempting to confirm the possibility that apnea could be related to such deaths.

Rees et al[113] studied eight diabetic patients with autonomic neuropathy. They reported that 3 had more than 30 apneas per night (range: 38–73). Two had predomi-nantly central apneas while the other patient suffered predominantly obstructive apneas. Age may have contributed to these findings as two of the apneic patients were older than any of the controls. Guilleminault[114] reported four diabetics with autonomic neuropathy. Two had obstructive apneas with a frequency of 9 and 11 per hour and desaturation to 81 and 77 percent respectively. One had six central apneas per hour with desaturation to 84 percent. Other evidence conflicts with these find-ings. Catterall[115] studied 8 diabetics with autonomic neuropathy finding no statisti-cal significance between apnea frequency (no more than 11 per night in either group) in them compared to age, weight matched diabetics without autonomic neuropathies. Such conflicting studies make it difficult to say whether or not apneas are more common among diabetics with autonomic neuropathy and cast doubt upon apnea activity as a major contributor to sudden death in this population.

Shy-Drager syndrome is a progressive disease, which in its extreme form, con-sists of variable deficits of autonomic function combined with Parkinsonian like pyramidal and extrapyramidal motor signs. Although a rare disease, there are several reports of sleep apnea and nocturnal breathing abnormalities related to this syn-drome.

Briskin et al[116] studied three patients with Shy-Drager syndrome. Symptoms of hypersomnolence, mental confusion, and snoring were present. One patient died abruptly during sleep before studies were carried out. The other 2 were found to have apnea frequencies of 75 and 79 per hour of sleep (>450 per night), over 70 percent of which were obstructive. One of the two surviving patients died from a respiratory arrest during sleep in the hospital despite medical treatment, and the other under-went tracheostomy. His symptoms improved, but he developed increasing central apnea thereafter and expired four months after surgery. Of interest in this report are the hemodynamic monitoring studies performed during sleep in two of the patients. While pulmonary artery pressure continued to show cyclic elevations during the hypoxemia associated with apnea, systemic pressure showed no such variation (cyclic elevation of systemic pressure is commonly seen in apneics with normal autonomic function). This agrees well with our knowledge that the acute elevation of pulmonary artery pressure is a direct, local response to hypoxia while the systemic pressure elevation in response to hypoxemia is most likely mediated by the autonomic nervous system.[117]

Lehrman[118] reported a case of Shy-Drager syndrome with apnea, remarkably similar to the above cases. Monitoring revealed approximately 450 apneas per night, over 90 percent of which were obstructive. The patient was scheduled for elective permanent tracheostomy, but despite medical therapy, he expired from respiratory difficulties during the night. McNicholas et al[105] examined 2 patients with Shy-Drager syndrome whose apneas were less severe, with only 60–80 apneas per night, all central in origin. There was no accompanying arterial O_2 desaturation.

Both central and obstructive apneas appear to be more prevalent among patients suffering from Shy-Drager syndrome. On the basis of various case reports, they also appear to be at great risk for morbidity and mortality associated with nocturnal breathing abnormalities. Sleep apnea may account for daytime symptoms of hypersomnolence, confusion, and decreased intellectual function. Polysomnography should be performed and aggressive therapy should be instituted. Therapy should then be monitored, checking for any increase in central apnea. In some cases, both tracheostomy and ventilator or diaphragmatic pacing may be necessary to preserve nocturnal oxygenation.[116]

Patients with acquired and familial dysautonomia show variable signs and symptoms of autonomic nervous system dysfunction. These include dilated, nonreactive pupils, decreased tearing and sweating, abnormal temperature and cardiovascular control, absence of deep tendon reflexes, motor incoordination, and some sensory deficits. A rare disease, only a few reports of sleep studies exist in these patients. In an extensive case report that includes autopsy findings, Frank et al[119] describe a 6-year-old girl who eventually died of respiratory insufficiency experienced mainly at night. With the finding of both central and obstructive apneas, tracheostomy initially helped, but persistent central apnea and hypopnea required treatment by a positive pressure ventilator during sleep. Death followed accidental disconnection from the ventilator. Nocturnal respiratory abnormalities are more complex than just an increased incidence of sleep apnea, however. Irregular respirations have been seen in one patient during sleep stages 3 and 4, usually the most regular period of the night.[114] In another, nocturnal sleep disturbance was attributed to documented esophageal reflux during sleep.[114]

DISORDERED BREATHING RELATED TO ENDOCRINE DISEASE

Hypothyroidism

Several case reports[120-124] have appeared in the medical literature describing sleep apnea syndrome in patients with myxedema. This association was difficult to make because many of the symptoms and physical findings (hypersomnolence, drowsiness, lethargy, mental deterioration, hypoventilation, obesity, and personality changes) were common to both diseases. Although the apneas are predominantly obstructive,[125] some cases of nearly pure central apneas have also been reported.[126,127] Seemingly diverse apnea types appearing in the same patient and reversed by the same form of therapy has prompted investigators to postulate "that all apneic episodes, whether they be obstructive, mixed, or central, are all 'central' in origin, even though mechanisms behind their development might be different."[127]

There are multiple reasons why hypothyroidism could predispose to obstructive apnea. Myxedematous swelling of skeletal muscle may involve the pharyngeal musculature, especially the tongue, thereby causing narrowing of the upper airway. In addition, contractile properties of such muscles are interfered with causing slow, sustained contractions, which may make inspiratory pharyngeal-diaphragmatic coordination difficult. Neural conduction may be interfered with as well, perhaps affecting upper airway muscle coordination. Finally, ventilatory responses to hypoxia and hypercarbia are abnormal, perhaps contributing to abnormal nocturnal respiratory control.[125,128] Both types of apnea are reported to disappear with L-thyroxine therapy when the patient returns to a euthyroid state. Skatraud et al[128] report successful treatment of obstructive apnea with medroxyprogesterone acetate in hypothyroidism. Awake ventilatory control also improved.

The incidence and frequency of sleep apnea among persons with hypothyroidism may be generally underestimated by most practitioners. A recent study[125] found 9 of 11 patients diagnosed with hypothyroidism to have sleep apnea. Their apnea indices ranged from 17 to 176 apneas per hour. There was a significant correlation with body weight. However, both obese and nonobese patients showed significant improvement with thyroxine therapy even without change in body weight after therapy. Since the signs and symptoms of hypothyroidism may be masked by the presence of obesity, mental dullness, and hypersomnolence often associated with sleep apnea, it is advisable to order thyroid function studies in all sleep apnea patients to rule out this treatable, underlying cause.

Acromegaly

Patients with acromegaly often develop macroglossia, increased hypopharyngeal soft tissue, and macroagnathia related to their abnormally high levels of growth hormone. The presence of these anatomic changes of the upper airway would certainly place them at increased risk for obstructive sleep apnea, which has been reported previously[129–132] and associated with such anatomic changes.[133–136] Recent reports have confirmed that there is a greater association between *active* acromegaly and sleep apnea, which appears to be related to the level of growth hormone.[137,138] Acromegalic patients with predominant central apneas have been reported but such patients are rare and the predominant form of apnea appears to be obstructive.

Hart et al[138] found 4 out of 10 patients whom they studied with active acromegaly to have the apnea syndrome. The mean growth hormone level (ng/mL) in these 4 was 83.1 ± 53.9 as opposed to 43 ± 41.2 in the 6 without apnea. Among 11 patients with inactive acromegaly (growth hormone level 3.2 ± 2.2 ng/mL), none were found to have sleep apnea.

Although the number of patients with acromegaly who have been studied is small, it appears that treatment of the acromegaly may be adequate to eliminate the sleep apnea syndrome. For example, Mezon[130] mentions a patient who had classic symptoms of sleep apnea associated with her active illness (acromegaly) but which disappeared following radiation of her pituitary gland. However, in the face of untreated, long-standing acromegaly, Guilleminault and van den Hoed[129] have suggested that if permanent facial bone or cartilaginous changes have occurred, the sleep apnea syndrome may not be reversible, and tracheostomy or other treatment may be necessary.

In patients with active acromegaly, nocturnal polysomnography is indicated when any symptoms of daytime somnolence or excessive snoring are present. Otolaryngologic evaluation may be indicated as hypertrophy of the laryngeal muscle and fixation of the vocal cords have been reported along with other upper airway abnormalities.

Testosterone

Several recent reports have related exogenous testosterone administration to the development of obstructive sleep apnea in males. Sandblom et al[139] report a patient in whom symptoms and polysomnographic evidence of sleep apnea appeared in conjunction with the use of exogenous testosterone administration initially and on rechallenge. Johnson et al[140] report a similar case in which classic obstructive apnea developed with the use of androgen for anemia of chronic renal failure in a 54-year-old woman. The apnea syndrome disappeared with discontinuation of the medication, reappeared with rechallenge, and again disappeared with discontinuation of the androgen. Harmon et al,[141] investigating the relationship of morbid obesity to apnea found desaturation or disordered breathing in six of seven men. The only obese subject that did not show desaturation and disordered breathing was a man with hypogonadism. Sleep apnea syndrome occurring at the time of puberty may impair sexual maturation.[142] This is believed to be due to a disturbance in sleep cycle that interferes with the sleep related elevation in luteinizing hormone secretion, which in turn stimulates testosterone secretion.

Progesterone

The increase in mininute ventilation associated with pregnancy and the luteal phase of the menstrual cycle has been attributed to the excess of progestin hormones present and their stimulatory effect on ventilation has been known for many years.[143] At one time or another, medroxyprogesterone has been used with variable success to increase or improve ventilation in chronic moutain polycythemia,[144] in COPD while awake[145,146] and asleep,[147] in sleep apnea,[148,149] and in obesity-hypoventilation syndrome.[150,151] Block et al[152] has demonstrated that apnea and sleep-disordered breathing is much more common among postmenopausal than premenopausal women. However, having treated 11 postmenopausal females with sleep-disordered breathing with exogenous progesterone, he was unable to demonstrate significant reduction in apnea frequency.[153] Thus, the exact role of these agents remains undefined.

DISORDERED BREATHING RELATED TO MISCELLANEOUS DISEASE STATES

Chronic Maintenance Hemodialysis

Millman et al[154] have recently reported an increased incidence of sleep apnea among a population of chronic maintenance hemodialysis patients. Because many chronic hemodialysis patients receive testosterone to stimulate erythropoiesis, this previously documented risk factor for apnea was carefully evaluated as a possible etiology. Of 29 chronic hemodialysis patients, 12 (41 percent) had clinical symptoms compatible with sleep apnea syndrome including hypersomnolence, nocturnal arousals, snoring, morning headaches, and excessive movement during sleep. Eight were studied with formal nocturnal polysomnography and 6 were found to have obstructive apneas and hypopneas ranging from 34 to 95 per hour. Studies were compared both on and off of weekly testosterone administration and showed little change, suggesting that testosterone was not the major factor causing disordered breathing. A relationship between the severity of azotemia and sleep-disordered breathing index existed. In addition, all had severe anemia, a factor shown to enhance the peripheral chemoreceptor-mediated response to transient hypoxia.

Cardiac Disease

The incidence of obstructive apnea has been reported to be increased in patients with coronary artery disease. De Olazabal[155] studied 17 middle-age males with symptomatic coronary artery disease (documented by angiography) using nocturnal polysomnography. Thirteen had breathing abnormalities during sleep, two of which were Cheyne-Stokes breathing and the remainder, obstructive sleep apnea. The apnea index among the 13 was 20 per hour. Oxygen desaturation occurred in 10 of the patients with a mean fall in saturation of 11 percent.

Along with Cheyne-Stokes respiration, central apnea is now a reported nocturnal breathing dysrhythmia among patients with left ventricular failure. Dark et al[156] reports 2 of 9 patients with compensated left ventricular failure to have greater than 30 apneas per night. The same group[157] has related this finding to the state of ventricular compensation. In 2 of 4 subjects studied, the frequency of central apneas decreased from 230 and 50 per night to 42 and 0 respectively, following treatment of the congestive heart failure. The clinical significance of these findings remains unknown.

Obesity-Hypoventilation Syndrome

A muddled and somewhat confusing picture of what is called "Pickwickian Syndrome" has emerged since its description by Burwell et al.[158] The original description included such characteristics as marked obesity, hypersomnolence, periodic breathing during naps, hypoxemia and hypercarbia due to alveolar hypoventilation, polycythemia, and cor pulmonale. Unfortunately, this eponym is often used synonymously with sleep apnea in the presence of obesity. Actually, massive obesity may be accompanied by a variety of ventilatory patterns.[159] First, the awake and asleep ventilatory pattern as well as pulmonary function and blood gases may be normal, the appropriate term being "simple obesity." Massive obesity with nocturnal periodic breathing or obstructive apnea may be seen with normal daytime blood gases, the appropriate term being "sleep apnea syndrome with obesity." Or, the obese, apnea patient may have daytime alveolar hypoventilation with hypoxemia and hypercarbia (and normal lungs) thus displaying "sleep apnea syndrome with obesity-hypoventilation" (probably the most common cause of "Pickwickian Syndrome"). Finally, the patient may display marked obesity and daytime alveolar hypoventilation but have little or no apnea during sleep. This can truely be labeled "obesity-hypoventilation syndrome" as nocturnal apneas have little to do with the patient's symptoms or eventual development of cor pulmonale (most likely the least common cause of "Pickwickian Syndrome"). The separation of these categories is of some importance for proper understanding of the pathophysiology as well as treatment. A simple obesity patient needs no treatment. An obese sleep apnea patient without daytime alveolar hypoventilation is unlikely to develop full blown "Pickwickian Syndrome" although he may be symptomatic with snoring and hypersomnolence. An obese apnea patient with daytime alveolar hypoventilation is much more likely to develop cor pulmonale and become Pickwickian. This is because of the additional hypoxemia present during the day, which may add to the pulmonary hypertension already experienced at night, hastening the onset of right ventricular failure.[160] Both types of apnea subjects may benefit symptomatically and hemodynamically from tracheostomy but the latter form is more likely to need aggressive therapy because of hemodynamic compromise. Thus far, tracheostomy has not been shown to benefit obesity-hypoventilation patients who do not have disordered breathing at night.

The factors that may contribute to the development of hypoxemia, hypoventilation and eventual cardiopulmonary dysfunction in obesity-hypoventilation syndrome have been nicely summarized by Rochester and Enson and include: (1) decreased thoracic wall and lung compliance; (2) increased mechanical work of breathing, inefficiency, and oxygen cost of breathing; (3) abnormal gas exchange; and (4) abnormal chemosensitivity and ventilatory response.[161]

Obesity adds a mass load to the chest, which may alone reduce thoracic compliance (in some studies up to 60 percent). But it has been observed that weight loss in some patients with obesity-hypoventilation may not improve chest wall compliance and abnormal respiratory muscle tone has also been postulated as a contributing factor.[162] Lung compliance was also observed to be reduced 40 percent and has been attributed in part to closure of alveolar units, increased pulmonary blood volume, and possibly increased pulmonary extravascular water.

The mechanical work of breathing in simple obesity is 40–50 percent greater than in normals[161] and nearly three times normal in obesity-hypoventilation syndrome subjects.[163] Several authors have shown that the oxygen cost of breathing is increased in obese subjects,[164,165] is directly correlated with the degree of hypercarbia, and may be decreased with weight reduction.[162] The increased energy cost may exceed the increased mechanical work of breathing thus rendering the respiratory muscle efficiency low.[162] Rochester observed moderate weakness of inspiratory muscles in three patients with obesity-hypoventilation, all of whom were hypercapnic.

The lower lung volumes associated with massive obesity may predispose to microatelectasis, ventilation/perfusion mismatch, and shunt thereby causing hypoxemia through abnormal gas exchange in the absence of hypoventilation. Many authors report abnormalities in $\dot{V}/\dot{Q}$ in obese subjects[166-168] and several have documented improvement in hypoxemia following weight loss.[169]

Finally, the role of central chemosensitivity and respiratory drive in obesity-hypoventilation must be considered. It appears that simple obesity requires a central respiratory output (measured as change in integrated EMG output versus change in CO_2) that is three to four times higher than normal to maintain adequate levels of ventilation.[170] However, patients with obesity-hypoventilation exhibit diminished EMG-CO_2 response either because of impaired diaphragmatic function or decreased neural diaphragmatic drive. This could theoretically be due to reapportionment of neural drive to other muscles of respiration such as the chest wall. Recently, Lopata and Onal[159] observed that abdominal mass loaded controls and eucapnic obese patients are able to increase respiratory muscle output ($P_{0.15}$) and drive above normal. Eucapnic obese patients with sleep apnea and hypercapnic obese patients with sleep apnea exhibit equally diminished respiratory muscle output ($P_{0.15}$) even though diaphragmatic EMG (drive) was equivalent to that of controls.

In summary, there may be an overall balance of respiratory drive and output combating the mass-loading effect of obesity that is finally overcome by excessive weight, nocturnal hypoxemia resulting from apnea, and pulmonary decompensation accompanying cor pulmonale.

The relationship between sleep apnea and obesity-hypoventilation as well as their combined prevalence remain unclear. While sleep apnea is suspected of being a frequent contributing factor in obesity-hypoventilation, this theory cannot be settled until a better understanding of pathogenesis and mechanisms is reached. Patients with obesity-hypoventilation should have nocturnal polysomnography to rule out the presence of obstructive sleep apnea. If obstructive sleep apnea is present, curative treatment will often convert hypoventilating subjects to eucapnia.[171-173] Treatment for obesity-hypoventilation without nocturnal apnea includes weight loss, treatment of associated problems such as COPD or cor pulmonale, and the administration of respiratory stimulants such as progesterone, acetazolamide, diaphragmatic pacing or mechanical ventilators (see Chapter 5).

REFERENCES

1. Bye TP, Issa F, Berthon-Jones M, Sullivan CE: Studies of oxygenation during sleep in patients with interstitial lung disease. Am Rev Respir Dis 129:27–32, 1984
2. Stokes D, McBride J, Wall M, et al: Sleep hypoxemia in young adults with cystic fibrosis. Am J Dis Child 134:741–743, 1980
3. Francis PWJ, Muller NL, Gurwitz D, et al: Hemoglobin desaturation: Its occurrence during sleep in patients with cystic fibrosis. Am J Dis Child 134:734–740, 1980
4. Muller NL, Francis PW, Gurwitz D, et al: Mechanism of hemoglobin desaturation during rapid-eye-movement sleep in normal subjects and in patients with cystic fibrosis. Am Rev Respir Dis 121:463–469, 1980
5. Tepper RS, Skatrud JB, Dempsey JA: Ventilation and oxygenation changes during sleep in cystic fibrosis. Chest 84(4):388–393, 1983
6. Spier S, Rivlin J, Hughes D, Levison H: The effect of oxygen on sleep, blood gases, and ventilation in cystic fibrosis. Am Rev Respir Dis 129:712–718, 1984
7. Ghannam RD, Schreier L, Vanselow NA: Fatal bronchial asthma: An analysis of terminal treatment in twenty cases. Ann Allergy 26:194–205, 1968
8. Cochrane GM, Clark TJH: A survey of asthma mortality in patients between ages 35 and 64 years in the Greater London hospitals in 1971. Thorax 30:300–305, 1975
9. Hetzel MR, Clark TJH, Branthwaite MA:

Asthma: analysis of sudden deaths and ventilatory arrests in hospital. Br Med J 1(6064):808–811, 1977

10. Leeder SR, Callaghan AF, Hensley MJ, Hardes GR: Preventing death from asthma. Aust Fam Physician 10:194–200, 1981

11. Cardell BS, Pearson RSB: Death in asthmatics. Thorax 14:341–352, 1959

12. Lopez-Vidriero MT, Reid L: Pathologic change in asthma, in Clark TJH, Godfrey S (eds): Asthma. London, Chapman and Hall, pp 79–95, 1984

13. Messer JW, Peters GA, Bennett WA: Causes of death and pathologic findings in 304 cases of bronchial asthma. Dis Chest 38:616–624, 1960

14. James OF, Mills RM, Allen KM: Severe bronchial asthma: factors influencing intensive care management and outcome. Anaesth Int Care 5:11–18, 1977

15. Mellis CM, Phelan PD: Asthma deaths in children: A continuing problem. Thorax 32:29–34, 1977

16. Clark TJH, Hetzel MR: Diurnal variation of asthma. Br J Dis Chest 71:87–92, 1977

17. Hudgel DW, Kellum R, Martin RJ, Johnson B: Depressed arousal response to airflow obstruction: A possible factor in near-fatal nocturnal asthma. Am Rev Resp Dis 125(S):202, 1982

18. Kales A, Kales JD, Sly RM, et al: Sleep patterns of asthmatic children: All-night electroencephalographic studies. J Allergy 46:300–308, 1970

19. Turner-Warwick M: On observing patterns of airflow obstruction in chronic asthma. Br J Dis Chest 71:73–86, 1977

20. Soutar CA, Costello J, Ijaduola O, Turner-Warwick M: Nocturnal and morning asthma: Relationship to plasma corticosteroids and response to cortisol infusion. Thorax 436–40, 1975

21. Hetzel MR, Clark TJH: Does sleep cause nocturnal asthma? Thorax 34:749–754, 1979

22. Connolly CK: Diurnal rhythms in airway obstruction. Br J Dis Chest 73:357–366, 1979

23. Hetzel MR, Clark TJH, Brown D: Normal circadian rhythms in peak expiratory flow rate. Thorax 33:668, 1978

24. Olson LG, Hensley MJ, Saunders NA, Sullivan CE: Sleep, Breathing and Lung Disease, in Saunders NA, Sullivan CE (ed): Sleep and Breathing. New York, Marcel Dekker Inc., 1984, pp 517–58

25. Lewinsohn HC, Capel LH, Smart J: Changes in forced expiratory volumes throughout the day. Br Med J 1:462–464, 1960

26. Kales A, Beall GN, Bajor GF, et al: Sleep studies in asthmatic adults: Relationship of attacks to sleep stage and time of night. J Allergy 41:164–173, 1968

27. Montplasir J, Walsh J, Malo JL: Nocturnal asthma: features of attacks, sleep and breathing patterns. Am Rev Respir Dis 125:18–22, 1982

28. Catterall JR, Douglas NJ, Calverley PMA, et al: Irregular breathing and hypoxaemia during sleep in chronic stable asthma. Lancet 1:301–304, 1982

29. Barnes P, Fitzgerald G, Brown M, Dollery C: Nocturnal asthma and changes in circulating epinephrine, histamine and cortisol. New Engl J Med 303:263–267, 1980

30. Maunsell K, Wraith DG, Cunningham AM: Mites and house dust allergy in bronchial asthma. Lancet 1:1267–1270, 1968

31. Davies RJ, Green M, Schofield N McC: Recurrent nocturnal asthma after exposure to grain dust. Am Rev Respir Dis 114:1011–1019, 1976

32. Taylor AJ, Davies RJ, Hendrick DJ, Pepys J: Recurrent nocturnal asthmatic reactions to bronchial provocation tests. Clin Allergy 9:213–219, 1979

33. Gandevia B, Milne J: Occupational asthma and rhinitis due to Western Red Cedar. Br J Indust Med 27:235–244, 1970

34. Chen WY, Chai H: Airway cooling and nocturnal asthma. Chest 81:675–680, 1982

35. Martin RJ: Nocturnal Asthma, in Martin RJ: Cardiorespiratory Disorders During Sleep. New York, Futura Publishing Company, pp 119–45, 1984

36. Overholt RH, Voorhees RJ: Esophageal reflux as a trigger in asthma. Dis Chest 49:464–466, 1966

37. Urschel HC Jr, Paulson DL: Gastroesophageal reflux and hiatal hernia. Complications and therapy. J Thorac Cardiov Surg 53:21–32, 1967

38. Davis MV: Evolving concepts regarding hiatal hernia and gastroesophageal reflux. Ann Thorac Surg 7:120–133, 1969

39. Mays EE: Intrinsic asthma in adults. Association with gastroesophageal reflux. J Am Med Assoc 236:2626–2628, 1976

40. Goodall RJ, Earis JE, Copper DN, et al: Relationship between asthma and gastro-oesophageal reflux. Thorax 36:116–121, 1981

41. Mansfield LE, Stein MR: Gastro-oesophageal reflux and asthma: A possible reflex mechanism. Ann Allergy 41:224–226, 1978

42. Davis RS, Larsen GL, Grunstein MM: Esopha-

geal acid infusion during sleep in asthmatic children with gastroesophageal reflux. Am Rev Respir Dis 125(S):190, 1982

43. Soutar CA, Carruthers M, Pickering CAC: Nocturnal asthma and urinary adrenaline and noradrenaline excretion. Thorax 32: 677–683, 1977

44. Simon RA, Stevenson DD, Arroyave CM, Tan EM: The relationship of plasma histamine to the activity of bronchial asthma. J Allergy Clin Immunol 60:312–316, 1977

45. Charles TJ, Williams SJ, Seaton A, et al: Histamines, basophils and eosinophils in severe asthma. Clin Sci 57:39–45, 1979

46. Brown R, Ingram RH Jr, Wellman JJ, McFadden ER Jr: Effects of intravenous histamine on pulmonary mechanics in nonasthmatic and asthmatic subjects. J Appl Physiol 42:221–227, 1977

47. Barnes PJ, Greening AP, Neville L, et al: Single dose slow-release aminophylline at night prevents nocturnal asthma. Lancet 1:299–301, 1982

48. Cole RB, Al-Khader A: Effect of slow-release oral aminophylline on circadian variation in airflow obstruction in asthmatics. J Int Med Res 7(Suppl 1):40–44, 1979

49. Milledge JS, Morris J: A comparison of slow-release salbutamol with slow-release aminophylline in nocturnal asthma. J Int Med Res 7(Suppl 1):106–110, 1979

50. Fairfax AJ, McNabb WR, Davies HJ, Spiro SG: Slow-release oral salbutamol and aminophylline in nocturnal asthma: Relation of overnight changes in lung function and plasma drug levels. Thorax 35:526–530, 1980

51. Kreitzer SM, Feldman NT, Saunders NA, Ingram Jr RH: Bilateral diaphragmatic paralysis with hypercapnic respiratory failure: A physiologic assessment. Am J Med 65:89–95, 1978

52. Skatrud J, Iber C, McHugh W, et al: Determinants of hypoventilation during wakefulness and sleep in diaphragmatic paralysis. Am Rev Respir Dis 121:587–593, 1980

53. Thorpy MJ, Schmidt-Nowara WW, Pollak CP, Weitzman ED: Sleep-induced nonobstructive hypoventilation associated with diaphragmatic paralysis. Ann Neurol 12:308–311, 1982

54. Newsom-Davis J, Goldman DM, Loh L, Casson M: Diaphragm function and alveolar hypoventilation. Quart J Med (new series) XLV:87–100, 1976

55. Secker-Walker RH, Ho JE, Gill IS: Observations on regional ventilation and perfusion in kyphoscoliosis. Respiration 38:194–203, 1979

56. Kafer ER: Respiratory function in paralytic scoliosis. Am Rev Respir Dis 110:450–457, 1974

57. Mezon BL, West P, Israels J, Kryger M: Sleep breathing abnormalities in kyphoscoliosis. Am Rev Respir Dis 122:617–621, 1980

58. Guilleminault C, Kurland G, Winkle R, Miles LE: Severe kyphoscoliosis breathing, and sleep. Chest 79(6):626–630, 1981

59. Spire JP, Hsu L, Holmes K, Rosenberg R: Sleep patterns in myasthenia gravis. Neurol 32:A123, 1982

60. Martin RJ: Neuromuscular and skeletal abnormalities with nocturnal respiratory disorders, in Cardiorespiratory Disorders During Sleep. New York, Futura Publishing Co. Mount Kisko, 1984, pp 177–215

61. Martin RJ, Sufit RL, Ringel SP, et al: Respiratory improvement by muscle training in adult-onset acied maltase deficiency. Muscle and Nerve 6:201–203, 1983

62. Buchsbaum HW, Martin WA, Turino GM, et al: Chronic alveolar hypoventilation due to muscular dystrophy. Neurol 18:319–327, 1968

63. Perloff JK, Stevenson WG, Roberts NK, et al: Cardiac involvement in myotonic muscular dystrophy (Steinert's Disease): A prospective study of 25 patients. Am J Cardiol 54:1074–1081, 1984

64. Grigg LE, Chan W, Mond HG, et al: Ventricular tachycardia and sudden death in myotonic dystrophy: clinical, electrophysiologic and pathologic features. J Am Coll Cardiol 6:254–256, 1958

65. Adie WJ, Greenfield JG: Dystrophica myotonica. Brain 46:73–127, 1923

66. Thomasen E. Myotonia: Thomsen's Disease (Myotonia Congenita), Paramyotonia, and Dystrophic Myotonica: A clinical and heredobiologic investigation. Aarhus, Denmark, Universitetsforlaget I Aarhus, 1948, p 251

67. Benaim S, Worster-Drought C: Dystrophica myotonia with myotonia of the diaphragm causing pulmonary hypoventilation with anoxaemia and secondary polycythaemia. Med Illus 8:221–226, 1954

68. Kohn NN, Faires JS, Rodman T: Unusual manifestations due to involvement of involuntary muscle in dystrophia myotonica. N Engl J Med 1179–1183, 1964

69. Kilburn KH, Eagan JT, Heyman A: Cardiopulmonary insufficiency associated with myotonic dystrophy. Am J Med 26:929–935, 1959

70. Begin R, Bureau MA, Lupien L, et al: Pathogenesis of respiratory insufficiency in myotonic dystrophy. Am Rev Respir Dis 125:312–317, 1982

71. Carroll JE, Zwillich CW, Weil JV: Ventilatory response in myotonic dystrophy. Neurol 27:1125–1128, 1977

72. Serisier DE, Mastaglia FL, Gibson GJ: Respiratory muscle function in motor neuron disease and myotonic dystrophy. Q J Med 51:205–226, 1982

73. Tsueda K, Shibutani K, Lefkowitz M: Postoperative ventilatory failure in an obese, myopathic woman with periodic somnolence: A case report. Anesth and Analg Cur Research 54:523–526, 1975

74. Kaufman L: Anaesthesia in dystrophia myotonica. Proc Roy Soc Med 53:183–187, 1959

75. Gilliam PMS, Heaf PJD, Kaufman L, Lucas BGB: Respiration in dystrophia myotonica. Thorax 19:112–120, 1964

76. Coccagna G, Mantovani M, Parchi C, et al: Alveolar hypoventilation and hypersomnia in myotonic dystrophy. J Neurol, Neurosurg, Psychiatry 38:977–984, 1975

77. Cummiskey J, Lynne-Davies P, Guilleminault C: Sleep study and respiratory function in myotonic dystrophy, in Sleep Apnea Syndromes. New York, Alan R. Liss, Inc., 1978, pp 295–308

78. Plum F, Posner JB: The Diagnosis of Stupor and Coma. Philadelphia, FA Davis Co., 1980, pp 35–36

79. Bulow K: Respiration and wakefulness in man. Acta Physiol Scand 37:899–903, 1963

80. Power WR, Mosko SS, Sassin JF: Sleep-stage-dependent Cheyne-Stokes respiration after cerebral infarct: A case study. Neurology 32:763–766, 1982

81. Freemon FR: Sleep in patients with organic disease of the nervous system, in Williams RL, Karacan I (eds): Sleep Disorders: Diagnosis and Treatment. New York, Wiley, 1978, pp 261–283

82. Paulson GW: Neurological Examination in Dementia, in Wells CE (ed): Dementia (2 ed). Philadelphia, F.A. Davis Co., 1977

83. Prinz PN, Peskind ER, Vitaliano PP, et al: Changes in the sleep and waking EEGs of nondemented and demented elderly subjects. J Am Geriatr 30:86–93, 1982

84. Smallwood RG, Vitiello MV, Giblin EC, Prinz PN: Sleep apnea: relationship to age, sex, and Alzheimer's dementia. Sleep 6:16–22, 1983

85. Smirne S, Franceshi M, Bareggi S, Comi G, et al: Sleep apneas in Alzheimer's disease, in Sleep, 5th European Congress of Sleep Research. Basel: Karger, 1980, 442–444

86. Reynolds CF, Kupfer DJ, Taska LS, et al: Sleep Apnea in Alzheimer's Dementia: Correlation with mental deterioration. J Clin Psychiatry 46:257–261, 1985

87. Moldofsky H, Goldstein R, McNicholas WT, et al: Disordered breathing during sleep and overnight intellectual deterioration in patients with pathological aging, in Guilleminault C, Lugaresi E (eds): Sleep/Wake Disorders: Natural History, Epidemiology, and Long-Term Evolution. New York, Raven Press, 1983

88. Cohn JE, Hiroshi K: Primary alveolar hypoventilation with western equine encephalitis. Ann Intern Med 56:633–644, 1962

89. White DP, Miller F, Erickson RW: Sleep apnea and nocturnal hypoventilation after western equine encephalitis. Am Rev Respir Dis 127:132–133, 1983

90. Devereaux MW, Kean JR, Davis RL: Automatic respiratory failure associated with infarction of the medulla. Arch Neurol 29:46–52, 1973

91. Levin BE, Margolis G: Acute failure of automatic respirations secondary to a unilateral brainstem infarct. Ann Neurol 1:583–586, 1977

92. Chaudhary BA, Elguindi AS, King DW: Obstructive sleep apnea after lateral medullary syndrome. S Med J 75:65–67, 1982

93. Guilleminault C, Motta J: Sleep Apnea Syndrome as a Long-Term Sequela of Poliomyelitis, in Guilleminault C, Dement WC: Sleep Apnea Syndromes. New York, Alan R. Liss, 1978, pp 309–315

94. Plum G, Swanson AG: Abnormalities in central regulation of respiration in acute and convalescent poliomyelitis. Arch Neurol Psychiat 80:267–285, 1958

95. Solliday NH, Gaensler EA, Schwaber JR, Parker TF: Impaired central chemoreceptor function and chronic hypoventilation many years following poliomyelitis. Respiration 31:177–192, 1974

96. Turino GM, Goldring RM, Fishman AP: Cor pulmonale in musculo-skeletal abnormalities of the thorax. Bull NY Acad Med 41:959–980, 1965

97. Lane DJ, Hazelman B, Nichols PJR: Late onset respiratory failure in patients with previous poliomyelitis. Q J Med 172:551–568, 1974

98. Hill R, Robbins AW, Messing R, Arora NS:

Sleep Apnea Syndrome after Poliomyelitis. Am Rev Respir Dis 127:129–131, 1983

99. Minz M, Autret A, Laffont F, et al: A Study on Sleep in Amyotrophic Lateral Sclerosis. Biomedicine 30:40–46, 1979

100. Krieger AJ, Rosomoff HL: Sleep-induced apnea. (parts 1 & 2) J Neurosurg 40:181–185, 1974

101. Krieger AJ, Standish MS, Rosomoff HL: Respiratory and autonomic dysfunction following percutaneous cervical cordotomy. Crit Care Med 2:91–95, 1974

102. Krieger AJ: Sleep apnea produced by cervical cordotomy and other neurosurgical lesions in man, in Guilleminault C, Dement WC (eds): Sleep Apnea Syndromes. New York, Alan R. Liss, Inc., 1978, pp 273–294

103. Williams A, Hanson D, Calne DB: Vocal cord paralysis in the Shy-Drager syndrome. J Neurol Neurosurg Psychiatry 42:151–153, 1979

104. Bannister R, Gibson W, Michaels L, Oppenheimer DR: Laryngeal abductor paralysis in multiple system atrophy. Brain 104:351–368, 1981

105. McNicholas WT, Rutherford R, Grossman R, et al: Abnormal Respiratory Pattern Generation during Sleep in Patients with Autonomic Dysfunction. Am Rev Respir Dis 128:429–433, 1983

106. Eisele JH, Cross CE, Rausch DC, et al: Abnormal respiratory control in acquired dysautonomia. N Engl J Med 285:366–368, 1971

107. Edelman NH, Cherniack NS, Lahiri S, et al: The effects of abnormal sympathetic nervous function upon the ventilatory response to hypoxia. J Clin Invest 49:1153–1165, 1970

108. Chokroverty S, Barron KD, Fatz FH, et al: The syndrome of primary orthostatic hypotension. Brain 92:743–768, 1969

109. Page MMB, Watkins PJ: Cardiorespiratory arrest and diabetic autonomic neuropathy. Lancet 1:14–16, 1978

110. Garcia-Bunuel L: Cardiorespiratory arrest in diabetic autonomic neuropathy. Lancet 1:935–936, 1978

111. Ewing DJ, Campbell IW, Clarke BF: The natural history of diabetic autonomic neuropathy. Q J Med 49:95–108, 1980

112. Ewing DJ, Borsey DQ, Travis P, et al: Abnormalities of ambulatory 24-hour heart rate in diabetes mellitus. Diabetes 32:101–105, 1983

113. Rees PJ, Cochrane GM, Prior JG, Clark TJH: Sleep apnoea in diabetic patients with auto-

nomic neuropathy. J Roy Med 74:192–195, 1981

114. Guilleminault C, Briskin JG, Geenfield MS, Silvestri R: The impact of autonomic nervous system dysfunction on breathing during sleep. Sleep 4(3):263–278, 1981

115. Catterall JR, Calverley PMA, Ewing DJ, et al: Breathing, sleep, and diabetic autonomic neuropathy. Diabetes 33:1025–1027, 1984

116. Briskin JG, Lehrman KL, Guilleminault C: Shy-Drager Syndrome and Sleep Apnea, in Guilleminault C, Dement WC (eds): Sleep Apnea Syndromes. New York, Alan R. Liss, 1978, pp 317–322

117. Fletcher EC, Schaaf JW, Miller J, Fletcher JG: Urinary catecholamines in patients with obstructive sleep apnea. Sleep Res 114:154, 1985

118. Lehrman KL, Guilleminault C, Schroeder JS, et al: Sleep apnea syndrome in a patient with Shy-Drager Syndrome. Arch Intern Med 138:206–209, 1978

119. Frank Y, Kravath RE, Inoue K, et al: Sleep apnea and hypoventilation syndrome associated with acquired nonprogressive dysautonomia: clinical and pathological studies in a child. Ann Neurol 10:18–27, 1981

120. Sanders V: Neurologic manifestations of myxedema. N Engl J Med 266:547–552, 1961

121. Massumi RA, Winnacker JL: Severe depression of the respiratory center in myxedema. Am J Med 36:876–882, 1964

122. Duron B, Quinchard J, Fullana N: Nouvelles recherches sur le mechanisme des apnees du syndrome de Pickwick. Bull Physiopathol Respir 8:1277–1288, 1972

123. Yamamoto T, Hirose N, Miyoshi K: Polygraphic study of periodic breathing and hypersomnolence in a patient with severe hypothyroidism. Eur Neurol 15:188–193, 1977

124. Orr WC, Males JL, Imes NK, et al: Myxedema and obstructive sleep apnea. Am J Med 70:1061–1066, 1981

125. Rajagopal KR, Abbrecht PH, Derderian SS, et al: Obstructive sleep apnea in hypothyroidism. Arch Int Med 101:491–494, 1984

126. Millman RP, Bevilacqua J, Peterson DD, Pack AI: Central sleep apnea in hypothyroidism. Am Rev Resp Dis 127:504–507, 1983

127. Onal E, Lopata M: Central sleep apnea in hypothyroidism. Am Rev Respir Dis 127:504–507, 1983

128. Skatrud J, Iber C, Ewart R, et al: Disordered breathing during sleep in hypothyroidism. Am Rev Respir Dis 124:325–329, 1981

129. Guilleminault C, van den Hoed J, Mitler MM:

Clinical overview of the sleep apnea syndromes, in Guilleminault C, Dement WC (eds): Sleep Apnea Syndromes. New York, Alan R. Liss, 1978, pp 1–12

130. Mezon BJ, West P, Maclean JP, Kryger MH: Sleep apnea in acromegaly. Am J Med 69:615–618, 1980

131. Romanczuk BJ, Potsic WP, Atkins JP: Hypersomnia with period breathing (an acromegalic Pickwickian). J Otolaryngol 86:897–903, 1978

132. Cadieux RJ, Kales A, Santeen RJ, et al: Endoscopic findings in sleep apnea associated with acromegaly. J Clin Endocrinol Metabol 55:18–22, 1982

133. Siegler J: Acromegaly associated with laryngeal obstruction. J Laryngol 66:620–621, 1952

134. Bhatia ML, Misra SC, Prakash J: Laryngeal manifestations in acromegaly. J Laryngol 80:412–417, 1966

135. Southwick JP, Katz J: Unusual airway difficulty in the acromegalic patient-indications for tracheostomy. Anesthesiology 51:72–73, 1979

136. Ovassapian A, Doka JC, Romsa DE: Acromegaly-use of fiberoptic laryngoscopy to avoid tracheostomy. Anesthesiology 54:429–430, 1981

137. Perks WH, Horrocks PM, Cooper RA, et al: Sleep apnoea in acromegaly. Br Med J 280i:894–897, 1980

138. Hart TB, Radow SK, Blackard WG, et al: Sleep apnea in active acromegaly. Arch Int Med 145:865–866, 1985

139. Sandblom RE, Matsumoto AM, Schoene RB, et al: Obstructive sleep apnea syndrome induced by testosterone administration. N Engl J Med 308:508–510, 1983

140. Johnson MW, Anch AM, Remmers JE: Induction of the obstructive sleep apnea syndrome in a woman by exogenous androgen administration. Am Rev Respir Dis 129:1023–1025, 1984

141. Harmon EM, Wynne JW, Block AJ: The effect of weight loss on sleep disordered breathing and oxygen desaturation in morbidly obese men. Chest 82:291–294, 1982

142. Mosko S, Lewis E, Sassin JF: Impaired sexual maturation associated with sleep apnea syndrome during puberty: A case study. Sleep 3:13–22, 1980

143. Heerhaber I, Loeschoke HH, Westphal U: Eine Wirkung des Progesterons auf die Atmug. Plfugers Arch 250:42–55, 1948

144. Kryger M, Glas R, Jackson D, et al: Impaired oxygenation during sleep in excessive polycythemia of high altitude: Improvement with respiratory stimulation. Sleep 1:3–17, 1978

145. Tyler JM: The effect of progesterone on the respiration of patients with emphysema and hypercapnia. J Clin Invest 39:34–41, 1960

146. Skatrud JB, Dempsey JA, Bhansali P, Irvin C: Determinants of chronic carbon dioxide retention and its correction in humans. J Clin Invest 65:813–821, 1980

147. Skatrud JB, Dempsey JA, Iber C, Berssenbrugge A: Correction of CO_2 retention during sleep in patients with chronic obstructive pulmonary disease. Am Rev Respir Dis 124:260–268, 1980

148. Orr WC, Imes NK, Martin RJ: Progesterone therapy in obese patients with sleep apnea. Arch Intern Med 139:109–111, 1979

149. Strohl KP, Hensley MJ, Saunders NA, et al: Progesterone administration and progressive sleep apneas. JAMA 245:1230–1232, 1981

150. Sutton FD Jr, Zwillich CW, Creagh CE, et al: Progesterone for outpatient treatment of Pickwickian syndrome. Ann Intern Med 83:476–79, 1975

151. Lyons HA, Huang CT: Therapeutic use of progesterone in alveolar hypoventilation associated with obesity. Am J Med 44:881–888, 1968

152. Block AJ, Wynne JW, Boysen PG: Sleep-disordered breathing and nocturnal oxygen desaturation in postmenopausal women. Am J Med 69:75–79, 1980

153. Block AJ, Wynne JW, Boysen PG, et al: Menopause, medroxyprogesterone and breathing during sleep. Am J Med 70:506–510, 1981

154. Millman RP, Kimmel PL, Shore ET, Wasserstein AG: Sleep apnea in hemodialysis patients: The lack of testosterone effect on its pathogenesis. Nephron 40:407–410, 1985

155. De Olazabal JR, Miller MJ, Cook WR, Mithoefer JC: Disordered breathing and hypoxia during sleep in coronary artery disease. Chest 82:548–552, 1982

156. Dark DS, Pingleton SK, Drieling R, et al: Sleep disordered breathing and desaturation in stable severe congestive heart failure. Am Rev Respir Dis 129:A58, 1984

157. Crabb JE, Pingleton SK, Gollub S, et al: Sleep disordered breathing in decompensated and compensated congestive heart failure. Am Rev Respir Dis 131:A104, 1985

158. Burwell CS, Robin ED, Whaley RD, Bickelmann AG: Extreme obesity associated with

alveolar hypoventilation. A Pickwickian syndrome. Am J Med 21:811–818, 1956

159. Lopata M, Onal E: Mass loading, sleep apnea, and the pathogenesis of obesity hypoventilation. Am Rev Respir Dis 126:640–645, 1982

160. Bradley TD, Rutherford R, Grossman RF, et al: Role of daytime hypoxemia in the pathogenesis of right heart failure in the obstructive sleep apnea syndrome. Am Rev Respir Dis 131:835–839, 1985

161. Cherniack RM, Guenter CA: The efficiency of the respiratory muscles in obesity. Can J Biochem Physiol 39:1215–1222, 1961

162. Rochester DF, Enson Y: Current concepts in the pathogenesis of the obesity-hypoventilation syndrome: mechanical and circulatory factors. Am J Med 57:402–420, 1974

163. Sharp JT, Henry JP, Sweany SK, et al: The total work of breathing in normal and obese men. J Clin Invest 43:728–739, 1964

164. Kaufman BJ, Ferguson MH, Cherniack RM: Hypoventilation in obesity. J Clin Invest 38:500–507, 1959

165. Fritts HW Jr, Filler J, Fishman AP, Cournand A: The efficiency of ventilation during voluntary hyperpnea: Studies in normal subjects and in dyspneic patients with either chronic pulmonary emphysema or obesity. J Clin Invest 38:1339–1348, 1959

166. Holley HS, Milic-Emili J, Becklake MR, Bates DV: Regional distribution of pulmonary ventilation and perfusion in obesity. J Clin Invest 46:475–481, 1967

167. Vaughan RW, Cork RC, Hollander D: The effect of massive weight loss on arterial oxygenation and pulmonary function tests. Anesthesiology 54:325–328, 1981

168. Barrera F, Hillyer P, Ascanio G, Bechtel J: The distribution of ventilation, diffusion, and blood flow in obese patients with normal and abnormal blood gases. Am Rev Respir Dis 108:819–830, 1973

169. Emirgil C, Sobol BJ: The effects of weight reduction on pulmonary function and the sensitivity of the respiratory center in obesity. Am Rev Respir Dis 108:831–842, 1973

170. Lourenco RV: Diaphragm activity in obesity. J Clin Invest 48:1609–1614, 1969

171. Guilleminault C, Cummiskey J: Progressive improvement of apnea index and ventilatory response to CO_2 after tracheostomy in obstructive sleep apnea syndrome. Am Rev Respir Dis 126:14–20, 1982

172. Sullivan CE, Berthon-Jones M, Issa FG: Remission of severe obesity-hypoventilation syndrome after short-term treatment during sleep with nasal continuous positive airway pressure. Am Rev Respir Dis 128:177–181, 1983

173. Fletcher EC, Schaaf JW, Miller J, Fletcher JG: Long term cardiopulmonary sequellae in patients with sleep apnea and chronic lung disease. Chest 88:545, 1985

Mary Anne McCaffree

11

Sudden Infant Death Syndrome: Respiratory Mechanisms

Sudden Infant Death Syndrome (SIDS), the leading cause of death for infants between 1 month and 1 year of age in the United States, accounts for approximately 2 deaths per 1000 live births yearly; more than 5500 reported deaths due to SIDS[1] occur annually. The Sudden Infant Death Syndrome Act of 1974 (PL 93-270) helped inaugurate a program of research and family services for SIDS.

Criteria for the diagnosis of SIDS were established in 1969 at the Second International SIDS Research Conference. Since then many investigators have reported somewhat conflicting data regarding postmortem findings in infants with SIDS. Although a plethora of theories regarding the pathogenesis of SIDS has emerged, no single theory has explained all SIDS deaths.

This lack of concensus has prompted some researchers to hypothesize that SIDS occurs because of an imbalance in autonomic regulation of cardiorespiratory control during early infancy (2 to 6 months).[2] Potential respiratory mechanisms for SIDS and their imbalance will be the focus of this review.

DEFINITION

SIDS is defined as "the sudden death of any infant or young child which is unexpected by history and in which a thorough post-mortem examination fails to demonstrate an adequate cause for death."[3] Theoretically, a suspected abnormality in cardiorespiratory control might have been initiated by a stimulus, such as an upper respiratory tract infection. Two characteristics unique to SIDS are its age distribution and relation to sleep. Most infants die between 2 and 4 months of age with sparing of the first 3 weeks and a decrease in SIDS after the fifth month of life. They are usually found between midnight and 6 A.M.[1]

ABNORMALITIES OF RESPIRATION DURING SLEEP
ISBN 0-8089-1812-5

Copyright © 1986 by Grune & Stratton, Inc.
All rights of reproduction in any form reserved.

PATHOLOGY

Although the postmortem exam fails to identify a cause of the infants death, a constellation of findings typify the necropsy results in the SIDS infant. The child, apparently well developed and nourished, has a small amount of fluid at the nares (bloody or watery) and is cyanotic. Internal examination reveals thymic, pleural, and intrathoracic petechiae, minor inflammatory reaction of the upper respiratory tract with focal necrosis of the larynx, full expansion of the lungs with pulmonary congestion and edema, prominence of lymphoid structures, and an empty urinary bladder.[4]

Considerable controversy has recently occurred between pathologists regarding "subtle alterations in structure" in certain organs[2] indicating that chronic hypoxia occurred prior to the infant's sudden demise. Theoretically, altered regulation of alveolar ventilation could result in hypoxia, with the occurrence of a secondary increase in pulmonary arteriolar pressure and astroglial growth in the brain stem. This chronic hypoxia hypothesis reported by Naeye,[5] has been inconsistently supported by findings of other pathologists.

Naeye's report of muscular hypertrophy noted in the small pulmonary arteries of SIDS infants, thought to be secondary to chronic hypoxia,[5] has not been confirmed by others.[6–8] Other tissues reported to be markers for hypoxia, i.e., brown fat retention, or right ventricular hypertrophy[9] were not substantiated by other pathologists.[10,11] Tissues identified as abnormal in SIDS patients by Naeye have been reevaluated. Adrenal gland weight, reportedly decreased in SIDS infants[9] has recently been found to be similar to that of controls.[12,13] Persistent extra medullary hepatic hematopoesis, once thought to indicate chronic hypoxia, was not confirmed by Valdes-Dapena.[14] Carotid body size and function has been investigated in SIDS infants. Naeye reported a low carotid body volume in some infants with SIDS.[15] Others have found no difference in volume of glomus cells in the carotid body[16] of infants with SIDS.

The morphology of the central nervous system, however, is abnormal in the infants with SIDS. Naeye identified increased gliosis in the brainstem of SIDS infants compared to controls.[17] Further work by Takashima noted astroglial growth in the solitary tract nucleus, dorsal vagal nuclei, the nucleus ambigius and retroambigius and the reticular formation, all essential sites for respiratory control.[18] Kinney noted increased numbers of "reactive astrocytes" in the medulla oblongata in SIDS compared to controls in six individual anatomical regions of the medulla.[19]

In summary, the hypoxic marker theory has yet to be established regarding histologic evidence for long-standing hypoxemia causing SIDS. Central nervous system gliosis, particularly in the brain stem areas regulating respiration is increased. The significance of brainstem gliosis in the pathogenesis of SIDS has yet to be determined. The brainstem contains afferent and efferent fibers important in respiratory control. Neurons responsible for respiratory rhythm include inspiratory and expiratory neurons found in the medulla.[20] Although these brainstem neurons receive signals from the pons and forebrain, the main influence on respiration is from pulmonary afferents via the vagus nerve. Stretch receptors regulate the rate and volume of respiration in the infant via the vagal and glossopharyngeal nerves.[21] Further investigation of these abnormalities of gliosis and astrocytes by immunohistochemistry will provide more data regarding changes in the respiratory control center and their potential effect on respiration.

Based upon recent experimental, clinical, and pathological data it can be suggested that at least one mechanism of SIDS is upper airway obstruction. Finding intrathoracic petechiae at postmortem exam in SIDS infants prompted Beckwith to suggest that a markedly increased negative pressure occurred within the thorax prior to death.[3] Krous noted petechiae microscopically in the epimyocardium (69 percent) and outer thymus (56 percent) but rarely in the endomyocardium or inner thymus (16 percent) in 103 autopsied cases of SIDS. Central parenchymal petechiae occurred only when the subserosa was involved.[22] Theoretically, these petechiae could have been produced by gasping against an obstructed airway, which would significantly increase negative intrathoracic pressure (the Mueller maneuver). Such a maneuver lowers pressure around the heart, increases systemic venous return, and distends the right ventricle.[23,24]

The effect of hypoxia during upper airway obstruction would result in decreased cardiac contractility. Increased pulmonary wedge pressures have been documented in adults with obstructive sleep apnea[23] and during the Mueller maneuver.[24] Farber et al have demonstrated left ventricular failure in rabbits breathing against an obstructed airway. Numerous pulmonary petechiae were identified when animals were sacrificed after they had reached significant pressure differences between pulmonary wedge and intratracheal pressures. When the differences of these pressures exceeded 25 torr during inspiration and 10 torr during expiration, congestive lung edema and petechiae were noted, and the animals developed bradycardia.[25]

Anatomic features of the nasopharynx in the infant, particularly the soft palate and the base of the skull, make the patient more susceptible, at this age, to upper airway obstruction due to airway occlusion with muscle relaxation. Tonkin demonstrated the mobility of the mandible in infants.[26] Muscle relaxation of the nasopharynx was noted during rapid-eye-movement (REM) sleep by Reed et al.[27] Considerable expansion of the pharyngeal airway has been demonstrated during inspiration with constriction during expiration in the young infant.[28]

Considering the relatively compromised narrow upper airway of the infant, upper respiratory infections may be associated with enhanced muscle relaxation during sleep and further narrow the airway. Mucosal edema associated with such infections could further compromise the already small diameter of the airway. Reed and colleagues demonstrated, in infant cadavers, that normal inspiratory pressures (-1.5 to -12 cm H_2O) precipitate pharyngeal closure by inward movements of the lateral pharyngeal walls and posterior tongue movement.[27]

Obstruction of the upper airway of the infant can occur secondary to a number of anatomical abnormalities, i.e., cleft palate, micrognathia with glossoptosis, tracheomalacia, etc. and is associated with noisey breathing (snoring, stridor). However, "silent" asymptomatic obstructions that occur during sleep may be significant. Airflow itself may be essential to the patency of the airways in the infant. Thach et al in a rabbit model demonstrated pharyngeal collapse when the airway was not stimulated by airflow.[29] Mathew and coworkers have identified a high pharyngeal obstruction in one infant with congenital stridor who later died of SIDS.[30] Obstructive apnea has been associated with greater oxygen desaturation,[31] and deserves further investigation.

The infant may be more vulnerable to airway obstruction because of seemingly minor changes in muscle tone. Phillipson cited several factors that may be associated with altered ventilation. During active sleep, skeletal muscle tone from gamma motor-neurons may be inhibited.[32] Tongue recession and relaxation of pharyngeal constricting muscles may result in airway obstruction.[33] The infant has a shallow hypopharynx, more cephalad tongue and epiglottis and a mobile mandible[26] with a more compliant rib cage than the older child, predisposing the infant to inadequate ventilation.[34]

Several alterations in respiratory physiology may theoretically predispose infants to airway closure. Loss of muscle tone in the upper airway could narrow the nasopharynx resulting in obstruction with increased airway resistance. Decreased intercostal muscle tone during sleep could lead to a decreased functional residual capacity with resultant hypoxemia and central apnea.[34]

EPIDEMIOLOGY

A variety of minor abnormalities have been retrospectively identified in infants who have died of SIDS. Many epidemiological studies have focused on this group of infants. The risk of SIDS is increased in the offspring of young (<20 yrs.), poor, unmarried, smoking women who receive little or no prenatal care or experienced previous fetal loss, illness during gestation, or abused narcotics.[34–38] Paternal factors that are associated with increased risk of SIDS include low socioeconomic level or young age (<20 yrs).[39] Ethnic group incidences of SIDS varies; Asians have a low risk (0.51/1000),[40] whereas Alaskan natives (4.5/1000)[41] and economically disadvantaged blacks (5.04/1000)[42] have a high risk.

American Indians have been reported to have a higher SIDS rate than caucasians (5.93 to 6.56/1000).[40] Kaplan, Bauman, and Krous, however, noted that Oklahoma American Indians infants' rate of SIDS was not statistically different from caucasians (Indians 2.32/1000 versus whites 1.80/1000).[43] Variability in the incidence of SIDS, especially the inverse relationship of SIDS with maternal age, may be effected by maternal nutrition during pregnancy, as suggested by Peterson, Van Belee, and Chinn[44] as well as other factors.

In addition to ethic origin, male sex, preterm, and low birth weight increase the risk for SIDS. Yount reported a SIDS rate of 11/1000 live births in infants with low birth weight (1000–1500 grams).[45] Infants who are products of multiple births, especially twins, also have a higher rate of SIDS (42/1000),[46] and simultaneous deaths in twins have been reported.[39,46]

Infants with SIDS were noted to have lower 5 minute Apgar scores[47] and required resuscitation. The incidence of SIDS in infants with bronchopulmonary dysplasia is significantly increased. Werthammer reported that 11 percent of infants with bronchopulmonary dysplasia died from SIDS compared to 1.5 percent (1/64) in infants of similar low birth weight without chronic lung disease.[48] SIDS occurs more frequently in the winter months.[39]

Infection

SIDS may be potentiated by infection and is associated with a mild upper respiratory tract infection in 40–75 percent of the cases.[49] However, evidence of systemic infection has not been documented at necropsy. The frequency of specific organisms associated with SIDS, such as respiratory syncytial virus (RSV) or *Clostridium bolulinum* has recently been reviewed. Bruhn reported that significant apnea occurred in 20 percent of infants with RSV.[50] Hall and colleagues reported the sudden death of two infants recovering from RSV.[51] Premature infants with RSV infection have been noted to have apnea requiring mechanical ventilation.[52] The mechanism of virus-induced altered respiratory control remains unclear and needs to be investigated.

Approximately 5 percent of California infants with SIDS had evidence of botulism.[53–55] Reports from other states[56] and Austria[57] confirmed the presence of *C. botulinum* in the intestinal wall of SIDS patients. The role of this pathogen in SIDS is unclear. However, because honey frequently contains *C. botulinum* spores, its use is contraindicated for children under 1 year of age.[54] The effect of this curtailment of honey consumption on the incidence of botulism or SIDS needs to be determined.

Immunizations

Concern about the possible link of immunizations of infants with Diphtheria-tetanus toxoid-pertussis (DTP) oral polio vaccine and SIDS was raised following the deaths of four infants in Tennessee.[58] A review of SIDS deaths in that state by the CDC revealed no differences in SIDS rates in the intervals prior to and following the reported four deaths.[59] Preliminary data from the NIH sponsored multicenter epidemiologic case control study on SIDS and DTP vaccinated infants also showed no increased SIDS frequency in vaccinated infants compared with matched controls.[60] Keens and colleagues evaluated the ventilatory pattern of control infants, siblings of SIDS, and infants with apnea prior to and following immunization by the pneumogram technique. Periodic breathing was decreased, and there was no increase in central apnea in these patients.[61] These data support the recommendation of complete immunizations for all infants at 2, 4, and 6 months of age.

Respiratory

Respiratory differences in parents of SIDS infants have been compared to normal controls in order to determine familial responses that might contribute to a sudden demise in their offspring. A decreased respiratory response to CO_2 challenge was noted in 12 pairs of parents of infants with SIDS compared to adult controls by Shiffman et al. The slope of SIDS parents' response to hypercarbia and the change in mouth occlusion pressure $(P_{0.1})$ divided by the change in alveolar P_aCO_2 was lower than control subjects. Normal increases in respiratory drive $(P_{0.1}/P_aCO_2)$ were demonstrated in controls when inspiratory resistance was added whereas parents of SIDS infants failed to respond.[62] However, Zwillich and coworkers were unable to detect differences in hypoxic ventilatory drive among 8 parents of SIDS infants compared to controls.[63] Normal ventilatory responses to CO_2[64,65] and hypoxia[64] were demonstrated in parents of SIDS infants. Berman noted less of an increase in heart rate in response to CO_2 and O_2 in SIDS parents compared to controls.[64]

Parents of infants with a diminished response to CO_2 were evaluated by Kanarek et al; four of the infants with the blunted CO_2 response later died of SIDS.[66] Ventilatory responses to hypoxia and hypercarbia were normal among these parents.

These studies indicate that respiratory control in the parents of SIDS infants is not consistently altered and support the suggestion that factors other than genetics are important in the occurrence of SIDS.

Sleep

The majority of infants with SIDS have been found after a period of sleep (between midnight and 6 A.M.). The relationship of sleep to SIDS was hypothesized by Steinschneider after excessive amounts of apnea were documented in sleeping infants who later had SIDS.[67] Gould has suggested the theory that sleep "unmasks faulty respiratory control mechanisms that are sleep specific,"[68] such as those noted in Ondines curse.[69]

Newborns enter sleep in the "active phase" with rapid eye and body movements, irregular cardiorespiratory rates, with low voltage, rapid wave EEG activity for 40–60 minutes. A "quiet state" of sleep follows with high voltage slow wave EEG and regular cardiorespiratory rates, without body movements.[65] Indeterminate sleep periods occur when the infant manifests a combination of phasic features characteristic of rapid movements and tonic features of quiet sleep. As the infant develops in the first 3 months of life, sleep states mature so that, at 3 months, infant sleep has a predominate quiet sleep pattern.

Sleep differences between siblings of SIDS (SSIDS) and control infants have been characterized. Longer active sleep epochs, fewer waking periods,[69–71] increased respiratory and heart rates while asleep[72] have been reported in this group of infants. Differences in quiet sleep maturation were noted in infants with apnea compared to controls.[70,73] During active sleep, arousal response threshold is increased.[71] Lacey evaluated EEG's of infants with recurrent apnea, "near-miss SIDS" and SSIDS, excessive frequent variability of sleep spindles were detected in infants with apnea and "near-miss" SIDS.[74] These data support developmental differences in sleep organization for certain infants in the first 2–3 months of age that normalize at 6 months. Theoretically, the inability of an infant to respond to a noxious event such as gastroesophageal reflux during active sleep,[75] could result in apnea or bradycardia.

INFANTS "AT RISK"

Apnea, SSIDS, Preterm Infants

SIDS occurs associated with sleep; it is possible that physiologic abnormalities associated with sleep at this age (2–6 months) would identify infants susceptible to airway closure (upper airway obstruction) or breathing pauses (central apnea). Theoretically, the population of at risk infants (SSIDS, apnea, preterms) may be unable to change tonic and phasic activity of skeletal muscles of respiration in response to various stimuli[33] that could result in periodic breathing or central apnea. Posterior pharyngeal muscle relaxation[27] in these patients could lead to compromise of the already narrow upper airway and result in airway obstruction.

Antecedent Events

Parents of infants with SIDS have reported antecedent respiratory events prior to their child's demise. Mandell noted symptoms of apnea, cyanotic episodes, wheezing, and irregular respirations reported by parents of infants with SIDS in 37 percent of the cases compared to parents of infants without SIDS.[76] Beal noted that 16 percent of Australian parents had identified a previous episode prior to the SIDS event.[77] These data prompt many investigators to recommend that infants who are symptomatic with apnea, cyanosis, and irregular breathing, represent a population of patients to be evaluated.

Siblings of SIDS

Siblings of SIDS (SSIDS) have an increased risk (5.6/1000) of SIDS.[78] Respiratory control has been evaluated in SSIDS; conclusions from these studies have been divergent. Normal end tidal PCO_2 and response to 5 percent CO_2 and 100 percent O_2 was demonstrated by Fagenholz in 14 subsequent SIDS.[79] Higher respiratory rates at 3 months of age were noted in 35 subsequent SIDS compared to controls by Hoppenbowers.[80] SSIDS have more periodic breathing than normal infants.[81]

Infantile Apnea

Infants with apnea, found by their parents to be "limp, unresponsive, cyanotic" and not breathing have been referred to as "near miss for SIDS." Steinschneider reported an increase in short (>6 sec.) apnea in infants who later died of SIDS.[67] Later studies by Steinschneider noted that infants with prolonged apnea during sleep had an increased frequency and duration of brief (>6 sec.) apnea and increased periodic breathing during a daytime nap.[82] Prolonged central apnea (>15 sec.) has been documented in infants with apnea and in patients who later died of SIDS.[31,67,82,83] Infants with apnea have demonstrated excessive short central apnea (3–6 sec),[84,85] periodic breathing,[67,81,82,84] and mixed apnea.[85,86] Some infants have a decreased respiratory drive to hypercapnia[87,88] or hypoxia,[89,90] or increased short (3–6 sec.) upper airway obstruction.[85,91,92] Guilleminault and colleagues found that infants with apnea had an increase in mixed and obstructive events compared to controls.[86,93] Vander Hal and colleagues identified that only 38 percent of infants with apnea had arousal to hypoxic challenge, and subsequently had more severe apnea episodes than controls. Infants with apnea had a higher PCO_2 at arousal than control infants.[94] These studies indicate some respiratory abnormalities in this population of infants.

Prematures

Premature infants frequently develop central apnea or bradycardia in the nursery. Gehardt and Bancalari evaluated premature infants with apnea compared to similar patients without apnea. Symptomatic infants had a decreased ventilatory response to CO_2 compared to control patients.[95] Their poor response to inspiratory loads indicated a decreased ability to compensate compared to controls.[96] These data support immature reflex responses and poor regulation of breathing in preterm infants with apnea. Methylxanthines have been used by some investigators when infants have excessive periodic breathing or central apnea.[96,97] Hunt and colleagues documented improved pneumogram studies in infants after its use.[98] Others, however have identified infants who failed to respond.[99,100] Use of xanthines is contraindicated in infants with gastroesophageal reflux since it promotes reflux.

Evaluation

The clinical evaluation of the *symptomatic child* with a history of apnea (or "near-miss") should include: a careful history, inpatient cardiorespiratory monitoring, and detection of associated abnormalities that might explain the symptoms. The detailed history about the event, whether it occurred while awake or asleep may provide some clues regarding likely diagnoses. Evaluations for gastroesophageal reflux, seizures, cardiac arrhythmias, and electrolyte imbalance should be performed. If clinically indicated, the possibility of sepsis or viremia may be investigated.[97]

Two different types of cardiorespiratory evaluations can be performed; polysomnography (PSG) and pneumocardiogram. Polysomnographic studies in infants have been reported in sibling of SIDS, controls, and symptomatic infants.[67,69,72,73,80,82,84–86] A relatively small number of control infants have been studied; however, similar results have been reported from several laboratories.[90,92] Patients with gastroesophageal reflux and apnea will benefit from continuous distal esophageal pH evaluation[101] simultaneous with PSG to determine the relationship of reflux to apnea and desaturation.

Pneumogram techniques have been developed to evaluate infants, both in the laboratory and at home. Stein and Shannon initially reported that continuous cardiorespiratory trend event recordings in preterm infants were helpful in identifying the frequency of central apnea.[102] Respiratory rates are recorded by chest wall impedance; QRS signals are detected for the heart rate. Periodic breathing, frequent in preterm infants, and defined as "three or more central pauses of three or more seconds with a duration of respiration of 20 seconds or less," can be scored and reported as episodes per 100 minutes.[103] Values for controls, SSIDS, and symptomatic infants have been reported.[81,103]

The main advantage of the pneumocardiogram technique is its versatility. It can be performed at the patient's bedside, whether as an inpatient or in the home. Current home cardiorespiratory monitors have a cassette tape attachment for recording the pneumogram from which a hard copy can be printed and incidences of central apnea, bradycardia, and periodic breathing scored.

However, since airflow is not detected using this technique, upper airway obstruction (UAO) cannot be identified. Episodes of obstructive apnea can only be inferred from episodes of bradycardia occurring without central apnea. Several studies indicate that UAO is common (15–40 percent) in symptomatic infants.[85,91,92] Modification of the pneumogram technique, by addition of an airflow channel, would provide more complete evaluation of these patients. Development of home monitors that can detect air flow signals will improve the current technology. Inpatient evaluation can be improved by utilizing oximetry as well as airflow detection.

RECOMMENDATIONS

Symptomatic infants with apnea represent a heterogeneous group of patients. Since the symptom of apnea is nonspecific, conditions associated with apnea must be investigated (gastroesophageal, seizures). Infants with abnormal respiratory studies (PSG or pneumogram) should be placed on home cardiorespiratory monitors[104] following careful instruction of the parents in infant CPR and equipment use. Cain et al noted that parental anxiety regarding their apneic infant decreased after thorough testing, instruction in equipment and CPR, and a parent support group.[105] A visiting nurse referral is recommended by Wasserman.[106] Cardiorespiratory monitoring should be continued until the infant is alarm free for 2 months. During this time, usually 4.5 months, immunizations (DTP and polio) should be completed. Frequently the infant has experienced at least one upper respiratory infection during this time.

Parents with a SSIDS frequently request evaluation of their infant. Periodic breathing is increased in this group of patients.[81] Home cardiorespiratory monitoring is recommended until the anniversary date of the SIDS sibling. CPR instructions, parent support groups, and visiting nurse referrals are indicated for these families.

Premature infants can be evaluated prior to hospital discharge. Patients with increased periodic breathing, central or obstructive apnea benefit from home cardiorespiratory monitors. Some investigators recommend methylxanthine treatment for these infants until the respiratory pattern normalizes (2–6 months).

REFERENCES

1. Merritt T, Valdes-Dapena M: SIDS research update. Ped Ann 13:193–207, 1984
2. Shannon D, Kelly D: SIDS and Near SIDS. NEJM 306:959–965, 1982
3. Beckwith J: The Sudden Infant Death Syndrome. Curr Prob Pediatr 3:1–36, 1973
4. Valdes-Dapena M: The morphology of the Sudden Infant Death Syndrome: An overview, in J Tildon, L Roedes, A Steinschneider: Sudden Infant Death Syndrome. New York, Academic Press, 1983, pp 169–182
5. Naeye R: Pulmonary arterial abnormalities in the Sudden Infant Death Syndrome. NEJM 289:1167–1170, 1973
6. Mason J, Mason L, Jackson M, et al: Pulmonary vessels in SIDS. NEJM 292:479, 1975
7. Phat V, Durigon M: Mort subite du nourrisson: etude morphometrique des arteres pulmonaires. Rev Electroencephalogr Neurophysiol Clin 6:93–96, 1976
8. Kendell S, Ferris J: Apparent hypoxic changes in pulmonary arterioles and small arteries in infancy. J Clin Pathol 30:481–485, 1977
9. Naeye R: Hypoxemia and the Sudden Infant Death Syndrome. Science 186:837–838, 1974
10. Williams A, Vawter G, Reid L: Increased muscularity of the pulmonary circulation in victims of sudden infant death syndrome. Pediatr 63:18–23, 1979
11. Valdes-Dapena M, Amazon K, Gillave M, et al: The question of right ventricular hypertrophy in sudden infant death syndrome. Arch Pathol Lab Med 104:84–86, 1980
12. Valdes-Dapena M, Gillane M, Catheman R: Brown fat retention in sudden infant death syndrome. Arch Pathol Lab Med 100:547–549, 1976
13. Emery J, Dinsdale F: Structure of periadrenal brown fat in childhood in both expected and cat deaths. Arch Dis Child 53:154–158, 1978
14. Valdes-Dapena M, Gillane M, Ross D, Catherman R: Extramedullary hematopoesis in the liver in sudden infant death syndrome. Arch Pathol Lab Med 103:513–515, 1979
15. Naeye R, Fisher R, Ryser M, Whalen P: Carotid body in the sudden infant death syndrome. Science 191:567–569, 1976
16. Dinsdale F, Emery J, Gadsdon D: The carotid body—a quantitative assessment in children. Histopathology 1:179–187, 1977
17. Naeye R: Brainstem and adrenal abnormalities in the sudden infant death syndrome. Amer J Clin Pathol 66:526–530, 1976
18. Takashima S, Armstrong D, Becker L, et al: Cerebral hypoperfusion in the sudden infant death syndrome? Brain gliosis and vasculature. Ann Neurol 4:257–262, 1976
19. Kinney H, Burger P, Harrell F, Hudson R: Reactive gliosis in the medulla oblongata of victims of the sudden infant death syndrome. Pediatr 72:181–186, 1983
20. Kalia MP: Anatomical organization of central respiratory neurons. Ann Rev Physiol 43:105–120, 1981
21. Olinsky A, Bryan MH, Bryan AC: Influence of lung inflation on respiratory control in neonates. J Appl Physiol 36:426–429, 1974
22. Krous H: Microscopic topography of intrathoracic petechial hemorrhages in sudden infant death syndrome. Arch Pathol Lab Med 108:77–79, 1984
23. Buda A, Schroeder J, Guillimault C: Abnormalities of pulmonary artery wedge pressures in sleep induced apnea. Internat J Cardiol 1:67, 1981

24. Buda A, Pinsky M, Ingels N, et al: Effect of intrathoracic pressure on left ventricular performance. NEJM 301:453–459, 1979

25. Farber J, Catron A, Krous H: Pulmonary petechiae: Ventilatory-circulatory interactions. Pediatr Res 17:230–233, 1983

26. Tonkin S, Partridge J, Beach D, Whiteney S: The pharyngeal effect of partial nasal obstruction. Pediatr 63:261–271, 1979

27. Reed W, Roberts B, Thach B: Role of inspiratory suction and muscle hypotonia in obstructive sleep apnea. Presented at the International Research Conference on Sudden Infant Death Syndrome. Baltimore, 1982

28. Bosma J: Evaluation of the infant mouth and pharynx pertinent to feeding, in A Nowak, A Erenberg (eds): Factors influencing orofacial development in the ill, preterm, low birth weight and term neonate. Iowa City, University of Iowa, 1984, pp 55–58

29. Abu-Osba Y, Mathew O, Thach B: An animal model for airway sensory deprivation producing obstructive apnea with postmortem findings of sudden infant death syndrome. Pediatr 68:796–801, 1981

30. Mathew O, Roberts J, Thach B: Pharyngeal airway obstruction in preterm infants during mixed and obstructive apnea. J Pediatr 100:964–968, 1982

31. Guilleminault C, Peraita R, Souquet M, Dement W: Apneas during sleep in infants: Possible relationship with sudden infant death syndrome. Science 190:677–679, 1975

32. Henderson-Smart D, Read D: Depression of intercostal and abdominal muscle activity and vulnerability to asphyxia during active sleep in the newborn, in C Guilleminault, W Dement (eds): Conference on sleep apnea syndrome. New York, Alan R. Liss, 1978, pp 93–118

33. Phillipson E: Control of breathing during sleep. Am Rev Respir Dis 118:909–939, 1978

34. Shannon D, Kelly D: SIDS and near-SIDS. NEJM 306:1022–1028, 1982

35. Peterson D, VanBelle G, Chinn N: Epidemiologic comparisons of the sudden infant death syndrome with other major components of infant mortality. Am J Epidemiol 110:699–707, 1979

36. Spiers P, Wang L: Short pregnancy interval, low birthweight and the sudden infant death syndrome. Am J Epidemiol 104:15–21, 1976

37. Rajcgowda B, Kendall S, Falciglia H: Sudden unexpected death in infants of narcotic dependent mothers. Early Human Development 2:219–225, 1978

38. Chavez C, Ostrea E, Stryker J, Smialek Q: Sudden infant death syndrome among infants of drug dependent mothers. J Pediatr 95:407–409, 1979

39. Froggatt P, Lynas M, Marshall T: Sudden unexpected death in infants ("cot death"): Report of a collaborative study in Northern Ireland. Ulster Med J 40:116–135, 1971

40. Kraus J, Borhani N: Post neonatal sudden unexplained death in Calif: A cohort study. Am J Epidemiol 95:497–510, 1972

41. Fleshman J, Peterson D: The sudden infant death syndrome among Alaskan natives. Am J Epidemiol 105:555–558, 1977

42. Valdes-Dapena M, Birle L, McGovern J, et al: Sudden unexpected death in infancy: A statistical analysis of certain socioeconomic factors. J Pediatr 73:387–394, 1968

43. Kaplan D, Bauman A, Krous H: Epidemiology of sudden infant death syndrome in American Indians. Pediatr 74:1041–1046, 1984

44. Peterson D, Van Belee G, Chinn N: Sudden infant death syndrome and maternal age. Etiologic implications. JAMA 247:2250–2252, 1982

45. Yount J, Flanagan W, Dingley E, et al: Evidence for an exponentially increasing incidence of sudden infant death syndrome (SIDS) with decreasing birth weight (BW). Pediatr Res 13:510, 1979

46. Arsenault P: Maternal and antenatal factors in the risk of sudden infant death syndrome. Am J Epidemiol 111:278–284, 1980

47. Standfast S, Jereb S, Tarrerich D: The epidemiology of sudden infant death of upstate New York: Birth characteristics. Am J Public Health 70:1061–1067, 1980

48. Werthammer J, Brown E, Neff R, Taeusch H: Sudden infant death syndrome in infants with bronchopulmonary dysplasia. Pediatr 69:301–304, 1982

49. Beckwith JB: Observations of the pathological anatomy of the sudden infant death syndrome, in A Bergman, J Beckwith, C Ray (eds): Sudden infant death syndrome: Proceedings of the second international conference on causes of sudden infant death in infants. Seattle: University of Washington Press, 1970, pp 83–102

50. Bruhn F, Mokrohisky S, McIntosh K: Apnea associated with respiratory syncytial virus infection in young infants. Pediatr 90:382–386, 1977

51. Hall C, Kopelman A, Douglas R, et al: Neonatal respiratory syncytial virus infection. NEJM 300:393–396, 1979

52. Anas N, Boettrich C, Hall C, et al: The associ-

ation of apnea and respiratory syncytial virus infection in infants. J Pediatr 101:65–68, 1982

53. California Morbidity Department of Health Services. State of California. 1982, No. 18, May 14

54. Arnon S, Medura T, Damus K: Intestinal infection and toxin production by clostridium botulinum as one cause of sudden infant death syndrome. Lancet 1:1273, 1978

55. Arnon S, Midura T, Damus K, et al: Honey and other environmental risk factors for infant botulism. J Pediatr 94:331–336, 1979

56. Thompson J, Glasgow L, Warpinski J, Olson C: Infant botulism: Clinical spectrum and epidemiology. Pediatr 66:936–942, 1980

57. Sonnabend O, Sonnabend W, Heinzle R, et al: Isolation of clostridium botulinum type G botulinum toxin in humans. Report of 5 sudden unexpected deaths. J Infect Dis 143:22, 1981

58. Centers for Disease Control. DTP vaccination and sudden infant deaths. Tennessee. MMWR 28:131, 1982

59. Bernier R, Frank J, Dondero T, et al: Diphtheria-tetanus toxoids-pertussis vaccination and sudden infant death syndrome in Tennessee. J Pediatr 101:419–421, 1982

60. Preliminary report of the National Institute of Child Health and Human Development multicenter epidemiologic study: Presented before the Society for Pediatric Research. Washington D.C., May 1982

61. Keens T, Ward S, Gates E, et al: Ventilatory pattern following diphtheria-tetanus-pertussis immunizations in infants at risk for sudden infant death syndrome. Am J Dis Child 139:991–994, 1985

62. Schiffman P, Westlake R, Santiago T, Edelman N: Ventilatory control in parents of victims of sudden infant death syndrome. NEJM 302:486–491, 1980

63. Zwillich C, McCullough R, Guilleminault C, et al: Respiratory control in the parents of sudden infant death syndrome victims: ventilatory control in SIDS parents. Pediatr Res 14:762–764, 1980

64. Berman T, Bartlett M, Westgate H, et al: Attenuated responses to CO_2 and hypoxia. Chest 79:536–538, 1981

65. Couriel JM, Olinsky A: Response to acute hypercapnia in the parents of threatened sudden infant death syndrome infants. Pediatrics 75(5):652–655, 1984

66. Kanarek D, Kelly D, Shannon D: Ventilatory chemoreceptor response in parents of children at risk for sudden infant death syndrome. Pediatr Res 15:1402–1405, 1981

67. Steinschneider A: Prolonged apnea and the sudden infant death syndrome: Clinical and laboratory observations. Pediatr 50:646–654, 1972

68. Gould J: SIDS, a sleep hypothesis, in J Tildon, L Roeder, A Steinschneider (eds): Sudden Infant Death Syndrome. Academic Press, New York, 1983, pp 443–452

69. Harper R, Leake B, Hoffman H, et al: Periodicity of sleep states is altered in infants at risk for sudden infant death syndrome. Science 213:1030–1032, 1981

70. Navelet Y, Payan C, Guilhaume A, Benoit O: Nocturnal sleep organization in infants at risk for sudden infant death syndrome. Pediatr Res 18:654–657, 1984

71. Hoppenbrowers T: Ontogenesis of sleep and waking, in C Stark, H Hoffman (eds): Ontogeny of Sleep and Cardiopulmonary Regulation: Factors Related to Risk for the Sudden Infant Death Syndrome. Washington D.C., National Institutes Child Health and Development, 1982; Sect. II, Chapter 2

72. Hoppenbrowers T, Hodgman J, McGinty D, et al: Sudden infant death syndrome. The emergence of a circadian pattern in respiratory rates: Comparison between control infants and subsequent siblings of SIDS. Pediatr Res 14:345–351, 1980

73. Gould J, Lee A, James L, et al: The sleep state characteristics of apnea during infancy. Pediatr 59:182–194, 1977

74. Lacey D: Sleep EEG abnormalities in children with near-miss sudden infant death syndrome, in siblings, and in infants with recurrent apnea. J Pediatr 102:855–859, 1983

75. Kenigsberg K, Griswold P, Buckley B, et al: Cardiac effects of esophageal stimulation: Possible relationship between gastroesophageal reflux and sudden infant death syndrome. J Ped Surg 18:542–545, 1983

76. Mandell F: Cot death among children of nurses: Observations of breathing patterns. Arch Dis Child 56:312–314, 1981

77. Beal S: Some epidemiological factors about sudden infant death syndrome in South Australia, in J Tildon, L Roeder, A Steinscheider (eds): Sudden infant death syndrome. Academic Press, New York, 1983, pp 15–28

78. Irgens L, Skjaerven R, Peterson D: Prospective assessment of recurrence risk in sudden infant death syndrome siblings. J Pediatr 104:349–351, 1984

79. Fagenholz S, O'Connell K, Shannon D:

Chemoreceptor function and sleep state in apnea. Pediatr 58:31–36, 1976

80. Hoppenbowers T, Hodgman J, McGinty D: Sudden infant death syndrome. Sleep apnea and respiration in subsequent siblings. Pediatr 66:205–214, 1980

81. Kelly D, Walker A, Cohen L, Shannon D: Periodic breathing in siblings of sudden infant death syndrome victims. Pediatr 66:515–520, 1980

82. Steinschneider A: Prolonged sleep apnea and respiratory instability. A discriminative study. Pediatr 59:962–970, 1977

83. Southall D, Richards J, Brown D, et al: 24-hour tape recordings of ECG and respiration in the newborn infant with findings related to sudden infant death and unexplained brain damage in infancy. Arch Dis Child 55:7–16, 1980

84. Monod N, Curzi-Dascalova L, Guidasci S, Valenzuela S: Pauses respiratoires et sommeil chez le nouveau-ne' et le nourrisson. Rev Electroencephalogr Neurophysiol Clin 6:105–110, 1976

85. Guilleminault C, Ariagno R, Korobkin R, et al: Mixed and obstructive sleep apnea and near-miss for sudden infant death syndrome. 2. Comparison of near-miss and normal control infants by age. Pediatr 64:882–891, 1979

86. Guilleminault C, Ariagno R, Souquet M, et al: Abnormal polygraphic recordings in near-miss sudden infant death. Lancet 1:1326–1327, 1976

87. Shannon D, Marsland D, Gould J, et al: Central hypoventilation during quiet sleep in two infants. Pediatr 57:343–346, 1976

88. Shannon D, Kelly D, O'Connell K: Abnormal regulation of ventilation in infants at risk for sudden infant death syndrome. NEJM 297:747–750, 1977

89. Brady J, Arigno R, Wats J, et al: Apnea hypoxemia and aborted sudden infant death syndrome. Pediatr 62:686–691, 1978

90. Hunt C, McCulloch K, Brouillette R: Diminished hypoxic ventilatory responses in near miss SIDS. J Appl Physiol 50:1313–1317, 1981

91. Dransfield D, Spitzer A, Fox W: Episodic airway obstruction in premature infants. Am J Dis Child 137:441–443, 1983

92. McCaffree MA, Toubas PL, Orr WC, et al: Ef-

fect of sleep state and position on the incidence of obstructive and central apnea in infants. Pediatr 75:832–835, 1985

93. Guilleminault C, Ariagno R, Korobin R: Sleep parameters and respiratory variables in near-miss SIDS infants. Pediatr 68:354–360, 1981

94. VanderHal A, Redriquez A, Sargent C, et al: Hypoxic and hypercapneic arousal responses and prediction of subsequent apnea in apnea of infancy. Pediatr 75:848–854, 1985

95. Gerhardt T, Bancalari E: Apnea of prematurity. Lung function and regulation of breathing. Pediatr 74:58–62, 1984

96. Gerhardt T, Bancalari E: Apnea of prematurity. Respiratory reflexes. Pediatr 74:63–66, 1984

97. Brooks J: Apnea of infancy and sudden infant death syndrome. Amer J Dis Child 136:1012–1023, 1982

98. Hunt C, Brouillette R, Hanson D: Theophylline improves pneumogram abnormalities in infants at risk for sudden infant death syndrome. J Pediatr 106:969–974, 1983

99. Eyal F, Alpan G, Sagi E, et al: Aminophylline versus doxapram in idiopathic apnea of prematurity: A double blind controlled study. Pediatr 75:709–713, 1985

100. Roberts J, Mathew O, Thach B: Failure of theophylline to prevent apnea and bradycardia in low birth weight infants. J Pediatr 100:968–970, 1982

101. Jolley S, Johnson D, Herbst J, et al: An assessment of gastroesophageal reflux in children by extended pH monitoring of the distal esophagus. Surgery 84:16–24, 1978

102. Stein I, Shannon D: The pediatric pneumogram: A new method for detecting and quantitating apnea in infants. Pediatr 55:599–603, 1975

103. Kelly D, Shannon D: Periodic breathing in infants with near-miss sudden infant death syndrome. Pediatr 63:335–360, 1979

104. Southall D: Home monitoring and its role in the sudden infant death syndrome. Pediatr 72:133–138, 1983

105. Cain L, Kelly D, Shannon D: Parents' perceptions of the psychological and social impact of home monitoring. Pediatr 66:37–41, 1980

106. Wasserman A: Impact of home monitoring on the family. Pediatr 74:323–329, 1984

Index

Page numbers followed by (*f*) indicate figures. Page numbers followed by (*t*) indicate tables.